Politics of Occupation-Centred Practice

Politics of Occupation-Centred Practice

Reflections on Occupational Engagement across Cultures

Edited by

Nick Pollard

Senior Lecturer in Occupational Therapy
Faculty of Health and Wellbeing
Sheffield Hallam University
Sheffield, UK

Dikaios Sakellariou

Lecturer
School of Healthcare Studies
Cardiff University
Cardiff, UK

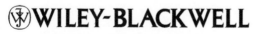

WILEY-BLACKWELL

A John Wiley & Sons, Ltd., Publication

This edition first published 2012
© 2012 by John Wiley & Sons Ltd

Wiley-Blackwell is an imprint of John Wiley & Sons, formed by the merger of Wiley's
global Scientific, Technical and Medical business with Blackwell Publishing.

Registered office: John Wiley & Sons, Ltd, The Atrium, Southern Gate, Chichester,
West Sussex, PO19 8SQ, UK

Editorial offices: 9600 Garsington Road, Oxford, OX4 2DQ, UK
The Atrium, Southern Gate, Chichester, West Sussex, PO19 8SQ, UK
2121 State Avenue, Ames, Iowa 50014-8300, USA

For details of our global editorial offices, for customer services and for information about how to
apply for permission to reuse the copyright material in this book please see our website at
www.wiley.com/wiley-blackwell.

The right of the author to be identified as the author of this work has been asserted in accordance
with the UK Copyright, Designs and Patents Act 1988.

Library of Congress Cataloging-in-Publication Data

Politics of occupation-centred practice : reflections on occupational
engagement across cultures / edited by Nick Pollard, Dikaios Sakellariou.
    p. ; cm.
  Includes bibliographical references and index.
  ISBN 978-1-4443-3698-6 (pbk.)
  I. Pollard, Nick, MSc(OT) II. Sakellariou, Dikaios.
  [DNLM: 1.   Occupational Therapy. 2.   Cross-Cultural Comparison. 3.
Occupations. 4.   Politics. 5.   Socioeconomic Factors. 6.   Work. WB 555]

  362.1′0425–dc23

                                                          2012002553

A catalogue record for this book is available from the British Library.

Wiley also publishes its books in a variety of electronic formats. Some content that appears
in print may not be available in electronic books.

Set in 10/12 pt Sabon by Thomson Digital, Noida, India

1   2012

Contents

List of Contributors

Marta Aoki
Occupational Therapist
Faculty of Medicine
University of São Paulo, São Paulo, Brazil

Mami Aoyama
Professor and Associate Dean
Faculty of Rehabilitation Sciences
Nishikyushu University, Kanzaki, Saga, Japan

Hope Block
Board Member
Autism National Committee
Rhode Island, USA

Pamela Block
Associate Professor
School of Health Technology and Management
Stony Brook University, Stony Brook, New York, USA

Neil Carver
Senior Lecturer
Faculty of Health and Wellbeing
Sheffield Hallam University, Sheffield, UK

Taísa Gomes Ferreira
Occupational Therapist
Health Science Center
Federal University of Santa Maria, Brazil

Sally Foster
Senior Lecturer
Faculty of Health and Social Sciences
Leeds Metropolitan University, Leeds, UK

Sandra Maria Galheigo
Senior Lecturer
Faculty of Medicine
University of São Paulo, São Paulo, Brazil

Sarah Kantartzis
PhD Candidate
Faculty of Health and Social Sciences
Leeds Metropolitan University, Leeds, UK

Devva Kasnitz
President, Society for Disability Studies
Devvaco Consulting/New Focus Partnerships, USA

Matthew Molineux
Director, Allied Health
Clinical Education and Training Queensland (ClinEdQ)
Brisbane, Australia
and
Adjunct Research Fellow
School of Occupational Therapy and Social Work
Curtin University, Perth, Australia

Fátima Corrêa Oliver
Senior Lecturer
Faculty of Medicine
University of São Paulo, São Paulo, Brazil

Jacob Pratt
Executive Director
Autism Spectrum Differences Institute of New England, Inc.
Connecticut, USA

Nick Pollard
Senior Lecturer
Faculty of Health and Wellbeing
Sheffield Hallam University, Sheffield, UK

Linda Rammler
Private Practice Consultant
Focusing on Autism, Positive Behavior Supports and Inclusion
Connecticut, USA

Dikaios Sakellariou
Lecturer
School of Healthcare Studies
Cardiff University, Cardiff, UK

Russell Shuttleworth
Senior Lecturer
Faculty of Health
School of Health and Social Development
Deakin University, Geelong Campus, Australia

Foreword

The occupational therapy profession's core concept of *occupation* ought never to be treated as if its defining characteristic ("meaningful and purposeful activity") were a property solely of patients or clients as individuals apart from their communal environments. Yet professional care in a clinic or hospital affords few clues to the interpersonal identities and communal lifestyles that occupations support. In this book, editors Nick Pollard and Dikaios Sakellariou lay a scholarly foundation for occupational therapy that treats the cultural, historical and political contexts of daily occupation within a unified worldview.

The book's contributors offer complementary perspectives from occupational therapy, anthropology, disabilities studies, folklore and folk life, and other key fields to promote a common cause. They link narrative (the most potent communicative link between the individual seeking treatment and the occupational therapist) back to wider material and social contexts. Such background contexts are too often merely supposed, or even overlooked, in the press of increasing technical core requirements of an occupational therapy curriculum. To understand how these complementary perspectives on occupation come together, I find it helpful to revisit the founding of the occupational therapy profession in the progressive era, circa 1890 to 1920, in the United States.

It is a truism that cultures are typically invisible to their members until a disruption occurs. For many observers today, global banking has shaped – and now disrupted – lives around the world on an unprecedented scale. Mass demonstrations, revolutions, and cries for democratic reform recall the progressive era, when so many reinventions and reinterpretations of everyday occupations emerged. Under the impact of unregulated industrial capitalism and massive displacements of populations, work and working conditions were redefined. Labourers left rural agricultural settings and small towns. Struggles for survival were drawn more sharply between new forces of 'labour' and 'capital'. New forms of cosmopolitan and pluralistic citizenship and political participation were envisioned and enacted. Traditional arts and crafts were reharnessed variously in movements to restore health and wellbeing, to provide vocational education, and to build utopian socialist communities. The occupational profession as an incorporated entity recognized under New York state laws also emerged this time. This incorporation of the profession, in 1917, marked a shift from an exclusively humanitarian and reformist use of occupations to ameliorate the lives of disabled people. The incorporated profession necessarily had also to become concerned with promoting the profession's own interests as a paid provider of services.

Occupational therapists in the United States, in 2003, adopted the rallying call: *We envision that occupational therapy is a powerful, widely recognized, science-driven, and evidence-based profession with a globally connected and diverse workforce meeting society's occupational needs.* This Centennial Vision issued by the American Occupational Therapy Association anticipates the completion of a hundred years of existence in 2017. The vision is ambitious, optimistic, and expansive. Yet it appears to embody an innocent faith in the background practices of global capitalism that have since brought the world's leading economies to the brink of collapse.

Perhaps an alternative Centennial Vision could be crafted in light of the global economic crisis. Countless families have been displaced from their homes; the value of stocks and savings have been sharply eroded; benefits and pensions are disappearing and thousands upon thousands of jobs have been eliminated on which individuals and families depended to survive with security and dignity. Speaking now just of the United States, the occupational therapy profession aims to gain a greater market share of a highly exclusionary health care system, while quality services become an ever more unaffordable dream for the 15% of the population that is uninsured. Roughly the same percentage of the population in the United States, about 50 million people, cannot put sufficient food on the table to maintain health. A million or more children go to bed at night hungry. The most vulnerable social programmes being cut concern services provided by occupational therapists and other rehabilitation professionals for people with disabilities.

This current volume, *Politics of Occupation-Centred Practice: Reflections on Occupational Engagement across Cultures*, offers an alternative vision of occupations, one that predates the reduction of occupational approaches into a profession shaped by a fee-for-service medical model. Pollard and Sakellariou restore a view of the occupations of everyday life embedded in their historical and political contexts, pointing us in the direction of cultures as collections of contested discourses and practices. They embody something of the progressive-era vision, when the realm of everyday life and daily labour was indeed being carved up in order to become the specialized, licensed province of competing profession, disciplines and academic societies.

We would not want to go back in time to the excesses and abuses of past. But we must and can encourage occupational therapists to treat the meaning and purpose of occupations in political and cultural contexts. Science and social justice must go forward hand in hand. Now, as a centenary ago, occupation must be reconceptualized in the broadest terms as a restorative dimension to assaults on the survival and communal lifestyles of 99% of the world's population in our own time. Read on!

Gelya Frank
Professor
Division of Occupational Science and Occupational Therapy
Herman Ostrow School of Dentistry
and Department of Anthropology
University of Southern California

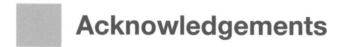

Acknowledgements

To my wife, Linda, and our children, for their patience during the times when I have been working on this project.

Thanks also to the support of my colleagues and students in the occupational therapy team here at Sheffield Hallam University, particularly Neil Carver and Janet Medforth with whom I've shared an office and who withstood my mess.

Nick Pollard

To my family. To Dimitra, Julia and Dean because they are here. To Erimo Okaasan because she greeted the man from Vladivostok. To Vagelio.

Thanks are also due to the School of Healthcare Studies in Cardiff University and in particular to the Department of Occupational Therapy for their support during the development of this and numerous other projects.

Dikaios Sakellariou

The editors would like to thank the proprietors and staff of The Eastend Café, Meriden Street, Birmingham, for their great service during our meetings there.

1 Introduction

Nick Pollard and Dikaios Sakellariou

Although the profession is a hundred years old, in some respects occupational therapy has a short academic pedigree, with the first degree programme in the subject offered in 1947 at the University of Southern California (Gordon, 2009). Although the 1989 Blom-Cooper report (1990) stated the College of Occupational Therapists 1981 diploma was at degree level, the first degree programmes in the UK did not begin until 1986. It was not until 1994 that the profession was all graduate entry (Paterson, 2008). In this short life, occupational therapy has reportedly already been through several paradigm changes (Gilfoyle, 1984) from an initial orientation around craft activities, to activities of daily living, to adaptation, to the idea of occupation as purposeful activity, and perhaps to the emergence of occupational science where the person is recognized as an occupational being. It has produced evidence on its effectiveness and has established a role for itself within the health and social care arena. Yet occupational therapists still have a problem explaining what exactly their profession is about.

Despite the development of an array of frameworks and models for practice there is an evident lack of a unifying conceptual framework that will chart the remit and the goals of the profession and provide a comprehensive overview of its processes. The purpose of such frameworks has been to ensure that professional activities are identifiable in order that payment can be made for occupational therapy services (e.g. American Occupational Therapy Association, 2002) and also that the profession remains relevant to the changing context of practice. An agreed framework might enable the goals and effectiveness of the profession to be communicated across a variety of audiences both within and outside the occupational therapy arena but it would also present challenges. The World Federation of Occupational Therapists has issued position papers and statements acknowledging the right of all people to occupation and the profession's responsibility to facilitate this right has become a reality (WFOT 2004, 2006). There has been a continuing debate about the remit of the profession and links between the underpinning concerns of occupational therapy with meaningful occupation with an assertion of occupation as a human right (Hammell, 2008; Galheigo, 2011).

Politics of Occupation-Centred Practice: Reflections on Occupational Engagement across Cultures,
First Edition. Edited by Nick Pollard and Dikaios Sakellariou.
© 2012 John Wiley & Sons, Ltd. Published 2012 by John Wiley & Sons, Ltd.

There have been debates concerning the universal applicability of Western concepts of occupational therapy in different cultural contexts (e.g. Iwama, 2006) and challenges to the holism that the profession claims. Hammell (2007, 2010) is amongst those who have challenged whether the profession is really client centred or concerned with its practitioners' own needs, as a critical exploration of the profession's values might suggest (Abberley, 1995).

Developing a clear understanding of what the occupation aspect of occupational therapy refers to might increase the recognition of the profession across different contexts but the same project might generate confusions. The American Occupational Therapy Association (2002) has made several revisions to its practice framework to take account of changes as the context of healthcare develops. Occupational therapy is not yet universally available as a profession. There are many countries where occupational therapists do not yet practise widely and there are many cultural contexts that therapists have yet to encounter. The profession, despite its holistic vision, operates within certain constraints of social class and gender as well as culture (Beagan, 2007; Sakellariou and Pollard, 2008; see Chapter 2) Those therapists who are dually qualified as anthropologists might be interested in the problems generated by the differences in perception observable in applications of a clinical or technical approach to wellbeing and the experiences of those to whom such interventions might be directed (see, for example, Park, 2008). Like Mattingly (1998) we have been concerned with the variety of possible interpretations of occupation and their connection with narratives of experience. This chapter explores some historical and cultural relationships to consider how occupational assumptions may be questioned in relation to power, and some of the implications this may have for the professional position of the therapist.

The Meaning of Occupation

The profession has its origins in an understanding of the need for meaningful and balanced access to occupation (Wilcock 1998, 2002, 2006; Turner 2002) in the sense of people deriving health benefits through purposeful individual and shared activity. While this may seem a fundamental concept, over the history of the profession its focus has shifted away from a broader understanding of occupation to one more connected with work and productivity and then back again to explorations of creativity (Hocking 2007). Thus in occupational therapy the term is not a narrow 'occupation' merely related to social function but to a political notion of having choice, participation and sharing in the community, making changes, and requiring 'social revolution' (Wilcock and Townsend, 2000: 85) to address issues of disadvantage, from individual through to political and organizational expression (Wilcock, 2007). Wilcock and Townsend apply 'meaningful occupation' as a 'practical means' for 'personal and community transformation' (2000: 85) – that is, for enabling and facilitating individuals in role change through challenging obstacles in the community and environment.

The meaning of occupation has not much been critically explored within the profession's literature. 'Meaningful' is an abstract value applied to occupation (see Chapter 8 for a critical discussion of the meaningfulness of occupation – also see Chapters 9, 11, 13 and 14). An occupation might be something that produces change; it could also be something that is concerned with maintenance, and it could also have negative results. Self-destructive behaviours or activities carried out while delusional, for example, are not meaningless. The occupations connected with eating disorders, such as the monitoring of weight or food intake to maintain a distorted body image, are not without meaning to the individual. Group activities such as football violence, communal drug use, or the occupations connected with religious cults might be challenging for other people to understand, but they are not without meaning. For those people who experience them they may be intensely meaningful (Foster, 1984; King, 2001; Klein, 2007). For example, Foster's (1984) discussion of Mormons, Shakers and the Oneida religious communities of the mid-nineteenth century reveals considerable reflection amongst members about the correctness of the paths they were following in responses to social developments around them. Klein's (2007) discussion of *khat* in the UK Somali community makes comparisons with other societies' use of drugs and notes the suggestion of a traditional aspect in which the drug is taken partly as an expression of cultural heritage, even though in the case of *khat* usage dates to recent times.

Occupational therapy, as it has only recently begun to grapple with ideas of cultural competency and has rarely engaged with concepts of social class or gender, has tended to assume an uncomplicated link between doing and productivity or perhaps with spirituality. It has not really considered how the meaningfulness of human occupation might be restricted or limited within a dominant ideology, or religious "cult" (Benjamin, 1996 [1921]: 288) of capitalism. Benjamin argued that capitalism was a parasitical development of Christianity and had become a dogma that relied on the same tools of guilt and anxiety to maintain order. The present hegemony represents a capitalist order serving global corporations, and so within this context what people do is determined by a market serving the needs of these organizations to sustain profits.

Despite the widespread idea of Western democracy, much of the social order is determined by the needs of capital, and so is ordered (not necessarily strictly controlled, although at times, for example through the conditions set out by the International Monetary Fund, this may be more evident) from the board room or shareholder meetings. Whether people engage in work, are unemployed, or are able to engage in leisure, their activities are free choices inasmuch as the options available to them are what is offered to them within the limits of what they can afford to do. Other societies might be more influenced by religion, in which what is meaningful is determined by adherence to religious principle. In others the relationship of a people with their environment shapes occupations which are ordained by the availability of natural resources, but the existence of such societies, perhaps as small indigenous groups, is very much on the periphery of global society.

The subservience of global society to capital and the assumption that all engagements have a monetary value of exchange has been questioned. For example, Max-Neef (2010) has devised a matrix of human development needs that cannot be quantified. His argument is that without people there would be no money; indeed much of what may be significant to people (although many of their activities will be underpinned by the exchange of capital through work and spending for leisure) does not involve transactions of monetary value but of occupational value.

On a day-to-day basis, the identification of forms of doing that are meaningful to individuals or to communities might be determined through interwoven and shared narratives. The autobiographical writing by English worker writers (see Chapter 11) produced in the last century showed that many people defined their lives in terms of the work they did, relationships, and the places in which they lived (Ikiugu and Pollard, in press). For example, many of the titles of these autobiographies would include the names of communities (Bailey, 1981; Peckham People's History, 1983; Thompson, 1987) or identify a form of work (Noakes, 1977; Harris, 1978; Beavis, 1980; Noble, 1984). Much of these autobiographical accounts celebrates aspects of work and community, but there are also stories of survival and hardship. While survival might be a particular feature of narratives written about the interwar period (e.g. Beavis, 1980), overcoming literacy difficulties (Shore, 1982), or about racism (e.g. Noble, 1984), there can also be a feature of more recent and prosperous times, for example due to the impact of disability (Irwin, 1995).

The development of this form of autobiographical writing is much concerned with the reflection of individual experience against a background of social change (Vincent, 1981; Morley and Worpole, 2009). In a movement of worker writers and community publishers it was part of a broader counter culture that, during the 1980s and 1990s, was documenting black, Asian, gay, women's, environmental and other expressions of critical consciousness (Woodin, 2009). More often than not, this writing was not expressly oppositional, yet, just like the long tradition of ballads and broadsheets to which it is linked, it contains distinctive perspectives of class, culture and social geography that have been marginalized, suppressed or treated dismissively (Lloyd, 1969, 1978; Morley and Worpole, 2009) (see Chapter 11 – this kind of reflection on meanings of occupation in relation to community narrative is evident in many cultures and Chapters 8–10 and 14 explore further examples).

Such a link between meaning and occupation carries a very different emphasis from the restorative or recovery oriented approach of a clinical profession. Thus when Mattingly (1998) describes how the therapist may be engaged in a technical solution to disability, yet a client interprets the loss of function she experiences in a personal way, it can be seen that a perspective of doing that comes from a therapeutic position might be very limited. It might fail to respect the expression of identity that the individual possesses outside the clinical setting: a social standing in the community; a network of informal relationships, which may not conform to a hierarchically determined work setting because they have been developed over years of familiarity; social roles derived from going to the local pub or hobby club (see Chapter 13), or which are dependent on the relationships between families (see Chapter 8).

Iwama's depiction of the Kawa or river model (2006) of occupation goes some way to facilitating the recognition of these issues by situating the individual's assets and difficulties in an environmental context, often as the 'floor' and 'banks of the river', which channel the individual's life flow. This model might be one means by which occupational therapists can gradually explain the right of all people to engage in occupations that correspond to their needs and desires and express their own professional responsibility to help make this right a reality, on an individual and community scale. The significance of the Kawa model is that it acknowledges a collective responsibility for occupation. The negotiation of what is to happen has to take account of the experiences that everyone brings into a situation, and questions whose meanings are being made operational (Iwama, Thomson and Macdonald, 2010).

The Term 'Occupation'

Given the frequency with which the term is used within the profession, 'occupation' has been notoriously hard to define in occupational therapy. According to Townsend (1997: 19) 'occupation is the active process of everyday living', while the *Concise Oxford Dictionary* (1999 edition) defines 'occupation' as 'the action, state, or period of occupying or being occupied; a job or profession; a way of spending time'. Significantly the *Chambers Twentieth Century Dictionary*'s (1983 edition) entry on 'occupation' emphasizes 'the act of occupying: possession: [...] the time during which a country, etc., is occupied by enemy forces...' This immense scope encompassed by its reference to human activity is an issue of definition, as several authors have recently acknowledged through their discussions of occupation in relation to complexity (do Rozario 1997; Creek, 2003; Molineux and Rickard, 2003; Whiteford, Klomp and Wright St Clair, 2005; Molineux and Whiteford, 2006). Like language, which has many uses and functions and may operate different forms of speech and expression to accommodate these even within a particular tongue, occupation is not one discrete aspect of human life but describes a form of engagement that reaches every area of human activity through its relationship to culture (Wilcock, 1998; Iwama, 2006). In professional literature occupation is described as basic to the experience of wellbeing (Wilcock, 2006). Occupation influences identity formation and is the means through which people perform the requirements of their multiple roles. Among other functions, occupation provides a sense of meaning, a time structure and a daily routine, can be a source of pleasure and of a sense of achievement, promotes interpersonal relationships and helps people to be aware of the capabilities of their bodies (Wilcock, 2006).

Efforts to delineate the meanings of the term accurately might be characterized as attempts to domesticate the term by assigning it a specific meaning, so as to exercise professional control over an area of human activity in multidisciplinary settings. Occupational therapists have a history of having to assert professional boundaries or reclaiming old professional territories (Whiteford, Townsend, and Hocking, 2000; Wilcock, 2002). Many professions concerned with human activities and health (for example psychology or nursing) continuously negotiate or even contest areas of their practice where role blurring creates problems in delivering care. Sometimes the arguments about definitions have more to do with one or other professional group's dominance over power and resources than abstract meanings (Wilcock, 2002, 2007; Hocking, 2007). As the concept of 'occupation' is bigger than its application in occupational therapy it presents a significant issue of classification and methodological appropriateness.

Seen briefly through the windows of an occupational therapy department, what goes on seems superficially simple – sitting down with a group of people and doing a crossword, baking scones, making a cup of tea (see Chapter 2). Anyone could do it – but all too often no-one gets the chance to as, without occupational therapists, the generic support worker is drawn into the tasks of physical care, or only providing activities that are supported by large numbers of clients.

Experientially, understood as components of a narrative in which the person is directly involved, these simple activities can be seen in the context of contributing to life quality. Breines (2004) points out that sometimes mundane activities contribute to occupational complexity in a set of reciprocities between individuals, their environments and their societies. Capturing these phenomena has proved difficult, especially in a way that would be recognized in a research hierarchy defined by biomedical paradigms. Consequently there may be some significant oversights in relation to research on meaningfulness and doing, such as the lack of exploration of the potential of hobbies (despite the anecdotes of Breines, 2004) for wellbeing (Bull, 2009; Burt and Atkinson, 2011; see Chapter 13). One reaction to biomedical dominance was to reconceptualize occupation in a biomedical frame, with activities such as bicycle fretsaw work administered in regulated sessions, but this resulted in a loss of professional identity (Turner, 2002; Hocking, 2007).

To occupational therapists and scientists, occupation is a symbol, a signifier assuming various meanings according to the context in which it appears (for a discussion of 'signifier' see Eco, 2000). The profession seems to accept that occupation refers to doing, being, becoming and belonging (Wilcock, 2006), terms that are associated with qualities of wellbeing, and the expression of which can be defined as components of good life quality (Phillips, 2006). Meaningful occupation (however this is defined) symbolizes a life of *good* qualities (Wilcock, 2007). Occupational therapy literature – if, for example, the covers of *OT News* are reviewed – frequently includes images of people engaged in activities such as cycling, painting, or gardening. The magazine, as a professional communication to members of the profession, reflects back a vision of itself as being concerned with positive images of people doing things with other people, being creative and active.

In its representation of arts and crafts, occupational therapy is no heroic upholder of a great principle of occupation. For all the splendid intentions of therapists to recapture the moral ground of activity as once described by moral therapy, the result has sometimes been rather hard to identify as having a value at all. Jokes about basket making and occupational therapy still occasionally surface, although they were wearying in the 1960s (Wilcock, 2002) while Mosey (1971) remarked that the idea that it was good for people to do things that they enjoyed seemed to have been abandoned in the 1960s in favour of treatments belonging to other disciplines.

Often this has arisen from the political context in which occupational therapists have operated (Hocking, 2007; Wilcock, 2007) – needing to be seen to be doing something, but lacking the real resources, or the power to challenge the lack of resources, or to make a case to do something worthwhile with some of the clients, rather than something worthless and boring with everyone – something that occupies but does not engage. In these situations of occupational absurdity, something that everyone may understand and recognize as an occupation is turned around and made into a therapy –something for 'doing you good' rather than something you feel good doing.

We should not overemphasize such criticisms against a professional history that is illuminated with numerous creative, innovative and inspirational examples. All therapists should own a copy of Estelle Breines' *Occupational Therapy: Activities for Practice and Teaching* (2004) to remind themselves of the value of serious play, the liberation to be gained from simple activities and enjoyments, and the celebration of life qualities combined with clinical assessments and therapeutic intervention. Posture work in the kitchen rolling dough for pastry can be identified in clinical reasoning, but it is also the setting for beginning conversations to investigate wider issues like, for example, whether the pastry should include free range eggs or battery eggs? (e.g. Fearnley-Whittingstall, 2010). The discussion of spatial freedom for chickens can lead to that of occupational justice for people, expressed perhaps for the right to a space in which to keep your own chickens, to become self-sufficient in developing food resources, and in the right of chickens (as well as humans) to do and be. Alternatively, there are many rich narratives to be explored through the experiences of cooking, the handing down of recipes and techniques that allow people to express themselves and their culture through the things they make.

However, as we have already discussed, the experience of doing, being, becoming and belonging is not necessarily an uncomplicated narrative of happy events. To return to the autobiographical narratives of worker-writers, one of the frequent defining characteristics of personal meaning in these accounts concerns the experience of overcoming hardships and dealing with difficulties. Such occupational narratives may also be shaped by such experiences as being a refugee or immigrant (Earl Marshall School, 1993), ill health and disability (Wiltshire, 1985; Irwin, 1995), bereavement, unemployment and conflict (Muckle, 1981; Sitzia and Thickett, 2002) and even imprisonment (Piper, 1995), all of which might be represented as assets in terms of the Kawa model of occupation (Iwama, 2006). Although people generally regard such experiences negatively, they are also a source of resiliency and personal strength, as is suggested in Chapters 9 and 10.

Occupational narratives carry a historical referent to not only who we are, but who we have been, and they anticipate who we will be. The concept of 'occupation' is a key to the way society is symbolized through the complex interaction of individual pasts, presents and possibilities and the resulting choices, opportunities, decisions, mistakes, and accidents (Mattingly, 1998; see Chapter 8). Occupation is therefore multidimensional. On one hand it represents an ontological flow developing over time through chronological narrative. Many occupations involve an unfolding process, such as the development of a skill or the creation of an object, in which certain steps of progression cannot be skipped in order to achieve a completed result. On another, while occupation measures time, it also telescopes time because it is through occupation that people anticipate the future and return to the past, as people can demonstrate through the breaks they may make in the telling of a narrative. The story that one person recounts to another is not necessarily linear – sense is made by interrupting chronological order to explain what was anticipated, or to explore earlier events before the current scene being described.

The richness of occupation presents a problem of developing a suitable means to adequately explore it and terms to describe it (Iwama, 2004; Molineux and Whiteford, 2006). Occupational therapists and scientists often generate theoretical terms by merely prefixing existing terms with 'occupation'. If this labelling endows them with a special meaning, the text that results is replete with jarring occupational concepts. Perhaps these fields of study need a wider range of terms for doing – a language of occupation; the development of a new vocabulary is part of any technical process. For example, a core problem in linguistics is that of classifying and analysing phenomena that are identified from a wide range of other disciplines. To do so requires a specific set of terms, and yet the difficulty with classifying what occurs in language is that it is in a continual state of flux, linked to the continuous social phenomenon of human interaction (Eco, 2000; see Chapter 8). Furthermore, in translating from one language to another, from one set of experiences to another, as in therapist-client interactions, the danger of misinterpretation is always imminent (Pollard and Sakellariou, 2008). An occupational perspective may claim to be holistic but it is only one perspective – and it is heavily influenced by one set of underpinning cultural ideas (Iwama, 2006).

The study of occupation, if it is concerned with people doing, being, becoming and belonging, has generally been constrained by the link to therapy and clinical practices. Although claims are made for occupational therapy's birth in social reform, the early identification with medical rehabilitation which made the practice into a profession (Frank and Zemke, 2008) may have diverted it from the critical engagements to which such origins might have led. As a clinical practice concerned with medical conditions the profession was less concerned with the social history of inequality, which contributed to the distribution and experience of illness and disability. The prescription of interventions for specific conditions is different from the development of practices for social change. Remarkably, given that the profession is based around engagement in activities from art to cooking, crafts to gardening, and forms of social interaction through games and dance to informal socializing, its perspective of occupation has neglected social history and cultural difference. There have been discussions of cultural competency, but little cultural analysis. Art, craft and cooking are seen as therapeutic media, taken out of the wider social context and developed in a clinical milieu. Were the profession to engage more deeply and seriously with these practices, practitioners might be able to advocate them more effectively.

The critical lens that the profession could have turned on human activity has also been denied its own practices. An emergent practice is ripe for investigation as it develops its own institutions and ways of constructing arguments in support of itself, but occupational therapy histories tend to hagiography rather than developing a critical perspective. In most countries where the occupational therapy profession has developed it has acquired a predominantly female membership that seems to replicate itself without admitting greater numbers of men. Such a marked gender imbalance combined with a remit to explore all human occupation suggests certain cultural characteristics amongst this exotic diaspora of 350,000 members that would be worthy of ethnographic or anthropological investigation.

Despite the fact that the profession relies on specialized social forms of language use to convey ideas about practice and other information (Detweiler and Peyton, 1999; Molineux and Rickard, 2003) occupational therapy has not concerned itself with the study of linguistics in relation to the description and interpretation of occupation. This is despite the fact that a key verb in many grammars is the term that equates with 'doing' and 'being', and the study of etymology may often reveal clues about the way words for doing particular occupations, tools, and familiar plants and animals have evolved in relation to human activity. To understand occupation, therapists need to develop the skills to read occupation and understand the instances where it is enabled or disabled – in effect to develop what Pollard (2008) has defined as 'occupational literacy' (see Chapter 3). Such a capacity is not finite but a continuous task of learning as the study of human activity is one of something that is always developing. This exposes a profession to challenges; its area of practice must shift boundaries, be subject to periodical negotiations as one activity eludes its remit and another is substituted, technologies give rise to new things to do, or new ways to do old things, human capacity for activity changes. The definition of what the profession is, and what it might refer to, is broadly constant but not fixed. Occupation is also concerned with territory and property, so it is not only associated with capacity, but prohibitions and proscriptions. The function of language as a means of social control or resistance has been documented (Mayr, 2004) but it has received little attention in occupational therapy and occupational science literature.

Therapists might be forgiven for remarking that they do not have time for all this. Indeed, there are many pressures on professionals' time originating in managerial procedures or the volume of cases – for example, many complain that they do not do the job for which they trained. For what purpose have professionals worked through three or four years of higher education, learning about ideals of practice that are so very different in the real clinical setting?

So, What Is Occupation?

In Chapter 8, Kantartzis, Molineux and Foster illustrate how doing is central to human life. Every day people orchestrate and perform numerous occupations. Some of them are responses to biological needs, such as eating or sleeping; some are socially required or expected (working, paying bills); some maintain the benefits of a social network and others may simply be fun whether alone or shared with others. A certain occupation is often performed for a combination of reasons and functions. To take one example, people engage in paid employment to maintain a social network, respond to social expectations, fulfil personal ambitions, escape poverty, or earn money. Work also gives access to resources, such as training and education opportunities, opportunities for travel, or access to facilities such as computer equipment and workshops. Work places may be located conveniently for other tasks such as collecting children from school, or enabling the worker to work from home. The same occupation can thus have significantly different effects on individuals and communities.

As *Chambers Twentieth Century Dictionary* (1983 edition) suggests, the meaning of the word 'occupation' refers to ownership of territory and the property relations that result. Military occupations are an obvious example. In a military occupation stakeholder involvements concern very different positions. No military occupation is permanent, although it may turn into or become an aspect of colonial possession that lasts hundreds of years and may involve many turns of conflict and cooperation between those who are occupying and those who are occupied (see Chapter 9).

Soldiers may be serving a tour of duty through a belief in defending a national interest, or because they have to fulfil national service obligations. Soldiering may be a vocation for some, and it may be a means to acquire experiences of adventure and travel, the income to obtain education, or purchase a house (Batistelli, 1997; Hedlund, 2011). As an occupation in itself, it is frequently the source of pride in the ability to present oneself smartly, put up with discomforts and stressful conditions, to develop technical and professional capacities. It is often represented as an entire way of life and, as it may encompass the stationing not only of the soldier but families and children in bases abroad with all the support and resources required to sustain social and community life, it can be so. Considerable efforts may be made to maintain the health and wellbeing of troops (Batistelli, 1997; Hedlund, 2011; see Chapter 13).

While soldiers are sending pay home, they are engaged in duties such as establishing law and order, maintaining peace or upholding colonial power, guarding the interests of some people and perhaps oppressing others; they may recognize that the military occupation in which they are engaged has complex outcomes, for example, because the rules of engagement impede them from preventing atrocities or returning fire (Weisaeth, 2003; Dandeker and Gow, 2004). It may limit or exacerbate conflict and the historical effects of the actions they are part of may continue for many years after they have returned home.

Civilians in an occupied area may also recognize very different positions. A military presence may represent a form of order, but it may encourage new forms of disorder, for example creating a market for drugs and prostitution or contraband goods, disrupting opportunities for sustainable work (Barr, 2010). There may be abuses of power that have to be weighed up against the abuses the troops are present to prevent. The troops may be suppressing an old corrupt regime but may not be able to prevent new forms of corruption that develop in the gaps which the former regime has left. When eventually the soldiers leave, as they inevitably must, there is a huge question of the stability of the society they will leave behind them, in which old scores can perhaps be settled.

Often as they are reported in the news such occupations are presented as political issues. It is difficult for outsiders to perceive how these politics are enacted and experienced by the people who pass each other in the street every day, on patrol or trying to go about their business, or follow the multiple objectives of officials, officers, politicians, entrepreneurs, and community leaders who each have their own occupational path to negotiate and whose daily decisions and actions impact on the people around them (Barr, 2010).

Some examples can be found in Gilmour's (1994) account of the life of Curzon, a prominent British politician of the late nineteenth and early twentieth century. Gilmour shows how the human failings and personal conflicts of key groups of powerful political figures and senior civil servants played an important part in determining the nature of some of the most important global conflicts of the later twentieth and early twenty-first centuries. Curzon's career was characterized by enmities where other politicians gave him the impression they were working with him while working against him. These souring friendships and personal disputes possibly exerted influences on the way Britain's colonial policy was carried out. There were, for example, attempts by Curzon's successors to reduce his influence and eradicate some of the projects he developed while Viceroy of India out of personal animosity. He tried to prevent a number of key political decisions because he felt they were made out of ignorance, but other politicians excluded or undermined his contributions. These decisions led to (amongst other things) the partition of India and Pakistan at independence in 1947, the dissolution of the Ottoman empire after the first world war and the formation of several middle eastern nations, including Israel, Syria, Iran and Iraq without proper regard to local ethnic interests. Gilmour notes that Curzon's views may have been borne out by history.

Thus different actors can use occupation for different purposes and occupation can be a means to exercise power, by validating one set of experiences whether this is of one culture, one class, or a perception of normality, over another. This is an unequal process, a long conflict with the odds stacked on the side of those with resources, but the outcome is not inevitable. Power can be evident in many ways, including decision making, agenda setting and manipulation (Barr, 2010). Foucault (2010) considered power as an dynamic, interactive process, and if we take a close look at instances of occupational injustice we will observe the following mechanisms: regulation (including total denial) of access to occupation, coercion for participation in certain occupations, regulation of resources necessary for access to occupation or manipulation and persuasion in exchange for other benefits.

Occupational Being

Doing things is, as Wilcock (2006, 2007) argues, what makes us healthy, or, which may be more important, feel healthy. Occupational therapy literature has discussed (e.g. Breines, 2004) but has rarely researched adult forms of recreation seriously as a contribution to wellbeing. Various forms of hunting and fishing are important in the lives of rural communities, and fishing is one of the most popular leisure activities in the UK, even in urban areas. The issue of poaching has a long history in

British culture as an element in the conflict between the gentry and nobility claiming ownership of the land and the things that grow upon it, and those labourers and farmers who lived off the land. The law, in supporting the rights of the gentry to reserve game for their shooting pleasures denied others what they felt was their right to God's bounty (Hopkins, 1986). At the heart of such activities is the occupational and spiritual relationship that people have with the natural and raw environment (Bull, 2009, and see Chapters 8 and 9) and which many poachers clearly viewed as their right: 'I am not going to be a Serf. They not only Stole the land from the People but they Stocked it with Game for Sport...' (Hawker, 1978: 62, *sic*). This relationship gave anglers an inner sense of wellbeing and contentment (Bull, 2009) – similar benefits to those obtained from other hobbies such as modelling, which may incorporate a more vicarious relationship with nature through the depiction of landscape (see Chapter 13).

Homo faber as an occupational being expresses a relationship with the world which is not merely vicarious, or a part time interest, or a way of being that is somehow dipped in and out of as if it was a commodity. Hawker's (1978) view of a fundamental right to the land was keenly felt; he was not a solitary example, but one in a long tradition. Hopkins (1986) links the long affray to the mass trespass of the ramblers association in 1932, an event still celebrated in the towns around the Peak District. In this people congregated on the grouse moors between the cities of Sheffield and Manchester to demand rights of way to enjoy the landscape, legal access to which continues to be an issue in England and Wales (Sheffield Campaign for Access to Moorland, 1988; Lowe and Shaw, 1993). Every occupational therapy walking group using the public footpaths exercises the rights won by events set in motion by the Mass Trespass. Similar sentiments concerning rights in relation to class equality and property were evident in the literature of English worker writers (some examples can be found in Morley and Worpole, 2009). Curzon expressed the view that he was merely a custodian of the properties he held, taking a deep interest in restoring them and giving them in his estate to the National Trust (Gilmour, 1994), although, as Hopkins (1986) points out, these arguments are fairly spurious given the effects of the control and power exercised in this relation. The theme of inequalities and health disparities arising from property ownership and land rights are repeated all over the world. Doing, being, becoming and belonging, may produce social transformation; the unequal social order is also a product of occupation.

Cultural Change and Acceptable Occupations

Lorretta Do Rozario (1994) has illustrated the importance of occupation in maintaining culture through key rituals. Archaeologists know that this is a feature of cultural exchange and transition. Pryor (2004) notes British made trade items amongst Native American grave goods, and Roman trade items in Late Iron Age graves in southern England. It is unreasonable to expect people to continue to uphold their traditional standards to satisfy a Western romance of the cultures its influence nearly destroyed, or to describe their failure to do so as a loss. Adopting or refusing these transitions is a right, just as Westerners expect to upgrade their mobile phones to the next generation and match their kitchen appliances to the latest colour scheme, which is progress. Pryor's claim (2004: 438) is that despite a couple of thousand years of considerable cultural change in the British Isles some values may have survived, and one of these is 'individual freedom'. Although this may have been imparted to many other cultures through the agency of colonial occupation, and to an extent this is what many colonial officials *believed* they were doing despite frequent failures to respond to the needs of the peoples they governed (Gilmour, 1994; Ferguson, 2004), Pryor asserts that it is an ancient value, one much more rooted in the people despite being suppressed by a succession of elites. The peacekeeping soldiers of various nationalities in Batistelli's (1997) and Hedlund's (2011) studies appear to have similar values and sometimes face similar problems in being able to respond (Dandeker and Gow, 2004).

All cultures change, but the political decision about which occupations are acceptable is an issue of power. Hopkins (1986) connects the rise of poaching as a source of social unrest with the rise of the rural poor. Like Linebaugh's (1991) depiction of the urban poor, he points to the removal of many of the opportunities that people had had to obtain payment in kind through their working practices, and which supplemented their wages. Linebaugh illustrates how eighteenth-century employers had allowed customs whereby a worker might keep spoiled produce or waste materials for their own use in lieu of higher wages, but these practices became criminalized. Consequently the eighteenth-century was a period where new distinctions of property and crime were being established to favour a wealthy elite, but a conflict over freedoms has continued. Much of the 2009 UK parliamentary expenses revelations show a similar difference between wealthy and poor social classes with regard to the expropriation of money from employers. Fiddling expenses is a crime but for many members of the UK parliament making false claims was until recently a way of supplementing their income, widely tolerated – just as labourers in the eighteenth century might acquire surplus or defective goods in the way of their work.

As we have seen, wealth and power have historically been key determinants of the occupational choices that are open to individuals, and social inequality based on relative affluence and poverty is a factor in producing health disparities (Thomas *et al.*, 2010). Due to their disposable income people may be able to afford treatment they have chosen over and above any that a state or more standard service may be able to support. There need not be any moral objection to this, as the individual is merely buying additional services (for a fuller discussion of these points see Tinghog *et al.*, 2010). A meritocratic argument for some of the disparities might be that it is reasonable that people should be encouraged to take responsibilities for reducing the costs of their healthcare to others. If people have the opportunity to eat healthily and exercise then it is their fault if they fail to do so, or if they decide to misuse substances or take other risks that injure their health.

Health and social care is often regarded as a form of commodity. In many countries people with sufficient resources can buy themselves care plans that ensure premium treatment that others cannot access. In such a system people may choose how much of their income they spend on health and receive a service according to the payments they make, but some groups of clients may not have many options, for example when they already have chronic mental health conditions. People who have experienced mental distress over a lifetime may have little economic power. However their condition creates considerable potential costs if they are brought into acute care because their situation is too chaotic for them to remain safely in the community. In the light of this possibility an egalitarian consideration about the distribution of healthcare resources might be that despite their choices everyone should have the same opportunity to access them when needed. It has often proved politically difficult, however, to determine how such equal opportunities can be provided when resources are limited (Tinghog *et al.*, 2010). Many governments are concerned about the rising cost of healthcare to meet people's expectations, not least in recent UK policy (Department of Health, 2006, 2010, 2011).

These concerns about cost place an emphasis on proving the value of services. Occupational therapists have a good fund of anecdotal and experiential knowledge of the benefits many therapeutic activities may have, but have lacked capacity in disseminating the evidence to support these claims (Taylor, 2007). Part of the problem of communicating this lies in the values of occupational therapy itself. If a key part of the goal of the therapist is to empower the client to own their individual achievements it can be difficult to standardize results. The outcome is reflected in what the client, not the therapist, has achieved. Craft activities with their easily realizable goals and capacity for building up strengths and ability in stages lend themselves to these enabling approaches if the client recognizes a purpose in them. However they can be difficult to facilitate in a replicable and generalizable way, and tend to involve small numbers of participants. This makes them difficult to represent in large-scale research studies. They have long been understood in health practices as being good for the soul, but have given way to work reablement or skills training, which is focussed on being better for the economy and for which evidence is stronger because standardized training techniques and measurable tools are being used. They can be assessed in larger numbers enabling randomized control trials (Gibson *et al.*, 2011).

Cost-effectiveness can be difficult to assess. We can determine the cost to one organization delivering healthcare, for example, of long-term mentally clients attending therapeutic sessions that may prevent their condition deteriorating and increasing their dependency on other services, or may reduce the risk of suicide. It is possible that the impact of providing this service reduces potential costs for other organizations running acute or community mental health services, but it may be difficult to ask them to pay towards it because it may be uncertain that the maintenance of relative health is due to this intervention rather than another factor affecting the group. However, there is often no real baseline against which nonevents arising from a policy of maintenance can be measured.

The therapist, who may struggle to identify the cost benefits of running traditional groups or individual programmes may instead become engaged in skills groups. However, a wealthy client can purchase premium occupational therapy treatments which can address the individual needs (perhaps those connected with lifestyle choices) a more cost conscious service may be unable to explore. The present policy of personalization of budgets in the UK has begun to generate a new range of services which service users can buy directly, such as attendance at craft groups for around £30 a session. These initiatives have been presented as a choice (Mandelstam, 2010) but their development is based on a calculation of what can be provided to generate a surplus for the organizations offering them, often operating from the voluntary sector. Thus, these choices are questions of occupation and power; but the question of who decides which occupations (in the form of lifestyles, life roles and health choices) are acceptable are essentially political questions that are determined by policy makers, and tend to be resolved by people who have access to power.

In the UK health professionals and service users are having to adapt to new conditions under which services are being provided. Perhaps these are the conditions that have already been established elsewhere in the world. The global spread of a market-led health philosophy may bring many practical benefits in containing the costs of health care and setting sensible limits to what a society may be expected to provide, but this does not mean that everything about it is right, simply because it is what many other people appear to accept. Many occupational activities are becoming standardized and delimited by these market forces.

Historically, human cultures of all scales reached a point where they were no longer sustainable. Often they used up the resources around them, and came into conflict with other groups, became too reliant on a narrow range of staple foods, or were weakened by diseases, reaching a point where they could not effect further adaptations to events around them (Fernandez-Armesto, 2000). On the other hand Willa Cather's *My Antonia* (1994 [1918]) set in Nebraska and Albert Facey's (1981) autobiography of settler life in Australia are reminders that the precarious origins of what may seem to their present members to be substantial modern societies and cultures are only a few generations away, only just out of living memory. The current urban interest in bushcraft, the popularity of activities like fishing and horticulture reveal that a relationship with the bounty of the raw landscape and a spiritual connection with nature remains as an important element of human expression of being and doing. The poacher's question concerning which person can really assert a right to the gifts of nature echoes the beliefs of the aboriginal hunter who maintains a symbiotic relationship with the environment, and is again reflected in the angler's experience of fishing (Bull, 2009). There is a tension between these direct personal engagements with the land and nature, and with the alienating forms of engagement that arise through human social development, the accumulation of property and patterns of consumption that reduce the environment, and therefore the things in it, including people, to objects.

Occupational Effect

The spectrum of human relationships with environment passes from the personal to the objective, and we do not intend to imply that a romantic quasi-aboriginal perspective of nature should be favoured over the evil mechanistic vision of a fallen humankind. Many of the examples we have so far discussed suggest that

Wilcock's (2006) mantra of doing, being, becoming and belonging is more than a series of pleasant sounding ideals. They concern acts of survival and determination, and express a mission (Wilcock, 2007) that, perhaps, is shared by the spiritual belief systems that people maintain. It is a particularly significant mission for occupational therapists because of their avowed concern with the facilitation of human activities. Despite this kind of vocation – after all the mantra occurs in many professional statements – few occupational therapists have yet (Wilcock, 2007: 19) 'to be true to their own rhetoric'. As Turner (2011) points out, the profession has rarely been able to exert powerful influence in law or policy, let alone the medical hegemony. The need for meaningful occupation as a right is continuously discussed in the professional literature, yet people with chronic conditions or in care homes often lack opportunities to express themselves, to escape the boredom or occupational alienation that might in others be a stimulus to action (e.g. Townsend and Wilcock, 2004). Wilcock (2007) points to the principle cause of this for a growing sector of the population – ageism. She argues that occupational therapists have to be active in confronting stigmatizations that lead to expectations of poor health and disability and to do so, Turner (2011) argues, therapists need to seek new alliances.

If occupational therapists are to uphold client centeredness or negotiate interventions in line with clients' needs, to form a rapport, then a different and more active politics of practice is required (Wilcock, 2007). Creating and maintaining professional status both establishes a boundary between the therapist from the client and identifies a separation of interest in the process of developing a client-centred practice. Professional status depends on the client relationship, which is used to justify the acquisition of specialist knowledge and forms of practice that have to be acquired through training and process. Professional education provides mechanisms for maintaining this distance, for example ethical principles that demand that this knowledge be employed in a professional way. The social construction of professionalization and its forms of intervention also creates parameters and boundaries between what is professional and unprofessional, formal and casual (Goffman, 1990; Abberley, 1995; Hammell, 2007, 2010; see Chapters 2, 10 and 15).

Client centredness also depends on a shared understanding of the benefits of intervention that empowers and informs the compliance of the client. The client has to feel that the intervention is enabling or facilitating an experience of doing and being in ways that relate to the client's existing or changing perception of what it is to do, be, become and belong, to occupy a role in society, to acquire social capital and experience the positive and affirming acknowledgement of others. Often this depends on a trust in the professional status of the therapist and this relationship sets boundaries to expectations that might otherwise produce role strain. Yet the professional relationship can also be constrained by the position occupational therapists occupy as stakeholders in issues such as clinical governance, the local implementation of health policies, through which they enact the decisions that others have taken concerning the clients with whom they work. The decisions they make or negotiate with other team members have an impact on how outcomes are delivered to the client; occupational therapists may espouse choice and client-centred practices but they often have to work within the limitations on those rights and choices set by their employers (Townsend and Wilcock, 2004; Hammell, 2007, 2010). Perhaps in these positions they accept a degree of powerlessness; perhaps they fear that if they raise the issues they will be squeezed out of the debate, such as it is. Some of the alliances that may be sought with client and carer lobbyists, but many do not have the power to influence care processes. In Chile, Alburquerque, Chana and CERTRAM Community (2010) have formed cooperative relationships between professionals and service users to build actions around occupational justice, and it is possible that such approaches can be adopted elsewhere, perhaps in the new context of healthcare emerging in the UK as new forms of organization become part of the framework of service delivery (Pollard, 2011).

These examples show how different actors operating in the same context have different motives and use different means to reach their goals. The resultant polyglossy refers to the different standpoints that people occupy and the means that these standpoints afford people to be recognized and their occupations legitimated. In such situations some groups of people, perhaps those with professional status such as occupational therapists, are legitimated through the law and the acceptance of practices, for example by the client.

However, a counter position can also be legitimated (even though it has no standing in law) because it is generally or widely accepted amongst a group of people. Poaching, because it concerns wild animals, has been popularly regarded as something other than theft. Gamekeepers upheld the law, while poachers questioned the law. In the arguments around the differences between these justifications each group had to afford the other some degree of recognition, even where poacher turned gamekeeper, and Hopkins (1986) reveals how both shared a keen interest in the phenomena concerning wild game. During the conflict between game preservers and poachers, each developed technologies, strategies and tactics to outmanoeuvre the other, and the justifications and legitimation altered.

Like occupational therapists, the gamekeepers were employed as professionals on behalf of a hegemony. They did not own the process although they had some power within it – they were servants to a particular social group who used the law to defend their interests. Occupational therapists are not employed as the defenders of a privileged minority but their position is still that of an intermediary at the frontline of a service operated by powerful groups. One of the hegemonic functions of this service is in ensuring social stability through the provision of adequate healthcare. As a consequence therapists have to be reactive as well as proactive if they are to maintain this position, keeping what Good (1994) termed a moving viewpoint, so as to capture all the different languages and voices that people use to express themselves in the environment of continuous change that they inhabit. In healthcare environments the health professional is often working with marginalized groups who do not belong to the normative ideal of society, who may be unable to access the changing language of the hegemony and whose needs often remain unmet. Changes which affect the way people are able to connect with services may have the effect of losing clients and threaten professional interests.

Being with the Others

Occupational polyglossy can lead to a healthy heterarchy of perspectives and cultures but the hegemonic group of a society often appropriates cultural discourse, while all other groups become problematized in varying degrees (see Chapters 2, 9 and 11). In the example of the game laws, which set the prevailing social structure of rural areas, a minority of powerful people wanted to reserve for themselves the right to exploit game. The consequence of laws that sequestered common land and the rights to the wildlife on it to protect this interest was that rural poverty increased. The threat to landowners' interests posed by the rural poor served as a reason to strengthen the law. The rural poor, marginalized from the land, became an 'other' (for a discussion of the concept of otherism see Kristeva, 1991), a problem calling for a solution.

The application of this process of otherness occurs across a range of margin-alizations, for example disabled people (see Chapters 10, 12 and 14), people who are refugees or asylum seekers, people who belong to ethnic minorities (see Chapter 9), who become objectified in the process. Often this has resulted in forms of state violence against people with disabilities, most notoriously in Nazi Germany, but also in democratic states, such as the US and the UK through forms of incarceration, forced sterilization and other medical treatments such as lobotomy carried out well into the postwar period (Breggin, 1993; Snyder and Mitchell, 2006). The least acceptable the diversity, the greater its problematization is likely to be. The consequence of idealizing the normal body and mind state is that it is always assumed to be the preferred state (see Chapters 12 and 14). Thus, as Siebers (2008) remarks, children with genital ambiguities or conditions such as adrenal hyperplasia are assigned the sexual organs the genitals they have most resemble. Irrespective of their gender, they will receive a surgical representation of a penis or vagina. Many people with disabilities have been denied the opportunity of a sexual life because of assumptions that they should somehow be debarred from exercising sexual func-tions, although, as Siebers illustrates through a number of examples, this is a fundamental human right (see Chapter 12).

Moreover, as Chapters 2, 10, 12 and 14 demonstrate, the battle over experiencing occupation your way or the normal way is something fought out with almost every human encounter, and as we have explored above, throughout much of the history of human society, expressed in many different ways. In some respects similar themes recur, although in different terminologies, but linked around aspects of the rela-tionship between human occupations and the social and physical environment in which these take place. Occupational therapists are part of a clinical apparatus and under the predominant medical framework of these forms of intervention are often expected to deal with discrete aspects of a process that is understood as the treatment of a condition, but the condition is often a product of the complex relationships between individual and a social context. The languages in which this relationship is expressed can take many forms, employing the terminologies and discourses of many knowledge disciplines, including the vernacular. These are further charged with issues of dominance and power. In order to understand the experiences of the individuals and communities they work with so that they can offer effective services, occupational therapists need to appreciate heteroglossia in their practice and develop an apparatus to navigate in it successfully (Sakellariou and Pollard, 2008).

Occupational therapists, by placing themselves as advocates for doing, being, becoming and belonging, represent part of the front line against the subtle expressions of occupational apartheid that arise in the discourses of power and use of knowledge, particularly in their facility to operate distinctions and categorizations that generate classes in which one group of people can call another 'other' (see Chapter 2). Snyder and Mitchell (2006) and Siebers (2008) make clear the link between perceptions of disability as disease and the biopolitics of racism. We might also add the biopolitics of class, which still has a tendency to be described in terms of disease and contamination such as 'feral underclass', 'breeds of violence', which have been repeatedly exploited in media discussions of social phenomena such as riots, violence and criminal activity amongst schoolchildren, benefit fraud and other evidence of social dysfunctionality (Cohen, 2002) and of course is the language of exclusion. In such a position, perhaps where they are working directly with people who are the objects of many forms of social exclusion, such as those experiencing chronic mental distress or long-term disability (do Rozario, 1994; Masterson and Owen 2006; see Chapters 10, 12, 14) occupational therapists need a combination of sensitivity and resiliency to withstand the crossfire and prove themselves worthy of the role they claim in facilitating expression through activity.

How this Book is Organized

The book is organized into three sections. In the first, consisting of Chapters 2–7, we consider how occupation may be structured through various metaphors concerning language, making connections with both occupational science and the practice of occupational therapy. Chapters 8–11 explore examples of occupation in the context of communities and environments and Chapters 12–14 consider individual aspects of occupational experience. Finally, in Chapter 15 these discussions are drawn together with a review of future directions in the field of occupation.

References

Abberley, P. (1995) Disabling Ideology in Health and Welfare – the case of occupational therapy. *Disability and Society* 10(2), 221–232.

Alburquerque, D., Chana, P., CERTRAM Community (2010) The CERTRAM community: building links for social change. In (eds) *Occupational Therapies without Borders (Volume 2): Towards an Ecology of Occupation-based Practices*. Edinburgh, Elsevier Science, 163–172.

American Occupational Therapy Association (2002) *Occupational Therapy Practice Framework Domain and Process*. Bethesday, American Occupational Therapy Association.

Bailey, D. (1981) *Children of the Green*. London, Stepney Books.

Barr, C. A. (2010) *How Civilians Survive Violence: A Preliminary Inventory*. Arlington, VA, The Cuny Centre.

Batistelli, F. (1997) Peacekeeping and the modern soldier. *Armed Forces and Society* 23(3), 467–484.

Beagan, B. L. (2007) The impact of social class: learning from occupational therapy students. *Canadian Journal of Occupational Therapy* 74(2), 125–133.

Beavis, D. (1980). *What Price Happiness? My Life from Coal Hewer to Shop Steward*. Whitley Bay, Strong Words.

Benjamin, W. (1996 [1921]) Capitalism as religion. In M. Bullock, M. W. Jennings (eds), *Walter Benjamin: Selected Writings. Volume 1: 1913-1926*. Cambridge, MA, The Belknap Press of Harvard University Press, pp. 288–291.

Blom-Cooper, L. (1990) *Occupational Therapy. An Emerging Profession in Health Care. Report of a Commission of Inquiry 1989*. London, Duckworth.

Breggin, P. (1993) *Toxic Psychiatry*. London, Fontana.

Breines, E. (2004) *Occupational Therapy: Activities for Practice and Teaching*. London, Whurr.

Bull, J. (2009) Watery masculinities: fly-fishing and the angling male in the south-west of England. *Gender, Place and Culture: A Journal of Feminist Geography* 16(4), 445–465.

Burt, E. L., Atkinson, J. (2011) The relationship between quilting and wellbeing. *Journal of Public Health* 33(2) doi: 10. 1093/pubmed/fdr041.

Cather, W. (1994 [1918]) *My Antonia*. New York, Dover.

Cohen, S. (2002) *Folk Devils and Moral Panics: The Creation of the Mods and Rockers*, 3rd edn. London, Routledge.

Creek, J. (2003) Occupational therapy defined as a complex intervention. London: College of Occupational Therapists.

Dandeker, C., Gow, J. (2004) Military culture and strategic peacekeeping. In J. Callahan, W. Schorborn,(eds) *Warriors in Peacekeeping: Points of Tension in Complex Cultural Encounters*. Piscataway, NJ, Transaction, pp. 11–27.

Department of Health (2006) *No Excuses. Embrace Partnership Now. Step Towards Change! Report of the Third Sector Commissioning Task Force*. London, Department of Health.

Department of Health (2010) *Equity and Excellence: Liberating the NHS*. London, Department of Health.

Department of Health (2011) *Health and Social Care Bill 2011*. London, Department of Health.

Detweiler, J., Peyton, C. (1999) Defining occupations: a chronotypic study of narrative genres in a health discipline's emergence. *Written Communication* 16, 412–468.

do Rozario, L. (1994) Ritual, meaning and transcendence: the role of occupation in modern life. *Journal of Occupational Science* 1(3), 46–53.

do Rozario, L. (1997) Shifting paradigms: the transpersonal dimensions of ecology and occupation. *Journal of Occupational Science* 4(3), 112–118.

Earl Marshall School (1993) *Lives of Love and Hope: A Sheffield Herstory*. Sheffield, Earl Marshall School.

Eco, U. (2000) *Kant and the Platypus; Essays on Language and Cognition*. New York, Mariner Books.

Facey, A. B. (1981) *A Fortunate Life*. Victoria, Penguin.

Fearnley-Whittingstall, H. (1997) *A Cook on the Wild Side*. London, Boxtree.

Fearnley-Whittingstall, H. (2010) Chicken Out! http://www.chickenout.tv/political.html accessed 12 October 2010.

Ferguson, N. (2004) *Empire. How Britain Made the Modern World*. London, Penguin.

Fernandez-Armesto, F. (2000) *Civilisations*. London, Macmillan.

Foster, L. (1984) *Religion and Sextuality. The Shakers, Mormons and the Oneida Community*. Illinois, University of Illinois.

Foucault, M. (1972) *The Archaeology of Knowledge*. Transl. A. M. Sheridan Smith. London, Routledge.

Foucault, M. (2010) *The Government of Self and Other; Lectures at the College de France*. Transl. G. Burchell. Basingstoke, Pallgrave Macmillan.

Frank, G., Zemke, R. (2008) Occupational therapy foundations for political engagement and social transformation. In N. Pollard, D. Sakellariou, F. Kronenberg (eds) *A Political Practice of Occupational Therapy*. Edinburgh, Elsevier/Churchill Livingstone, pp. 111–136.

Galheigo. S. M. (2011) What needs to be done? Occupational therapy responsibilities and challenges regarding human rights. *Australian Occupational Therapy Journal* 58, 60–66.

Gibson, R. W., D'Amico, M., Jaffe, L., Arbesman, M. (2011) Occupational Therapy Interventions for Recovery in the Areas of Community Integration and Normative Life Roles for Adults With Serious Mental Illness: A Systematic Review. *American Journal of Occupational Therapy* 65, 247–256.

Gilfoyle, E. M. (1984) Transformation of a profession. *American Journal of Occupational Therapy* 38, 575–584.

Gilmour, D. (1994) *Curzon*. London, John Murray.

Good, B. (1994). Medicine, rationality and experience. Cambridge: Cambridge University Press

Goffman, E. (1990) *The Presentation of Self in Everyday Life*. Harmondsworth, Penguin.

Gordon, D. (2009) The history of occupational therapy. In E. B. Crepeau, E. S. Cohn, B. A. Boyt-Schell (eds) *Willard and Spackman's Occupational Therapy*, 11th edn. Philadelphia, PA, Lipincott, Williams & Wilkins, pp. 202–215.

Hammell, K. W. (2007) Client-centred practice: ethical obligation or professional obfuscation? *British Journal of Occupational Therapy* 70(6), 264–266.

Hammell, K. W. (2008) Reflections on well-being and occupational rights. *Canadian Journal of Occupational Therapy* 75, 61–64.

Hammell, K. W. (2010) Contesting assumptions in occupational therapy. In (eds) *Occupational Therapy and Physical Dysfunction*. Edinburgh, Churchill Livingstone/Elsevier, pp. 39–54.

Harris, H. (1978) *Under Oars*. Hackney, Centerprise.

Hawker, J. (1978) *A Victorian Poacher: James Hawker's Journal*. Oxford, Oxford University Press.

Hedlund, E. (2011) What motivates Swedish soldiers to participate in peacekeeping missions: research note. *Armed Forces and Society* 37(1), 180–190.

Hocking, C. (2007) The romance of occupational therapy. In J. Creek, A. Lawson-Porter (eds) *Contemporary Issues in Occupational Therapy: Reasoning and Reflection*. Chichester, Wiley, pp. 23–40.

Hopkins, H. (1986) *The Long Affray: The Poaching Wars in Britain 1760–1914*. London, Papermac.

Ikiugu, M.N., Pollard, N. (in press). Meaningful living through occupation. London: Whiting and Birch.

Irwin, G. (1995) *The Sudden Change in My Life*. Brighton, QueenSpark. Iwama, M. (2004) Meaning and inclusion: revisiting culture in occupational therapy. Australian Occupational Therapy Journal 51(1) 1–2.

Iwama, M.K. (2006) *The Kawa Model: Culturally Relevant Occupational Therapy*. Edinburgh, Churchill Livingstone/Elsevier.

Iwama, M.K., Thomson, N.A., Macdonald. R.M. (2010) Cultural safety, inclusion and occupational therapy. In F. Kronenberg, N. Pollard, D. Sakellariou (eds) *Occupational Therapies without Borders*, Volume 2. Edinburgh, Elsevier/Churchill Livingstone, pp. 85–92.

King, A. (2001) Violent pasts: collective memory and football hooliganism. *The Sociological Review* 49(4), 568–585.

Klein, A. (2007) Khat and the creation of tradition in the Somali diaspora. In J. Fountain, D. J. Korf (eds) *Drugs in Society: European Perspectives*. Oxford, Radcliffe, pp. 51–61.

Kristeva, J. (1991) *Strangers to Ourselves*. New York, Columbia University Press.

Linebaugh, P. (1991) *The London Hanged*. Harmondsworth, Penguin.

Lloyd, A. L. (1969) *The Folksong of England*. London, Panther.

Lloyd, A. L. (1978) *Come All Ye Bold Miners: Ballads and Songs of the Coalfields*. London, Lawrence & Wishart.

Lowe, R., Shaw, W. (1993) *Voices of the New Age Nomads: Travellers*. London, Fourth Estate.

Mandelstam, M. (2010) Personalisation of social care: benefits and pitfalls for users of services and occupational therapists. *British Journal of Occupational Therapy* 73(8), 391–394.

Masterson, S., Owen, S. (2006) Mental health service users' social and individual empowerment: using theories of power to elucidate far-reaching strategies. *Journal of Mental Health* 15(1), 19–34.

Mattingly, C. (1998) *Healing Dramas and Clinical Plots. The Narrative Structure of Experience*. Cambridge, Cambridge University Press.

Max-Neef, M. (2010) The world on a collision course. *AMBIO* 39, 200–210.

Mayr A. (2004) *Prison Discourse: Language as a Means of Control and Resistance*. Hamphsire, Palgrave Macmillan.

Molineux, M., Rickard, W. (2003) Storied approaches to understanding occupation. Journal of Occupational Science 10(1), 52–60.

Molineux, M., Whiteford, G. (2006) Occupational science: Genesis, evolution and future contribution. In E.A.S. Duncan (ed) Foundation for practice in occupational therapy (4th ed). Edinburgh: Churchill Livingstone, pp 297–312.

Morley, D., Worpole, K. (2009) (eds) *The Republic of Letters*, 2nd edn. Philadelphia, New Cities Community Press/Syracuse University Press.

Mosey, A. C. (1971) Involvement in the rehabilitation movement – 1942 to 1960. *American Journal of Occupational Therapy* 25, 234–236.

Muckle, W. (1981) *No Regrets*. Newcastle upon Tyne, People's Publications.

Noakes, G. (1977) *To Be A Farmer's Boy*. Brighton, QueenSpark.

Noble, E. M. (1984) *Jamaica Airman, a Black Airman in Britain, 1943 and After*. London, New Beacon.

Park, M. (2008) Making scenes: imaginative practices of a child with autism in a sensory integration-based therapy. *Medical Anthropology Quarterly* 22(3), 234–256.

Paterson, C. F. (2008) A short history of occupational therapy in psychiatry. In J. Creek, L. Lougher (eds) *Occupational Therapy and Mental Health*, 4th edn. Edinburgh, Elsever/Churchill Livingstone, pp. 3–16.

Peckham People's History (1983) *The Times of Our Lives, Growing up in the Southwark Area 1900-1945*. Peckham, Peckham Publishing Project.

Phillips, D. (2006) Quality of Life, Concept, Policy and Practice. London, Routledge.

Piper, R., (1995) *Take Him Away*. Brighton, QueenSpark.

Pollard, N. (2008) When Adam Dalf and Eve Span: occupational literacy and democracy. In N. Pollard, D. Sakellariou, F. Kronenberg (eds) *A Political Practice of Occupational Therapy*. Edinburgh, Elsevier/Churchill Livingstone, pp. 39–51.

Pollard, N. (2011) Working in social enterprises. *International Journal of Physiotherapy and Rehabilitation*. 1(2), 30–37.

Pollard, N., Sakellariou, D. (2008) Facing the challenge: a compass for navigating the heteroglossic context. In N. Pollard, D. Sakellariou, F. Kronenberg (eds) *A Political Practice of Occupational Therapy*. Edinburgh, Elsevier/Churchill Livingstone, pp. 237–244.

Pryor, F. (2004) *Britain BC. Life in Britain and Ireland before the Romans*. London, Harper Perennial.

Sakellariou, D., Pollard, N. (2008) Three sites of conflict and co-operation: class, gender and sexuality. In N. Pollard, D. Sakellariou, F. Kronenberg (eds) *A Political Practice of Occupational Therapy*. Edinburgh, Elsevier/Churchill Livingstone, pp. 69–89.

Sheffield Campaign for Access to Moorland (1988) *Freedom of the Moors. Sheffield*, Sheffield, Campaign for Access to the Moorland.

Shore, L., (1982) *Pure Running, A Life Story*. Hackney, Hackney Reading Centre.

Sitzia, L., Thickett, A., (2002) *Seeking the Enemy*. London, wORking press

Siebers, T. (2008) *Disability Theory*. Ann Arbor, University of Michigan Press.

Snyder, S. L., Mitchell, D. T. (2006) *Cultural Locations of Disability*. Chicago, University of Chicago Press.

Taylor, M. C. (2007) *Evidence-based Practice for Occupational Therapists*. 2nd edn. Oxford, Blackwell.

Thomas, B., Dorling, D., Davey Smith, G. (2010) An observational study of health inequalities in Brita in: geographical divides returning to 1930s maxima by 2007. *British Medical Journal* 341 c3639 doi:10.1136/bmj.c3639.

Thompson, L., (1987) *Just a Cotchell, Tales from a Docklands' Childhood and Beyond*. London, Basement Writers.

Tinghog, G., Carlsson, P., Lyttkens, C. H. (2010) Individual responsibility for what? A conceptual framework for exploring the suitability of private financing in a publicly funded health-care system. *Health Economics, Policy and Law 5*, 201–223.

Townsend, E. (1997) Occupation: Potential for personal and social transformation. *Journal of Occupational Science* 4(1), 18–26.

Townsend, E., Wilcock, A. A. (2004) Occupational justice and client centred practice. *Canadian Journal of Occupational Therapy* 71(2), 75–87.

Turner, A. (2002) History and philosophy of occupational therapy. In A. Turner, M. Foster, S. Johnson (eds) *Occupational Therapy and Physical Dysfunction, Principles Skills and Practice*. Edinburgh, Churchill Livingstone, pp. 3–24.

Turner, A. (2011) The Elizabeth Casson Memorial Lecture 2011: occupational therapy – a profession in adolescence? *British Journal of Occupational Therapy* 74(7), 314–322.

Vincent, D. (1981) *Bread, Knowledge and Freedom, A Study of Ninteenth-Century Working Class Autobiography*. London, Europa Publications.

Weisaeth, L. (2003) The psychological challenge of peacekeeping operations. In T. W. Britt, A. B. Adler (eds) *The Psychology of the Peacekeeper: Lessons from the Field*. Wesport, CT, Praeger, pp. 207–222.

Whiteford, G., Townsend, E., Hocking, C. (2000) Reflections on a renaissance of occupation. *Canadian Journal of Occupational Therapy* 67(1), 61–69.

Whiteford, G., Klomp, N., Wright-St Clair (2005) Complexity theory: Understanding occupation, practice and context. In G. Whiteford and V. Wright-St Clair (eds) Occupation and practice in context. Sydney: Elsevier, pp. 3–15.

Wilcock A. A. (1998) Doing, being and becoming. *Canadian Journal of Occupational Therapy* 65, 248–257.

Wilcock A. A., Townsend, E. (2000) Occupational terminology interactive dialogue. *Journal of Occupational Science* 7(2), 84–86.

Wilcock A. A. (2002) Occupation for Health, Volume 2: A Journey from Prescription to Self Health. London, College of Occupational Therapists.

Wilcock, A. A. (2006) *An Occupational Perspective of Health*. Thorofare, NJ, Slack Inc.

Wilcock, A. A. (2007) Active ageing: dream or reality? *New Zealand Journal of Occupational Therapy* 54(1), 15–20.

Wiltshire, P. (1985) *Living and Winning*. Hackney, Centerprise.

Woodin, T. (2009) Rethinking society and culture. In D. Morley, K. Worpole,(eds) *The Republic of Letters: Working Class Writing and Local Publishing*. Philadelphia and Syracuse, New City Community Press/Syracuse University Press, pp. 240–256.

World Federation of Occupational Therapists (2004) Position paper on community based rehabilitation. Australia, WFOT.

World Federation of Occupational Therapists (2006) Position statement on human rights. Australia, WFOT.

2 The Language of Occupation

Nick Pollard and Dikaios Sakellariou

Occupational therapy has had to develop a professional discourse that objectivized occupation so that it could be explored. The reasons for this ranged from a need to codify the area of interest and the knowledge of the profession, to a survival tactic of allying with the scientific language (and by extension, the scientific ways and scientific language) of biomedicine. The continuously emerging vocabulary of occupational therapy encompasses several nouns that are qualified with the prefix 'occupational' and which are used to describe several aspects of the occupational therapy process or sphere of interest (e.g. occupational goals, occupational being, occupational justice, occupational trajectory, occupational adaptation). However, these terms have often been applied inconsistently (Hagedorn, 2001) and they may not make much sense outside of the realm of the profession, or else may be too close to lay language to be specific in their use.

Focusing on the use of language in occupational therapy, this chapter will offer a critical overview of the development of a professional language of occupation. This language not only acts to acculturate students and professionals in what occupational therapy is about but it also guides the interactions between professionals and service users and shapes, or enables the interpretation, of the different stories surrounding these interactions.

Language, Cultural Meanings and Nosologies

Language embeds occupation in cultural practices and maintains cultural hierarchy and notions of power through the use of various sociolinguistic codes. Thus we use different words (or 'signs') to refer to the same actions or persons according to context. The use for example of second person pronouns to denote familiarity or respect is widespread in many languages of Indo-European origin (e.g. French *tu/vous*; Spanish *tu/usted*; German *du/Sie*), although this distinction is mostly obsolete in modern English (*thou/you*) with the exception of some dialects. Different

Politics of Occupation-Centred Practice: Reflections on Occupational Engagement across Cultures, First Edition. Edited by Nick Pollard and Dikaios Sakellariou.
© 2012 John Wiley & Sons, Ltd. Published 2012 by John Wiley & Sons, Ltd.

languages and cultural contexts require context-appropriate use of language to maintain cultural hierarchy. In Japan, where language operates on the basis of an intricate nexus of social hierarchy, several first person pronouns are in use, and their use is stipulated by the relative position between the interlocutors, rather by a fixed position occupied by the speaker. Use of pronouns is just one of the ways that power is expressed through the use of language. The use of euphemisms, the distinctions between vernacular and formal expressions and the construction of professional languages, or jargon, are other ways through which the interplay between power and language can be witnessed.

Language, and the way nosological entities (i.e. the classifications of diseases) are being constructed, framed and described is also intricately connected to cultural meanings, associated not only with illness but with a 'normal' or expected way of living, in local or broader social worlds. The folk, the lay and the scientific explanatory models of illness all employ different terms to refer to disease, but also health seeking behaviour, aetiology and so forth. The advent of a discourse of normality, measuring normal behaviours and processes, led to the development of the concept of pathology (Canguilhem, 1989). Consequently, conditions that had been seen as legitimate ways of being were deemed not normal, and were subject to what Foucault (1989) called the medical gaze. The mechanisms through which pathologization occurs are many. Cultural meanings of pain and fatigue; availability of genetic testing; accurate and available diagnostic technologies; role of family and cultural images of the body can lead to the construction of behaviours as pathological, not normal, or in some way open them up to a notion of healthcare intervention, and to their regulation or management through the use of professional language.

Due to its very nature as a system of signs rather than symbols (the latter are related to their referents through a process of logical association, while the connection of signs to their referents is more abstract) (Eco, 2000), not only can one condition be constructed in different ways, with different terms to describe it, but often the same term will conjure many meanings and experiences, not all of them compatible. This of course depends on the context within which specific words are being used. Diagnostic terms like cerebral palsy (CP), amyotrophic lateral sclerosis (ALS) or dystonia refer to a specific set of symptoms, clinical signs and pathophysiological processes, and from that perspective, talking about ALS, for example, creates, or assumes, a shared understanding of the condition. On the other hand, research on the experience of living with chronic illness has shown that there is no template chronic illness experience, so that, in experiential terms, it may not be particularly useful to talk of CP or ALS. This is not to say that these terms do not have their use. In the following section we discuss the development of professional language in the case of occupational therapy, and its significance to the development of a professional identity.

Language, Occupation and Professional Status

Being a numerically small profession, one of the problems in the dissemination of occupational therapy knowledge, theory and practice is that many occupational therapy students have to study from texts in a second language. The profession, having developed in the English-speaking countries, is often reliant on English texts and journals. This situation is exacerbated by the use of English as the lingua franca of commerce. As a consequence knowledge of occupational therapy practice and theory has tended to flow from the West to other countries. Practitioners are generally interested in information that reflects their own cultural background and experience, so it is difficult to represent the potential that may be present in the practice of occupational therapy in non English speaking countries outside international conferences.

In order to become professionals occupational therapy students have to learn the codes of the profession, for example, the particular use of 'occupation' in English to denote human engagement in doing, being, becoming and belonging, rather than a more restricted application to forms of work, forms of assessment and analysis and the breaking down of actions into functional components. Students learn to describe actions in a technical vocabulary that objectifies these actions and makes them generalizable to other situations for assessment. They share an understanding of what 'occupation' refers to, even if the people they work with do not. As Iwama (2006) has indicated, the shared meaning of occupation and the individualist philosophy behind it may not always connect with the terms available in students' own culture.

Education in understanding and using these codes allows students to interpret events and phenomena in the formal languages of the occupational therapy and other clinical professions rather than employ the informal terms commonly used to describe everyday activities and tacit understandings of human actions. Through education, students learn to demonstrate their competences in the practice of human occupation through a professionalized discourse. This enables them to make the transition from a lay person into a professional. Their successful acquisition of these competences is demonstrated by a combination of assessments in practice and academic exercises using a specialized professional vocabulary, which is ceremonially recognized at graduation. With the assumption of a gown and mortar board, students enter the class of occupational therapists with a professional status that badges them as members of the middle classes (Sakellariou and Pollard, 2008).

Of course graduation is not really the marker of class status, for at the point of entry to their courses students begin to learn that in order to speak and behave as a professional it is necessary to adopt new codes of conduct and action that leave other behaviours, including the language that goes with them, behind. For example, common greetings in English such as 'whatcha, mate', 'wassup', or 'now then' might convey an impression of a lack of professionalism (although in some areas such as psychiatric work they might be used to maintain a friendly rapport with users of services). Even before this, in the process of school education, people are encouraged to acquire the rhetorical practices of presenting arguments in a way that recognize the cultural rules of dominance, the components of citizenship, the facilities with which a person can participate in a wider society and the rudiments of a literacy that will serve these governing principles (Cook-Gumperz, 1986). Education is overseen by government and generally serves the interests of political and socioeconomic, i.e. hegemonic, power, particularly under the present emphasis on vocational and business skills (Wright, 2011). It therefore serves to reinforce social class, even where policy might declare an intention to be socially inclusive (Beagan, 2007).

In Britain a social emphasis on literacy began to emerge in the eighteenth century (Cook-Gumperz, 1986), and as we explore in Chapter 3 this was expressed in the different uses of language operated by different social classes (Linebaugh, 1991). The introduction of mass schooling in the nineteenth century placed an emphasis on literacy that served the hegemony, favouring the knowledge that power requires and determines in the curriculum, rather than the forms of vernacular and tacit knowledge that exist amongst those with less power. Knowledge, language and literacy become stratified, and the forms that pertain to lesser levels of the hierarchical order are less regarded or are not recognized (Cook-Gumperz, 1986). A child who wrote 'watcha, mate' in a school essay would receive a correction such as 'this is not English', even though it was the language used in the playground or at home, just as, in colonial education systems, minority languages and the practices expressed through them were frequently dismissed or denied status (Romaine, 2002). As Ives (2009), Romaine (2002) and Crystal (2003) indicate, these issues are often influenced by complex social and environmental, we might say 'occupational' factors, which may operate beyond elements of policy and even in contradiction of, for example, attempts to preserve endangered languages. People with other linguistic heritages naturally need to acquire knowledge of dominant forms of languages such as English, Spanish, French, Mandarin or Russian where these are the lingua franca of particular societies. If they cannot, then they may be socially disenfranchised in the momentum of events because they do not have access to the medium in which leading social developments are being discussed. This has an impact both on less influential languages and on dialect, in that the tendency is to expand the influence of dominant forms. However, as Crystal (2003) points out, this is not a one-way exchange, because languages such as English contain numerous loan words, such as the German term that might be used to describe leading social developments: 'zeitgeist' – the spirit of the times. Although through such experiences people often learn to become multimodal, to change and suit their expression to the social circumstances, there remains a sense in which the tacit or vernacular forms of knowledge are of less value than those which are acquired formally. This is illustrated in Hines' (1969) novel *A Kestrel for a Knave* which has for years been popular school reading, and reflects the social disenfranchisement and division that existed in the UK's school system for children of average ability. Holbrook (1964) reported many damaging examples where, for their lack of formal knowledge, children's other abilities were ignored.

The legacy of this continues in the adult population today (Smart *et al.*, 2010, see Chapter 11). The majority of healthcare clients do not belong to the privileged classes. They have had restricted access to education and other opportunities due to regional economic and social differences. While 36% of the UK working population had a degree or equivalent in 2010, the highest proportion of these being in the south-east of England (Wright, 2011), other research suggests that 75% of the same population had numeracy skills and 56% had literacy skills below a good pass at GCSE level (General Certificate of Secondary Education) (House of Commons, 2009a). The lack of education and skills is one of the contributing factors to poverty, not only because of restricted employment opportunities but also because people are less equipped to understand and use information about finance, debt management, and access to services.

Holbrook (1964: 272) indicates how 'three eights of our whole population' (the children he referred to would now constitute those people currently reaching retirement age) were regarded as 'duds' even while they were in school, and learned this perfectly well by the time they left. At one level, people are simply unable to understand the terms in which this information is written because the language is not sufficiently clear. Another dimension of this is a long-established link between poverty in education, early involvement in crime and subsequent social deprivation, despite which the benefits of educational provision are ignored (Bynner, 2009). This socioeconomic problem exercises an influence far wider than those who are directly involved in criminal activity, affecting not only social conditions but also health. Essentially, as a number of headmasters and teachers critiqued by Holbrook (1964) indicated, educational opportunities are rationed. A limit to what is affordable is applied in all services, including health. That limit applied to each aspect of state provision produces multiple exclusions, but these often apply to the same group of people (House of Commons, 2009b).

Occupational therapists are often separated from the people they are working with, their 'clients'. The language they speak reflects their higher education and their professional status; they are expected to maintain a professional distance in the course of their work practice (Swain and French, 2009; College of Occupational Therapists, 2010). These distinctions underpin an economic difference through better security of tenure as public sector employees (Wright, 2011) in some countries and the better paid professional jobs and the privileges that go with their status. It is the higher education that determines the status, but the language that is used (forms of received pronunciation English in the UK, i.e. BBC announcers' English, augmented through regional accents) is one of the social markers through which this status is recognized. The vocabulary of occupational therapy is a recognizable feature that conveys the status of professional expertise.

Economic factors are another closely linked social marker; salaries give an approximate indication of these status differences. Most therapists with more than two or three years of experience are paid at a rate above the median UK male salary level (in 2010 this was £538 per week; £439 per week for women); the median for the public sector (where most UK occupational therapists are employed) was £544 (Office for National Statistics, 2011). Occupational therapist band 6, a level usually attained within 2–3 years, started at £24,931 to £33,436 and band 7 at £29,798 to £39,273 (£479–£643 and £573–£755 per week respectively, figures from Prospects, 2011).

Naturally, professional groups want to protect their status and advance their interests. Associations such as the World Federation of Occupational Therapists and professional bodies such as the UK's Health and Social Care Professions Council, or Australia's new registration scheme exist to regulate the profession. These establish, for example, guidelines for education and for fitness to practice, and to prevent other people who might simply call themselves occupational therapists from doing so without having undergone the appropriate training (Council of Occupational Therapists' Registration Boards (Australia and New Zealand)/OT Australia, (2010)). Such professional bodies celebrate their membership with their own events and ceremonies that are enacted regularly at conferences, formal dinners, elevated forms of membership given to mark the dedication of those who serve the profession and badges of office such as the insignia worn by their chairpersons. While these rituals are a way of recognizing and encouraging professional achievement, through such practices occupational therapists appear to leave 'secular' society and enter a 'priesthood' or sorority, just as in ancient times when healing was frequently part of the duties of priestly orders. Living in different accommodation, wearing different clothing, or communicating through cryptic codes were indicators of this distinctive role.

These distinctions are still maintained through therapy departments or offices, uniforms, and professional terminologies. The operation of codes through which everyday human activities are depicted as 'occupations' and are analysed to form a body of professional knowledge combines with other differences to afford occupational therapists a place in the hegemonic structures of power that operate over health and social care. Occupational therapists need to maintain boundaries not only to preserve their professional status with regard to the client or service user, but also with respect to the other elements of the hegemony within which they work and on which they depend for their status.

Whereas occupational therapy might be considered as working with people who are designated as 'other' through their experience of disabilities, at the same time, in order to define strategies to approach the resolution or the containment of otherness, occupational therapists must themselves be 'other'. However, because it is a profession that is connected to the shifting boundaries of tacit and formal knowledge, of changes in professional practice and policy with regard to provision of health and social care, and concerns about the legislation of practice (Council of Occupational Therapists' Registration Boards (Australia and New Zealand)/OT Australia, (2010)), occupational therapy is also preoccupied with the negotiation of 'indeterminate zones' of professional practice (Schon, 1987: 12). Consequently the profession has continuously been challenged to operate a core description of what it does (Mackey, 2006).

One of the difficulties in the negotiation of occupation is that having developed specialist knowledge and vocabulary about everyday 'doing', the professional encourages clients to achieve outcomes that they can recognize as their own. To do this, therapists have to reinterpret their language into terms that can be communicated back to and owned by the client but in the process the critical perspective is lost (Iwama, 2006; Pollard, 2010). Often clients and clinical colleagues hear 'common sense' solutions but do not recognize or value the process by which the solution is found. The resulting presumption is that 'anyone could do it', though often occupational therapists can identify situations where no-one else is doing it because the need for meaningful occupation is often overlooked (Wilcock, 2007). These perceptions combine with the historical craft orientation of the profession and its alliance to medicine to produce a general understanding of occupational therapy as a female profession (Hocking, 2007). This is replicated because the selection of occupational therapy activities is determined by its gendered membership – for example Denshire (2002) and Kinsella (2006) suggest that occupational therapists draw reflectively on their own living experience in establishing values, and necessarily incorporate a high degree of subjectivity in the representation of everyday life. The basis of the profession in everyday practicalities is its strength but is also its weakness. In the pursuit of professional status and values, occupational therapy has sought to move away from its gendered concern with secular creative and domestic values and align itself with dominant biomedical principles (Pollard and Walsh, 2000; Hocking, 2007).

If we consider that some of the origins of the profession are in the nineteenth-century Arts and Craft movement of Morris and Ruskin, there is a historical connection with the commodification of activities around the home, which might be reflected in this subjective replication of occupation. Morris in particular, through his concerns with home furnishings and design and quality of products may have been looking back to the renaissance era, but he was doing so at a time when new forms of mass consumerism were being vigorously developed (Haydon, 1994; Flanders, 2006; James, 2006). Zola's novel, *Au bonheur des dames* (*The Ladies Paradise*, 1883/1995) illustrates how the domestic arena, opportunities for leisure, for self-improvement and for self presentation were all being transformed by an industrial increase in the availability of things to furnish and adorn them with, things to do, places to go to. This was the era of the birth of popular tourism, spectator sports, mass media, mass entertainment, public transport, department stores and mail order. The language of what the profession might term as doing, being, becoming and belonging was full of new terms to describe new forms of activity with new products and as a consequence many new occupational identities (see, for example, Chapter 13). As Zola's novel and its companion *Pot bouille* (translated as *Pot Luck*, 1882/1999) in his depiction of nineteenth-century French society reveal, this largely middle-class pattern of consumption depended on low-paid hard work and extremely poor living conditions for an army of workers. It is perhaps no coincidence that, at the same time, attacks on the harsh factory conditions and human exploitation that served these consumer excesses were published, demanding a balance in work hours and better pay. While Larfargue's (1883/2000) critique sharply demanded a swing much more in favour of leisure than work, he did not propose very practical measures for change beyond a satirical revenge on the capitalists.

The improvements social reformers such as Octavia Hill aimed to make were often aspirational not only in a moral sense, but in the sense of altering or navigating patterns of consumption to suit a different moral environment, through, for example, opportunities for leisure (Wilcock, 1999). Despite their soulful and expressive values (Hocking, 2007) the reformism of Ruskin, Morris, Hill and many others was part of a middle-class reaction to these new patterns of consumption. In various ways the rising nineteenth-century middle class wanted to impose restrictions on working class idleness and dissolution and avoid social contamination (James, 2006), all the more so because poor and wealthy lived cheek by jowl in the sprawling cities and towns (Girouard, 1990; Haydon, 1994). Ruskin, despite his advice to men and women and despite his radical speech making, was at a distance from the poor whose rights he advocated. Ruskin may have abhorred many 'vulgar' aspects of mass consumerism, but in his advice on self-improvement and the acquisition of libraries, for example (1865/2002), he was as much a part of it as anyone else. In some respects, then, occupational therapy can regard itself as a product of the consumer era and the new opportunities this has brought to our contemporary cultures.

The idea that culture is lost is a romantic one but not necessarily true. It may be that, in many cases, consumerism both democratizes activities and assimilates new products into existing cultures, but many aspects remain unchanged (Sahlins, 1999; Pryor, 2004; see Chapter 13). As Kasnitz and Block discuss (Chapter 14), all people have a right to the benefits of the consumer culture they live in. At the same time, as Ikiugu (2008/2010) indicates, occupational therapists might take an occupational science approach to address the unsustainable issues these developments have generated. Such measures address the issues of unsustainability for everyone, and while Ikiugu seems to propose individual actions, there are also, as Max-Neef (2010) and others have suggested, fundamental concerns about the impossibility of continued economic growth and demand.

Despite this plethora of occupation the profession is constrained and contained by a male order of scientific paradigm within medical knowledge, and even more by that of the dominance of capital. The language of the health professions in the UK has increasingly become oriented to market concerns through the introduction of managerialism from the late 1980s and 1990s (Greer, 2010). Patients are now 'clients' who are not subject to interventions but can exercise choice in the treatments they access (although in practice the choice may be quite limited). Market values have had other effects, emphasizing productivity through rehabilitation toward work, speeding recovery or at least discharge times. Traditional creative occupational therapy interventions such as crafts became regarded as hobbies, and as having less economic value than skills training, for example (Hocking, 2007). As a consequence, authors such as Burt and Atkinson (2011) are able to remark that there is little literature on the value of hobbies in relation to wellbeing, and at a time when many Western countries have ageing populations who in facing longer retirements (because they will live longer than previous generations) may benefit from an emphasis on the creative and spiritual aspect of occupation rather than one on product.

Not only crafts may have suffered neglect, but other traditional male occupations may have also been overlooked, such as recreational angling, one of the most popular sports in the USA and UK (Bull, 2009), kit modelling or model engineering. Despite the fact that many of these can be done with basic equipment, they rarely feature as occupational therapy media (see Chapter 13). It is not so much that the language used within the profession does not afford the existence, or exploration, of a wide variety of occupational endeavours; it is rather the fact that despite holistic tools such as the model of human occupation or the recognition of the complexity of occupation, the profession has some difficulty making sense of or developing opportunities for such occupations. We are not suggesting that individual occupational therapists do not understand them but that, because of the professional context in which most therapists work, facilitating such occupations can be problematic. Aside from a tendency to interpret human occupation from a rather restricted conceptual basis of middle class, Western and gendered values, the working context of therapists in teams has been that certain professional values and commonalities have become emphasized over others (Hocking, 2007). To try and set such activities up within a department would involve taking them out of their usual sociocultural context and so deprive them of natural elements. Occupational therapists and occupational scientists are enmeshed in the disabling society against which they work with clients, educate students, and critique. Rather than working to a human dimension they are instead distanced from the production of what Illich 1975 calls 'conviviality' and Cruz, Stahel and Max-Neef (2009) might term an Aristotelian 'oikonomy' by the pervasive processes of capital and the effect this has on human activity.

Gesler's (1992: 735) discussion of 'therapeutic environments' suggests that there is a tension about ownership and definition of these spaces. Settings and activities can be defined as 'therapeutic' by those who use them in that way, thus fishing can be described as therapeutic or taking place in a therapeutic environment (Bull, 2009). However, translating activities into a clinical or an institutional environment in order to make them accountable is to reduce them and make them manageable, compromising creativity and spontaneity. An aspect of their containment concerns the risk constraints and budget in the occupational therapy department, so something about them is lost in translation. Clients have sometimes found that they are not stretched enough by what is available or that interventions offered to them have been infantile. Perhaps they also pose a threat to the ability of the therapist, who may be unable to translate client demands while at the same time being expected to coordinate and evaluate the activity.

This kind of difference in interpretation returns the argument to the question of whether informal or formal forms of knowledge are being privileged. Where they use activities occupational therapists have to choose those which offer multiple possibilities in order to meet a range of client determined outcomes but determining whether a person has obtained benefit from an activity is not up to the individual, despite the value they may give to it. The benefits experienced by the service user have to be formally translated into a professional language of categorization in order to be recognized by the therapist's other team members. Consequently there are many issues here about the codes or the codification of activities, the roles they suggest and their social implications, the person who is writing the narrative and whose terms are being used. The negotiation of values through this process becomes one in which terms are translated into the right words to use to obtain recognition, i.e. values are positioned in order to be effective in a clinical process. This may mean that they are removed somewhat from the service user's meaning, and from a sense of effectiveness that they might recognize as serving their needs (Pollard, 2010; see Chapters 12 and 14). Across such processes codes take on meanings of their own, since they are defined in practices which rely on a substantial amount of borrowed knowledge

(Hagedorn, 2001) and so are moved out of their original context. Whereas earlier we considered how one of the principles of occupational therapy is to enable clients to recognize their achievements but perhaps this means that therapy is devalued, here therapy is devalued because it is couched in terms that do not relate to tacit perceptions of common experience and vernacular expression, or mean quite the same thing as they do to others.

Having a narrow perspective of occupational values is professionally unsustainable. The language of health is often not merely the language of medicine; increasingly the balance in the mixed economy of state and market provision in health is favouring the market, and economics are determining the provision of health care. Since the early 1980s, UK governments have increasingly looked to market models for provision, and oriented themselves to how consumers can be involved in making choices about their own health needs, including the development of new business structures (Conservative Party, 2007, 2008; Department of Health, 2006, 2008, 2010, 2011; Marks and Hunter, 2007). This orientation to the market favours business conditions, stripping back state provision to open up the health sector for enterprise. In the UK new forms of social enterprise have been encouraged such as community interest companies (CICs), which closely resemble corporations. Some of these new organizations have included large hospital trusts, although it is anticipated that larger businesses will later swallow them up (Marks and Hunter, 2007; Greer, 2010), as even the Conservatives themselves admitted (2007).

As a relatively small profession, occupational therapists do not occupy enough executive posts in the NHS to be influential in issues of policy and market orientation. Although professions such as medicine have pointed to a lack of evidence to support the changes being made (Coombes, 2011; Godlee, 2011), the economic arguments that current levels of provision are unaffordable outweighs clinical perspectives. Perhaps a more significant factor on policy is that of public opinion (Milewa et al., 1999). During 2011 the government announced a pause in their pursuit of changes in health and social care, while in fact the measures continued to be implemented. Public opinion did not stop the programme, part of which was a continuation of decisions taken by the previous administration (Department of Health 2006; Marks and Hunter, 2007).

Many Western governments are experiencing dilemmas over demands for increasing expenditure on health care while recognizing a need for greater efficiency if an adequate service is to be afforded and maintained. Those who can afford to will often choose to pay for treatments rather than accept state provision because they can exercise choices in the care they buy (Srivasta and Zhao, 2008) and one of the political strategies adopted has been to emphasize personal decision making on behalf of the health consumer. Indeed, the Conservative government's 2010 White Paper borrowed the disability movement's mantra: 'no decisions about me, without me' (Department of Health, 2010) while appearing to echo the criticisms of health systems about responding to client needs. The language of choice and the language of the marketplace are features of most mixed economic approaches to healthcare. These argue that people have a right to choose the kinds of care they are prepared to pay for, rather than pay for everything for everybody, and that because of this right the state does not have to provide forms of care that people can pay for if they so choose.

However, criticisms of unresponsiveness, as explored elsewhere in this book (Chapters 1, 3, 6, and similar critiques in Chapters 12 and 14) have been made both of occupational therapy and from occupational therapists already working in private health care systems (Townsend 1998; Townsend *et al.*, 2003; Hammell, 2007, 2008, 2010). There are some contradictions between client-centred practice and some methods for limiting budgets, a concern with the productivity measures applied to hospital spaces, staff workloading and resources over the provision of care. Professionals may be concerned to uphold their codes of practice, but idealism is eroded when people consider their ability to pay their bills. The dominant force is marketplace economics, and everyone's life is conditioned by the principle that people can only choose what they can pay for when the market determines the price.

These issues are politicizing the practices of healthcare (Hammell, 2007, 2010; Rebeiro-Gruhl, 2009) but government is being selective about which professions it will listen to. Occupational therapy has no individual voice in the decisions being made in the UK at government level but is represented amongst a group of allied health professions, whereas in the arrangements for consulting over health commissioning processes one nurse per committee has a tokenistic presence. This is part of a pattern of excluding intermediaries out of the administrative process (Greer, 2010). Health services represent considerable business, given that the UK's NHS is one of the world's largest organizations (Gorsky, 2006), 'the closest thing the English have to a religion' (Lawson, 1992: 613). As health is a priority on every government agenda (e.g. Conservative Party, 2007, 2008) it was evident that the 2010 Conservative election campaign received substantial financial support from companies such as Care UK, who afterwards were in line for a £53 million contract for prison health services that had been formerly delivered through the NHS (*Daily Mirror*, 6 February 2011; *Guardian*, 8 March 2011).

These powerful economic forces are very difficult to resist (Srivasta and Zhao, 2008; Greer, 2010), despite the evidence that the models they adhere to generate inequalities and perpetuate different health experiences as part of their effect on life chances. Health problems are not generated by poverty itself but relative poverty in society with the consequent lack of access to amenities and opportunities (Phillips, 2006). Though government strategies over recent years had generally improved health in the UK, increasing disparity is evident (House of Commons, 2009b; Thomas, Dorling and Davey Smith, 2010) so that the difference in life expectancy is the same as in the 1930s (Pickett and Dorling, 2010). The critical House of Commons report (2009b) demanded cross departmental work, for example in government education and health departments to work on teaching children to prepare healthy meals and more effective food labelling. Improvements in health delivery tend to benefit the better off and better informed social groups, who can make more use of the resources. Top-down consumerist interventions to address obesity such as the promotion of gym membership were less significant than safer and more accessible routes to the gym and did not reach impoverished areas where people tended not to engage with services or information.

The Marmot Review (Marmot *et al.*, 2010) attempted to address these problems through strategies such as debt advice, generating work opportunities and small enterprises in the local economy and community development approaches. These engaged local community members in tackling the effects of low income on health but did not always directly involve health practitioners. Comparing this review to the 1980 Black Report on inequality, Pickett and Dorling (2010) saw little difference in the proposed strategies despite the 30 years between the two reports. Life expectancy has increased but it has increased much more for the wealthy. Echoing recognitions in the House of Commons Report (2009b), Pickett and Dorling (2010) conclude that better health for all may depend on some people giving up their access to good services. It is unlikely that they will be willing to do so. Pickett and Dorling's view is that the extremities of privilege are a threat to social stability.

Occupational therapy exhortations to 'do, be, become, belong' (Wilcock, 2006) are often cited as though occupational participation was merely a matter of getting up and going but, in fact, Wilcock calls for work towards social change (e.g. Wilcock, 2007). The discourse that the profession has developed and the definition of occupation as a specific field of scientific work is a story of the discipline narrated from within itself. It has often seemed independent of the social world around its practitioners, and some have argued, around the service users it works with (Swain and French, 2009). Occupational therapy models and concepts mostly concern the individual in the aseptic and scientifically reduced environment of the clinic with its focus on the carrying out of effective interventions. This may be good science, but the profession has made a number of claims to holism and complexity. As we explore in Chapter 6 (see also Chapter 10), clinicians have to think and collaborate outside the biomedical sphere.

Alburquerque *et al.* (2010) call for the development of participative networks and opportunities, including street demonstrations and theatre to confront and engage with a disabling society, something that may certainly raise a few eyebrows in the UK even where occupational therapists have been prominent in demonstrations against service cuts. A Chilean group of people with disabilities and health professionals and students, Colectivo Habilitar (see http://habilitar.cl/), uses nonviolent street action to voice demands for social change on the basis that irrespective of functionality and disability 'we are all equally different' and a revelation of their 'dreaming about the right to be' (Alburquerque *et al.*, 2010: 168). Max-Neef's reappraisal of economic values offers one model of how the complex interplay of cultural and structural socio-economic factors may contribute to the issues of wellbeing that occupational therapy aims to address, with a dimensional structure of 'being, having, doing and interacting' (Cruz *et al.*, 2009: 2026). This arrangement of terms may resonate well, and more thoroughly, than Wilcock's mantra, because it is a language that explores the relationship between these values and human cost. Perhaps occupational therapists need to find a way to articulate these values as 'permanent persuaders' (Gramsci, 1971:10; Pollard, 2010), through their emphasis on spontaneity and creativity as a focus for activism.

Conclusion

Language is not only about talking about things but also about how these things (behaviours, activities, diseases and symptoms) are being constructed, framed and lived. Many professions, for example, have created their own unique language, or jargon. These professional languages can serve various purposes. They can create a unified discourse on disease, distance the professional world from that of the client, prevent the client from understanding the professional process or context, or reduce ways of living with illness to physiological processes and to measurable pathology. In effect, professional languages are used to set out a territory that is the preserve of a particular profession as opposed to others in a similar field. An 'occupational' territory, as occupational therapy would put it.

However, in order to make sense of doing professional languages are not enough. The following chapter discusses occupational literacy and its use in making sense of a language of doing.

References

Alburquerque, D., Chana, P., CERTRAM Community (2010). The CERTRAM community: building links for social change. In F. Kronenberg, N. Pollard, D. Sakellariou (eds) *Occupational Therapies without Borders (Volume 2): Towards an Ecology of Occupation-Based Practices*. Edinburgh, Elsevier Science, 163–172.

Beagan, B. L. (2007) Experiences of social class: learning from occupational therapy students. *Canadian Journal of Occupational Therapy* 74, 125–133.

Bull, J. (2009) Watery masculinities: fly-fishing and the angling male in the South West of England. *Gender, Place and Culture: A Journal of Feminist Geography* 16(4), 445–465.

Burt, E. L., Atkinson, J. (2011) The relationship between quilting and wellbeing. *Journal of Public Health* 33(2) doi: 10. 1093/pubmed/fdr041.

Bynner, J. (2009) *Life-Long Learning and Crime: A Life-Course Perspective*. London, Institute of Education.

Canguilhem, G. (1989) *The Normal and the Pathological*. New York, Zone Books.

Chodorow, N. (1978) *The Reproduction of Mothering*. Berkley and Los Angeles, University of California.

College of Occupational Therapists (2010) *Code of Ethics and Professional Conduct*. London, College of Occupational Therapists.

Conservative Party (2007) NHS autonomy and accountability. A proposal for legislation. London, Conservative Party.

Conservative Party (2008) Delivering some of the best health in Europe. Outcomes, not targets. London, Conservative Party.

Cook-Gumperz, J. (1986) Literacy and schooling: an unchanging equation? In J. Cook-Gumperz (ed.), *The Social Construction of Literacy*. Cambridge, Cambridge University Press, pp. 16–44.

Coombes, R. (2011) Briefing: health and social care bill. *British Medical Journal* 342, d507.

Council of Occupational Therapists' Registration Boards (Australia and New Zealand)/OT Australia (2010) *Towards a National Safe System for Occupational Therapy Practice*.

Mile End, SA, Council of Occupational Therapists' Registration Boards (Australia and New Zealand) Fitzroy, Vic, OT Australia.

Cruz, I., Stahel, A., Max-Neef, M. (2009) Towards a systemic development approach: building on the Human-Scale Development paradigm. *Ecological Economics* 68, 2021–2030.

Crystal, D. (2003) *English as a Global Language*, 2nd edn. Cambridge, Cambridge University Press.

Denshire, S. (2002) Reflections on the confluence of personal and professional. *Australian Occupational Therapy Journal* 49, 212–216.

Department of Health (2006) *No Excuses. Embrace Partnership Now. Step Towards Change! Report of the Third Sector Commissioning Task Force*. London, Department of Health.

Department of Health (2008) *Putting People First: A Shared Vision and Commitment to the Ttransformation of Adult Social Care*. London, Department of Health.

Department of Health (2010) *Equity and Excellence: Liberating the NHS*. London, Department of Health.

Department of Health (2011) *Health and Social Care Bill 2011*. London, Department of Health.

Eco, U. (2000) *Kant and the Platypus; Essays on Language and Cognition*. New York, Mariner Books.

Flanders, J. (2006) *Consuming Passions. Leisure and Pleasure in Victorian Britain*. London, HarperCollins.

Foucault, M. (1989) *The Birth of the Clinic*. London, Routledge.

Gesler. W. M. (1992) Therapeutic landscapes: medical issues in light of the new cultural geography. *Social Science and Medicine* 34(7), 735–746.

Girouard, M. (1990) *The English Town*. London, Guild.

Godlee, F. (2011) NHS reforms – why now? *British Medical Journal* 342, d552.

Goffman, E. (1990 [1959]) *The Presentation of Self in Everyday Life*. London, Penguin.

Gorsky, M. (2006) Coalition policy towards the NHS: past contexts and current trajectories. History and policy, www.historyandpolicy.org/papers/policy-paper-111.html, accessed 15 March 2011.

Gramsci, A. (1971) *Selections from the Prison Notebooks*. Q. Hoare,(trans. and ed.) London, Lawrence & Wishart.

Greer, S. L. (2010) State authority and health care delivery in the United States and United Kingdom. University of Michigan, www.britishpoliticsgroup.org/greer%20bpg%20paper%201-4%20(Chicago%2015%20AD)pdf, accessed 16 March 2011.

Hagedorn, R. (2001) *Foundations for Practice in Occupational Therapy*, 3rd edn. Edinburgh, Churchill Livingstone/Elsevier.

Hammell, K. (2007) Reflection on a disability methodology for the client-centred practice of occupational therapy research. *Canadian Journal of Occupational Therapy* 74(5), 365–369.

Hammell, K. (2008) Reflections on well-being and occupational rights. *Canadian Journal of Occupational Therapy* 75(1), 61–64.

Hammell, K. (2010) Spinal cord injury rehabilitation research; patient priorities, current deficiencies and potential directions. *Disability and Rehabilitation* 32(14), 1209–1218.

Haydon, P. (1994) *The English Pub*. London, Robert Hale.

Hines, B. (1969) *A Kestrel for a Knave*. Harmondsworth, Penguin.

Hocking, C. (2007) The romance of occupational therapy. In J. Creek, A. Lawson-Porter (eds) *Contemporary Issues in Occupational Therapy: Reasoning and Reflection*. Chichester, John Wiley & Sons, Ltd, pp. 23–40.

Holbrook, D. (1964) English for the Rejected Training Literacy in the Lower Streams of Secondary School. Cambridge, Cambridge University Press.

House of Commons (2009a) *Skills for Life: Progress in Improving Adult Literacy and Numeracy. Third Report of Session 2008-09.* London, The Stationery Office.

House of Commons Health Committee (2009b) *Health Inequalities.* London, The Stationery Office.

Ikiugu, M. N. (2008) *Occupational Science in the Service of Gaia.* Baltimore, PublishAmerica.

Ikiugu, M. N. (2010) Influencing social challenges through occupational performance. In F. Kronenberg, N. Pollard, D. Sakellariou (eds) *Occupational Therapies without Borders*, Vol. 2 Edinburgh, Elsevier/Churchill Livingstone, pp. 113–122.

Illich, I. (1975) *Tools for Conviviality.* London, Fontana.

Ives, P. (2009) Global English, hegemony and education: lessons from Gramsci. *Educational Philosophy and Theory* 41(6), 661–683.

Iwama, M. (2006) *The Kawa Model; Culturally Relevant Occupational Therapy.* Edinburgh, Elsevier.

Jackson, S., Stevenson, C. (2000) What do people need psychiatric and mental health nurses for? *Journal of Advanced Nursing* 31(2), 378–388.

James, L. (2006) *The Middle Class. A History.* London, Little, Brown.

Kinsella, A. (2006) Poetic resistance: juxtaposing personal and professional discursive constructions in a practice context. *Journal for the Canadian Association for Curriculum Studies* 4(1), 35–59.

Lafargue, P. (1883 /2000) *The Right to be Lazy*, http://www.marxists.org/archive/lafargue/1883/lazy/, accessed 9 September 2011.

Lawson, N. (1992) *The View from No.11 Memoirs of a Tory Radical.* London, Bantam.

Linebaugh, P. (1991) *The London Hanged; Crime and Civil Society in the Eighteenth Century.* New York, Allen Lane Press.

Mace, J. (1998) *Playing with Time: Mothers and the Meaning of Literacy.* London, UCL Press.

Mackey, H. (2006) 'Do not ask me to remain the same': Foucault and the professional identities of occupational therapists. *Australian Occupational Therapy Journal* 54(2), 95–102.

Marks, L., Hunter, D. J. (2007) *Social Enterprises and the NHS Changing Patterns of Ownership and Accountability.* London, Unison.

Marmot, M., Allen, J., Goldblatt, P., Boyce, T., McNeish, D., Grady, M., Geddes, I. (2010) *Fair Society, Health Lives.* London, The Marmot Review, www.marmotreview.org/, accessed 29 July 2011.

Mattingly, C. (1998) *Healing Dramas and Clinical Plots: The Narrative Structures of Experience.* Cambridge, Cambridge University Press.

Mattingly, C. (2010) *The Paradox of Hope: Journeys through a Clinical Borderland.* Berkley, CA, University of California.

Max-Neef, M. (2010) The world on a collision course. *AMBIO* 39, 200–210.

Milewa, T., Vanetin, J., Calnan, M. (1999) Community participation and citizenship in British health care planning: narratives of power and involvement in the changing welfare state. *Sociology of Health and Illness* 21(4), 445–465.

Office for National Statistics (2011) Earnings: 2010 Survey of Hours and Earnings, www.statistics.gov.uk/cci/nugget.asp?id=285, accessed 3 May 2011.

Peck, E., Norman, I. J. (1999) Working together in adult community mental health services: exploring inter-professional role relations. *Journal of Mental Health.* 8(3), 231–242.

Perrin, T., May, H., Anderson, E. (2008) *Wellbeing in Dementia: An Occupational Approach for Therapists and Carers*, 2nd edn. Edinburgh, Churchill Livingstone/ Elsevier.

Phillips, D. (2006) *Quality of Life, Concept, Policy and Practice*. London, Routledge.

Pickett, K. E., Dorling, D. (2010) Against the organization of misery? The Marmot Review of health inequalities. *Social Science and Medicine* 71, 1231–1233.

Pollard, N. (2010) Occupational therapists – permanent persuaders in emerging roles. In F. Kronenberg, N. Pollard, D. Sakellariou (eds) *Occupational Therapies Without Borders*, vol. 2 Edinburgh, Elsevier/Churchill Livingstone, pp. 143–152.

Pollard, N., Walsh, S. (2000) Occupational therapy, gender and mental health: an inclusive perspective? *British Journal of Occupational Therapy* 63(9) 425–431.

Prospects (2011) Occupational Therapist Salaries and Conditions, ww2.prospects.ac.uk/p/types_of_job/occupational_therapist_salary.jsp, accessed 3 May 2011.

Pryor, F. (2004) *Britain BC. Life in Britain and Ireland before the Romans*. London, Harper Perennial.

Rebeiro-Gruhl, K. L. (2009) The politics of practice: strategies to secure our occupational claim and to address occupational injustice. *New Zealand Journal of Occupational Therapy* 56(1), 19–26.

Romaine, S. (2002) The impact of language policy on endangered languages. *International Journal on Multicultural Societies* 4(2), 194–212.

Rowles, G. D. (1991) Beyond performance: being in place as a compoent of occupational therapy. *American Journal of Occupational Therapy* 45(3), 265–271.

Ruskin, J. (1865 /2002) *Sesame and Lilies*. D. E. Nord (ed.). New Haven, Yale University Press.

Sahlins, M. (1999) What is anthropological enlightenment? Some lessons of the twentieth century. *Annual Review of Anthropology* 28, i–xxiii.

Sakellariou, D., Pollard, N. (2008) Class, gender and sexuality: three sites of conflict and cooperation. In N. Pollard, D. Sakellariou, F. Kronenberg (eds) *A Political Practice of Occupational Therapy*. Edinburgh, Elsevier.

Schon, D. A. (1987) *Educating the Reflective Practitioner*. San Franciso, Jossey Bass.

Smart, P., Frost, G., Nuffield, P., Pollard, N. (2010) Pecket Well Learning Community. In F. Kronenberg, N. Pollard, D. Sakellariou (eds) *Occupational Therapies without Borders*, Vol. 2 Edinburgh, Elsevier/Churchill Livingstone, pp. 19–25.

Srivasta, P., Zhao, X. (2008) *Impact of Private Health Insurance on the Choice of Public versus Private Hospital Services*. University of York, Health, Econometrics and Data Group. Working Paper 8/17.

Swain, J., French, S. (2009) Occupational therapy: a disability perspective. In M. Molineux, M. Curtin, J. Supyk (eds) *Occupational Therapy in Physical Dysfunction*, 6th edn. Edinburgh, Elsevier Science, pp. 27–38.

Thomas, B., Dorling, D., Davey Smith, G. (2010) An observational study of health inequalities in Britain: geographical divides returning to 1930s maxima by 2007. *British Medical Journal* doi:10. 1136/bmj.c3639.

Townsend, E. (1998) *Good Intentions Overruled: A Critique of Empowerment in the Routine Organization of Mental Health Services*. Toronto, ON, University of Toronto Press.

Townsend, E., Langille, L., Ripley, D. (2003) Professional tensions in client-centered practice: using institutional ethnography to generate understanding and transformation. *American Journal of Occupational Therapy*, 57, 17–28.

Wilcock, A. A. (1999) Creating self and shaping the world. *Australian Occupational Therapy Journal*. 46 77–88.

Wilcock, A. A. (2007) Active ageing: dream or reality? *New Zealand Journal of Occupational Therapy*, 54(1), 15–20.

Wright, J. (2011) *Cutting the Apron Strings? The Clustering of Young Graduates and the Role of the Public Sector*. London, The Work Foundation.

Zola, E. (1995 [1883]) *The Ladies' Paradise*. Brian Nelson (trans.). Oxford, Oxford University Press.

Zola, E. (1999 [1882]) *Pot Luck*. Brian Nelson (trans.). Oxford, Oxford University Press.

3 Occupational Literacy

Nick Pollard and Dikaios Sakellariou

Most professional disciplines develop a language of their own, a collection of terms and acronyms which refer to specific equipment and practices (see Chapter 2). However, a recent development in pedagogy has arisen from the ways in which knowledge needs to be applied in a diversifying global economy. This has led to an increased emphasis on professional literacies that enable adaption to change, flexibility and multidisciplinary. Such literacy offers an accuracy of understanding or use of defined terms but does not imply a fixed level of knowledge. It is instead a tool that offers access to a process of unravelling the challenges or problems encountered by different professions (Dowey, 2006). It gives a moving viewpoint that develops with increased access to knowledge and experience but which is contained within professional regulations which determine the limits of professional responsibility.

This viewpoint has to be periodically adjusted because the professional context from which it arises is heteroglossic (it involves the paroles of many different professional and tacit discourses that occur in that professional environment). Consequently, it has to be renegotiated continually at the borders of its territory where aspects of practice are positioned, bartered and exchanged with other professional groups and negotiated with clients, carers and service managers. As we suggested in Chapter 2, literacies of this sort have moved on from supporting professional power (although this issue certainly remains) through the abilities to classify and order depicted by Foucault (1972) to tools for collaborative and adaptive approaches to working (Dowey, 2006).

An occupational literacy might aim to be 'convivial' through aiming to be understandable not only to a professional group but to those with whom a profession works. Thus the usefulness of an occupational literacy is not restricted to a particular group of people but may have a general applicability through its utility in communicating and sharing, for example, aspects of practice. The vocabulary in which these shared practices are described may be dual. The previous chapter discussed some of the ways in which language not only supported professional power but was also an

Politics of Occupation-Centred Practice: Reflections on Occupational Engagement across Cultures,
First Edition. Edited by Nick Pollard and Dikaios Sakellariou.
© 2012 John Wiley & Sons, Ltd. Published 2012 by John Wiley & Sons, Ltd.

expression of cultural identity and belongingness and used by some marginalized groups to exclude outsiders.

Language is connected to identity and difference as well as cultural unity. The acquisition of language and the ability to use it is important in facilitating occupation and participation in knowledge sharing. The communities involved in many work and leisure activities develop specialist vocabularies to express common issues, perhaps tools, practices or components associated with them like for example 'weathering', 'super detail' or 'solid-scale modelling' (see Chapter 11). Such terms are usually understood between modellers but may have to be explained to nonmodellers, and they are also the means by which a modeller obtains a recognized and respected voice in modelling communities. Their use is evidence that the person 'knows what they are talking about'. As we have argued in Chapter 2, it may be challenging but useful to have a broadly understood occupational framework that values the capacity to express belonging through doing. Many occupations recognize different levels of expertise. Even in a leisure pursuit such as modelling there are not only distinctions between amateur and professional but also in the level of skill and interpretation available to the model maker. For example, Jenkinson (2001), Wylie (1987) and Simmons (1998) suggest that railway modellers avoid the mistake of being over ambitious in their initial projects by working from simple layouts to increasingly complex ones. Their books recommend that modellers join clubs to learn at first hand from more experienced hobbyists and contain technical suggestions and solutions that are based on the improvisations and bricolage worked out by others and passed on. Thus, although a model maker can read about techniques, an occupational literacy (in this case concerned with modelling) is not merely about reading and writing, but is interactive, requiring a community in which concepts, knowledge and products are exchanged between participants (see Chapter 13). Occupational literacy is a dialogical process or, following Paavola and Hakkarainen's (2005: 545) discussion of knowledge creation in their depiction of activity theory, trialogical, where 'trialogue means that by using various mediating artefacts (signs, concepts and tools) and mediating processes (such as practices, or the interaction between tacit and explicit knowledge) people are developing common objects of activity (such as conceptual artefacts, practices, products, etc.).' Without a demonstration of a practice using tools or producing particular artefacts it can be difficult to understand descriptions of activities or relate them to context.

Being Trialogical

In *The Pedagogy of the Oppressed*, one of the books that gave rise to the idea of reflective practice, which is widely encouraged in the health professions, Freire (1972) saw the promotion of literacy not simply as a measure to encourage people to be able to read and write so that they could follow instructions, but so that they could participate critically in a democratic process by questioning the status quo. Literacy, consequently, is not passive reading, but participatory, involving the discussion of synthesis and sharing of interpretation.

It is this trialogic sense of literacy that enables the questioning of practices, their origins and purpose that we wish to emphasize. However, there is no guarantee that by making the tools for an occupational literacy available that they will be used to convivial ends. The need for these tools arises because of the need for clarity about the nature of occupation, and the lack of clarity is often related to an imbalance of power in which knowledge is unevenly distributed. The facility with which to put knowledge into effect is also related to access to power. In an earlier discussion on the topic Pollard (2008) discussed how, in work situations, occupational literacy had not always produced a more democratic work process but instead had become a tool for managers to identify workers who were less effective. Occupational literacy is only one of a number of measures for change, and although it may provide one of the starting points in generating dialogue, it needs to be supported by other strategies.

The process of negotiating collaborative and adaptive approaches to working may develop according to the transient and contextual needs of local situations but the apparently temporary nature of these collaborations will often make reference to local interpretations of standing regulations, codes of practice or national guidance. They will also be driven by the desire of certain individuals or groups within the profession to develop innovations and others to resist change. This has led to both much more discussion of practice and more discursive practice – for example in the process of problem solving approaches or developing clinical pathways (Iedema and Scheeres, 2003).

Iedema and Scheeres (2003: 319) return to Foucault's later discussions (1980) to suggest that these negotiated practices can be empowering as they enable people to negotiate disruptions arising from changes, and become technologies for 'doing self'. Occupational therapists and their multidisciplinary colleagues working in the UK have experienced many structural changes in their working environment over the last 20 years. Occupational therapists have also been a mobile professional group, changing jobs in response to a strong demand for their skills (Moran *et al.*, 2005; Von Zweck and Burnett, 2006). Consequently a practitioner may find that patterns of interaction between occupational therapists and other professions may differ between one hospital and another. There will be differences in working practices between occupational therapists in one country and in others that have emerged as a result of local conditions, or legal institutions. In some countries occupational therapists have established a degree of professional autonomy in the services they can offer to clients, while in others the specific intervention and its duration may be prescribed by a doctor or perhaps even a financial administrator. Migrant occupational therapists taking up practice in other countries may have to take local examinations to ensure they understand the differences they will encounter in their new professional contexts.

If occupational therapy approaches are centred around client needs, then even where practices are similar there will be differences in what can be negotiated and achieved. The navigation of the individual therapist's own narrative thread in the tapestry of these interactions is supported or perhaps thwarted by other threads in the multiprofessional discourses of the work environment, such as conflict of opinion concerning treatment approaches, or the need to contain costs. Such exchanges may depend on knowledge and awareness of the evidence base but they are also based in human relationship dynamics such as the ability to conduct and win an argument, variations in mood and levels of confidence and interpersonal relations. The processes of human interaction are continuous and rapid, operating according to interpretations of action and circumstance which are often not developed into verbal articulation. These processes build up into an experiential model of the world, but personal experience is one dimension *of* and a limitation *to* the capacity for literacy. While it is possible to learn of and imagine other contexts and even convincingly represent them to others, this activity is not the same as participating in a lived experience of them. Because of this experience it is possible to 'read' occupations for others, but not as they would read them.

On the other hand there can be many interpretations of a narrative; the reader is the final writer of the story (Barthes, 1991). The way one person weaves their narrative threads may be read differently by other people according to their own experience. The distinction between the therapist's experience of a condition and its meaning and that of the client's experience of conditions and their meanings in terms of their own lives is one that Mattingly (1998) and writers on disability (e.g. Snyder and Mitchell, 2006; Siebers, 2008) have frequently pointed out (see Chapters 6, 10, 12 and 14).

Paavola and Hakkarainen's (2005) concept of trialogical learning recognizes the way that individual and communal exchanges of learning take place in an environment that changes through the products which are developed. All three – the individual pursuit of knowledge, the communal exchange of knowledge, and the environment where knowledge is applied – are interdependent elements of an engine of narrative. Thus although we have concerned ourselves with dialogue earlier on in the chapter, we have to recognize that the dialogue produces something in the way of conceptual and also physical change as new learning is applied in some way. Each application is read and in turn contributes to further knowledge. One of the 'artefacts' (Paavola and Hakkarainen, 2005: 546) of this revolution of literacy might be a narrative account.

Frank (1995, 2004) describes patients' narratives as belonging to three typologies: restitution, chaos and the quest. While healthcare narratives, often from the practitioner's perspective, talk of the patient's journey or care pathway implying a quest or restitution narrative, the experience can also be chaotic. The implications of different narrative interpretations in the power relationship between client and therapist have greater consequences for people living with disabilities. They may often be described as a 'client' or even a 'consumer' but what is offered to them is determined by the therapist or by a healthcare institution and the interpretation that has been made of the evidence base and affordability (or market) for intervention. In this respect occupational therapists are retailing a commodity within a catalogue of health interventions. If clients are aware of different needs but are not able to afford the costs of meeting them, they may not feel empowered to challenge these authorities, or they may recognize that their needs can only be met through further expenditure. The treatments an occupational therapist can offer may be evidenced, but they are also attached to a cost base that determines the market in which treatments are sold, as discussed in Chapter 1. However the market analogy, in which treatment is a commodity, is limited where the treatment is essential and the service user is a 'client' with little real choice except whether or not to engage with it. Treatment may not be successful and what is carried out may be unprofessional or unsatisfactory. There may be many things that the client feels unable to control or manage, and the experience of illness or disability can be very disruptive and traumatizing, without a sense of resolution.

There are, however, other constrictions. On one hand, professional vocabularies can be limited by the combination of evidence and experience. On the other hand they become extended through the problems encountered by professionals who use that vocabulary to define new phenomena. All narrative possibilities are contained by the experience that underpins what we are able to conceptualize. Despite the variety of human occupation, Frye (1951) claimed it is possible to reduce most narratives to the theme of the quest, around which the detail that fleshes out the story and characters is built up. In professional literature or the personal acquisition of expertise, i.e. a quest for further knowledge, these details are expanded as experience increases through time. People find names and classifications for the new phenomena they encounter, and if the terms are more widely useful they will enter the professional vocabulary.

Occupational literacy is therefore extended through experience, and this in itself is extended by meeting and resolving challenges and problems, whether or not the individual is successful or plays an effective role. It can be augmented by reading the experiences or evidence of others. It is underpinned by a vernacular of individual interpretation of experience worked out in concert with other people on a hetero-glossic basis, for example a combination of formal and informal relationships, professional and lay experience.

Making Sense of the World

Experience may affect how humans make sense of the world around them, but their capacity to do so is also facilitated and limited by their cognitive and physical resources, the ability they have to work with the community around them, and the community's preparedness to accommodate their needs (see Chapters 12 and 14). Experience depends on having a physical engagement with the world and may be developed further through social capital. Social capital depends on social skills acquired through successful social development, access to other people and an appropriate arena in which to practise these skills. Locally produced autobiographical texts are often centred on aspects of community combined with industrial or agricultural heritage, or geographical identity, conveyed through testimonies of experience. These books and accounts often contain close detail of former or different domestic or work-based practices, of struggles to achieve and sustain identities through the things that the authors have done. They have therefore been accounts of occupational literacy. They often correspond to the typologies that Frank (1995) identifies, although many are written because the authors have come to a point of restitution in looking back on their lives. This reflection may accommodate the events of the past in reminiscence, or present the narrative as a completed quest, such as an account of how a couple settle into their relationship or a person attains a particular stage in their working life. As a consequence of hindsight, the chaos of the 'narrative wreckage' (Frank 1995: 68) phase of their experience (illness, unemployment, breakup of home or relationships) is usually resolved, so it is possible to write the narrative because they have reintegrated themselves. However, many working-class writers choose to write poetry because the forms it offers can be worked on amidst the interruptions of other life demands (Morley and Worpole, 1982), suggesting that the experience of resolution and reintegration is in continual play against the potential of other influences to be disruptive. Such challenges may offer the opportunity to experience integration.

Although we will learn from chaotic and destructive events, they often teach us to be apprehensive and afraid; we are more likely to gain from positive experiences which reinforce our learning by rewarding it (Winnicott, 1971). This positive learning arena depends to a large extent on parenting. For the developing infant, the arena is first delineated through the interaction of the child with its mother, and the child becomes increasingly capable of independence, through the interactions it is able to achieve with others. Since social skills depend on the successful mastery of communication abilities first practiced with parents and siblings, perhaps first in the initial communication of mother and child through gaze and attention and in the cycle of feeding and attending to the child's needs (Winnicott, 1971), one of the elemental components of occupation and its literacy must be in early development.

Winnicott (1971) discussed how the child interacts with its mother in the early phases of development and learns to distinguish itself as an independent entity from her. Play occurs within a field bounded by the maternal gaze but which can be progressively expanded by the child. As a child grows and develops it pushes at the boundaries, checking with the mother to see what is permitted, touching forbidden objects or playing at the periphery of the maternally permitted space. The mother holds the child in the maternal space calling it back if it moves too far away from her, explaining events in it that the child does not understand to reassure it, and delineating what is possible and not possible according to the developing abilities of the child, incorporating elements of challenge and encouragement to allow the child scope to develop. Thus the mother encourages the child to develop its occupational literacy, but the child is predisposed to interpret the world around it in its own way.

Play replicates the child's other interactions with the environment. It is a field for experimentation and understanding, developing to incorporate the observed actions of others in the child's environment and to mimic or explore the roles of people that the child observes. Through play the child learns to read the actions of others and test whether it understands them correctly through parental approval. Often the model of the behaviour or role being played derives from parental behaviour and is actively encouraged through parental interaction, rewards and punishments. This accrues into an increasingly complex occupational vocabulary of behaviours and interpretations of others occupations, but the consequent occupational literacy is specific to the social and cultural context of the developing child. In Chapter 13 it is argued that play (although the description of the activity as play may be disguised and denied) may continue to have a value in adult life as a way of exploring the environment and occupational relationships in it.

Some aspects of social capital (as well as emotional, cultural, economic and political forms of capital) depend on the abilities individuals acquire in this way, as is suggested by the theories of Bourdieu (Bourdieu and Wacquant, 1992). Although there are a range of theories of social capital, and the social and economic situation in which a child is born will also be determining factors, a facility for networking and relating to others depends on experiences of relating to other people. Chapters 8, 11 and 13 discuss how certain activities offer both the means to engage in networking activities, and constitute a significant element of the enjoyment of participation. Not only that, but the focus of the interaction is largely concerned with sharing and finding out how to improve and develop skills (Paavola and Hakkarainen, 2005), whether they are the abilities one needs to navigate a community that one lives in, or, in the case of modelling, the facility to trade items or expand a collection.

These skills and abilities are also important components of tacit understanding and knowledge building with regard to how to survive, even in a negative environment. Bonfim's story (2005) of being a street child who eventually goes to university demonstrates this ability. He describes several occasions where his social abilities enabled him to emerge as a leader through finding a way to give others in his environment something they needed. Thus he navigated his progress despite the various obstacles he encountered.

Occupational Literacy as a Skill

The acquisition of occupational literacy depends on an individual being able to recognize and anticipate the needs of others. It can be a vital skill for survival where recognition of important issues, such as elements of risk, may be weighed against the need to continue existing in the here and now, as Bonfim (2005) illustrates. It may be difficult to read the consequences of actions taken in the present but individuals may anticipate that their actions will produce benefits and learn how to obtain further rewards. Even in the case of altruistic action, the motivation to help others may not necessarily be material, but in the form of knowledge or experience, or a positive view of a magical connection between good actions and indirect rewards. Occupational literacy is about knowing or having an understanding of what it is we have to do in a particular context.

Literacy is distinct from a fixed competence, and does not confer competence by itself. Knowing how to read is not necessarily the same as knowing how to do. It is not necessary for an occupational therapist to know how to do everything the client wants to do. It is enough for the therapist to be able to read the situations the client wants to experience in order to recover lost or new occupations sufficiently to be able to arrange the necessary opportunity. To offer appropriate encouragement to a client, occupational therapists do not need to be skilled in the activity but they do need the capacity of occupational literacy through which they recognize the value of the activity in which their client is interested. This understanding enables them to collaborate with other facilitators (for example a sports coach or adult educator) to identify the benefits the client obtains from the activity, such as confidence, physical coordination and strength, and working with others.

Occupational literacy thus operates like a minimalist program (see Chapter 4). In order to acquire a new language a learner has to see how the language is used and functions in context. This is difficult when learning from a book or a recorded programme. Language acquisition is much faster when learners are immersed in a situation where they immediately have to develop a usage of the language themselves. In immersion, the person observes how the language is used, learns to repeat words for significant objects and actions that take place with them, and in doing so makes the assumption that native speakers have correct knowledge of the language, just as we did when we learned to speak as children.

The capacity of anyone, even the most holistic occupational therapist, to truly acquire or understand everything is limited. Frank (1995) and Mattingly (1998) suggest that the practitioner's priority is the clinical aspect of the history. To negotiate an occupational literacy which approaches client centeredness the professional may be dependent on the knowledge possessed by clients, who may not need to be expert in their chosen occupations. For example, in Chapter 13 the accuracy or even an objective standard of finish of a model may not be as significant to the modeller as the enjoyment of making it. Similarly in community publishing (Chapter 11) and writing the process of exchanging narratives and enabling each others' participation might be more important to the individuals concerned than the literary quality of the writing produced. Such writing is perhaps a demonstration of occupational literacy with regard to a shared understanding of the authenticity of content as it pertains to occupational narratives, rather than the acquisition of a literacy, which is demonstrated through stylistic rules.

An occupational literacy is therefore a fluid concept, one that is not based in written knowledge (although it can be written down), but in the reading of experience. Some of this knowledge can literally be read from a written text, but it is also gained from experience of the world. It is the store of tacit knowledge, of shared vernacular practices, which enables people to work out how to do things. It can be informed by evidence and theory, but the way it is often applied is in the rapid deployment of skill and judgement in actions and interaction. There can be recognized methods and approaches, but there can also be innovations and adaptations and these can all be identified as technologies for 'doing self'.

A guitar, for example, can be played left or right handed and tuned in many different ways, learned formally and informally. There are correct, classical positions, which assist playing, but it can be played comfortably in others. The instrument can be used to play the same tune, but in endless variations in different hands. Like the modelling processes touched on earlier in this chapter, all these influences form a kind of bricolage from which a good enough result, at least, can be worked out. The guitar hanging on the wall of a bar will be subject to all these manipulations and differences when it is taken down and played by customers during a folk evening. Each player's performance will be recognized as their interpretation of a tune by the community around them. Perhaps they will show each other different fingerings, teach each other new songs or variants of old ones, and some of these exchanges will be incorporated into future music sessions. The doing of self will then progress to another chapter, the same self in some respects, but with a different ballad about another quest.

References

Barthes, R. (1991) *The Pleasure of the Text*. Oxford, Blackwell.

Bonfim, V. (2005) Once a street child, now a citizen of the world. In F. Kronenberg, S. Simo Algado, N. Pollard (2005) (eds), *Occupational Therapy without Borders – Learning from the Spirit of Survivors*. Oxford, Elsevier Science, pp. 19–30.

Bourdieu, P., Wacquant, L.J.D. (1992) *An Invitation to Reflexive Sociology*. Cambridge, Polity Press.

Dowey, T. (2006) What purposes, specifically? Rethinking purposes and specificity in the context of the 'new vocationalism'. *English for Specific Purposes* 25, 387–402.

Foucault, M. (1972) *The Archaelogy of Knowledge*. London, Routledge.

Foucault, M. (1980) *Power/Knowledge*. C. Gordon (ed.). New York, Pantheon.

Frank, A. W. (1995) *The Wounded Storyteller: Body Illness and Ethics*. Chicago, IL, University of Chicago.

Frank, A. W. (2004) Asking the right question about pain. *Literature and Medicine* 23(2), 209–225.

Freire, P. (1972) *Pedagogy of the Oppressed*, Harmondsworth, Penguin.

Frye, N. (1951) The archetypes of literature. *The Kenyon Review* 13(1), 92–110.

Iedema, R., Scheeres, H., (2003) From doing work to talking work: renegotiating knowing, doing and identity. *Applied Linguistics* (2003) 24(3), 316–337.

Jenkinson, D. (2001) *Historical Railway Modelling*, York, Pendragon.

Mattingly, C. (1998) *Healing Dramas and Clinical Plots. The Narrative Structure of Experience*. Cambridge, Cambridge University Press.

Moran, A., Nancarrow, S., Butler, A. (2005) 'There's no place like home.' A pilot study of perspectives of international health and social care professionals working in the UK. *Australia and New Zealand Health Policy* 2, 25.

Morley, D., Worpole, K. (eds.) (1982) *The Republic of Letters*. London, Comedia.

Paavola, S., Hakkarainen, K. (2005) The knowledge creation metaphor – an emergent epistemological approach to learning. *Science and Education* 14, 535–57.

Pollard, N. (2008). When Adam delf and Eve span: occupational literacy and democracy. In N. Pollard, D. Sakellariou, F. Kronenberg (eds), *A political practice of occupational therapy*. Edinburgh, Elsevier Science. 39–51.

Simmons, N. (1998) *Railway Modelling*, 8th edn. Sparkford, Patrick Stephens.

Siebers, T., (2008) *Disability Theory*. Ann Arbor, University of Michigan.

Snyder, S. L., Mitchell, D. T. (2006) *Cultural Locations of Disability*. Chicago, University of Chicago.

Von Zweck, C., Burnett, P. (2006) The acculturation of internationally educated health professionals in Canada. *Occupational Therapy Now* 8(3), 22–24.

Winnicott, D. W. (1971) *Playing and Reality*. London, Routledge.

Wylie, J. (1987) *The Professional Approach to Model Railways*. Sparkford, Patrick Stephens.

4 A Grammar for a Language of Occupation

Nick Pollard and Dikaios Sakellariou

In the language of occupation, grammar occupies a central role of allowing language to function. Grammar provides legibility and stabilizes meaning. It provides the structures that allow the components of doing to be understood, without being so rigid and inflexible as to distort the doing into something unrecognizable. It is the basis on which doing can be dynamic, directed and interconnected.

A grammar of doing is not something that is isolated from an interactive and social context. Over the course of their cognitive development people learn by observing and participating and are able to interpret the actions of others from their own experience, just as they are able to develop their use of language from its use in relation to social interaction and environmental cues. Human communication involves the simultaneous translation and exchange of many cues, only some of which are linguistic. Others involve posture, gesture and facial expression in addition to the use or display of objects. A concern with individual doing focuses on only a portion of this interaction and conceptualization of the world. The learning of a language is centred on the individual acquisition of verbal competences but, as anyone who has been educated in a second language knows, the experience of expressing themselves in a social situation outside the classroom is very different. Rapid interactions strain the limitations of a new vocabulary and grammatical rules that are not as embedded as those of a native language. Accent, facial expression, dialect words and other nuances that may not have occurred in the classroom have to be interpreted.

Despite these differences, most people can begin to make themselves understood when placed in a foreign social context. One of the most effective ways to learn a second language is immersion in an occupational context where words and actions are clearly related and opportunities to resort to a first language are restricted or denied. The consequence is often that, while the immersed learners develop a knowledge of new words, the vocabulary they acquire is built on the grammar of their first language. These features have become embedded in the various dialect forms of certain languages. Thus it has been claimed that Yorkshire dialect has strong

Politics of Occupation-Centred Practice: Reflections on Occupational Engagement across Cultures,
First Edition. Edited by Nick Pollard and Dikaios Sakellariou.
© 2012 John Wiley & Sons, Ltd. Published 2012 by John Wiley & Sons, Ltd.

elements of Old Norse and Danish amongst others (Kellett, 1994), Irish forms of English have a grammatical root in Irish (O Muirthe, 1977), and Caribbean patois contains grammatical structures that show their roots in African languages (McLaren, 2009). These differences can become important components of facility for literary expression and for cultural identity (O Muirthe, 1977). Through their use, they signify aspects of cultural identity and belongingness to a community of expression. Despite the recognizable differences and nuances in the usage of certain specific dialect words and grammatical forms that may not occur in other speakers' vocabularies, they share a sufficiently common range of components to be understood most of the time. This facility is due to linguistic competence which some linguistic theorists suggest is innate, and others suggest is learned. Linguistic competence allows individuals to interpret new words and employ them in speech.

Despite linguistic competence, the many regional variations in the use of words, again resulting from the influence of different languages, frequently give cause for confusion among native speakers. In English a fishcake can be either a mixture of fish and potatoes in a breadcrumb coating, or a sandwich of fish between slices of potato, encased in batter in different parts of the country. However, if asking for the former in a fish-and-chip shop, the customer may find that the item might also be called a fish rissole, or a fish patty. To confuse matters further, a fish patty might also turn out to be a Jamaican spicy fish mixture in turmeric-coloured short pastry. The incomprehension that can result from encountering these differences for the first time is partly resolved by their occurrence in a grammatical and social context, through which meaning can be inferred. Such variations may seem to be trivial but are socially significant in some circumstances. Such regional knowledge identifies local people from strangers, and is part of a complex of linguistic markers in the form of adjectives, verbs and idioms describing common events. These signify 'belongingness' to the identity connected with a particular locality or culture. In the field of community publishing, narratives frequently include dialect and patois as an expressive component of the local voice. This is often combined with reference to significant local events or landmarks (often those which have been demolished), and so give reference to a specific period to underpin the authenticity of the text. Language combines with geography and shared memory to locate occupational narrative with both individual and community identity.

Comprehension

Waterhouse makes much of this set of links in his novel *Billy Liar,* in which his protagonist, Billy Fisher, amuses his readership and exasperates his friends and family with compulsive lies and parodies of the small-town characters in his life. In one incident Billy Fisher encounters Councillor Duxbury, to whom he declares himself to be 'just about thraiped wi' Stradhoughton' (Waterhouse, 1962: 91). Billy has made this word up, although it roughly means fed up (it possibly derives from the word 'threeap', to grumble or complain (Kellett, 1994) and thus to be in a condition to complain). Despite the parodic context the reader is able to understand both the point of the humour and the literal meaning of the sentence, even though the word may not have been encountered before.

This capacity for comprehension is enabled by the linguistic structures that indicate the different parts of any utterance. They allow the content of speech to be mapped, and thus enable most of what people say to each other to be understood. The dystopian novel, *A Clockwork Orange* (Burgess, 1972), is a more developed example of how this facility operates. Burgess wrote the narrative using many Russian words to develop a distinctive argot, 'nadsat' (p. 24), for his teenage protagonist Alex and his 'droogs', or friends. The text is uncompromising from the first page but the reader soon becomes familiar with the new words without needing to refer to the glossary at the back. Had it been narrated in vernacular English, for example, the novel might not have been so notable, but the reader is drawn into the sociopathic world of Alex through the way Burgess uses a combination of familiar and unfamiliar language and plays on the way that language is learnt from context. *A Clockwork Orange* is a very violent novel, and the dense argot has the effect of amplifying the impact on the reader through the task of interpretation. His readers are made to comprehend an alienated society based on violence and empty consumption, perhaps to confront a set of moral values that are opposite to their own. The environment inhabited by Alex, in which the occupations of adolescent violence dominate, is constructed through the meeting of needs for social identity in lieu of any adult guidance. Although the reader is admitted into Alex's narrative, the language in which the key occupations are described suggests a teenage argot intended to obscure understanding. Often Alex's dialogue with adults departs into a painful parody of polite speech to beguile them into some form of empathy with him before committing violence.

A Clockwork Orange serves as a linguistic experiment through which it can be seen that language is a part of the means by which occupational relationships between people and objects in the environment are expressed. Some of the issues it raises will be returned to later, but first, we will explore the relationship of language structures and occupation.

Language Structures and Occupation

Occupation, like the language through which it is often expressed, necessarily has an active and dynamic structure. Take a sentence: 'I am making a scone'. This broadly breaks up into a noun phrase 'I am', which tells us who is doing (the subject); and the verb phrase 'making a scone', which tells us what is being done and the outcome expected (the object). All acts of human doing have this grammatical structure, since they require someone to do the doing, something that is to be done and the product. This structure can be compacted into one word, as might often be demonstrated by the Cuban singer, Compay Segundo: 'Hecha!': 'It (noun phrase) is done (verb phrase)!', while the person who has done the making, as the singer, is implied in this announcement. A scone cannot bake itself, nor a song sing itself; there must always be a relationship with a 'doer'. Similarly, at least in English, the word 'do' does not usually stand by itself; there is always something that is being done.

This underpinning occupational structure has to be simple enough to allow us to recognize a doing component in other people, or to satisfy a need 'to do' in ourselves. All the examples we have considered are, after all, occupational contexts that operate at several levels. Baking scones may be a simple task although aspects of the recipe might reflect elements of identity through traditions for the inclusion of fruit, ginger, or cheese. Billy Fisher and Alex represent aspects of adolescent occupations. Billy is very much a youth of the 1950s, straining against the confines of home and yearning for adult independence, exhibiting many of the features of young men in his irreverence and his gaucheness. Alex is meant to express a dystopian perspective of the development of youth cultures – in this case centred on violence, music, and drugs. Irreverent humour, the pangs of transition from adolescence to adulthood, violence, music and drugs are as much a part of the range of human occupations as any other activity in which people might indulge. Readers might distance themselves from Waterhouse's and Burgess's protagonists, but the readability of these popular novels depends on the narrative containing recognizable and even (despite Billy's lying and Alex's sociopathy) empathic elements of human occupations that relate to needs.

Perhaps this drive or instinct could be described as a 'minimalist program', a term that Chomsky (1995) uses to suggest a minimum linguistic syntax, a level of basic functioning that is programmed into the psychological functioning of the human being and on which verbal expression can be built. The concept of a minimalist program enables a link to be made between articulated sound and conceptual meaning. It is very complex because the program has to allow enormous flexibility, be operated at the early stages of language acquisition in infancy and yet maintain an essential integrity through simple to complex utterances. This flexibility depends in turn on the existence of building blocks of meaning within language, called morphemes. These can be combined in different ways to form a variety of words and enable reference to meaning with some constancy in different contexts. Humans have to be able to say an infinite number of things and yet what they say has to retain sufficient structure to be recognizable and interpretable for communication to take place. As we will consider, it is also possible that there are similar minimal components of 'doing'.

At a basic level, there is a relationship between the 'doer' and the 'doing' but it must soon be obvious that the relationship is not complete. Scones and songs are not spontaneous events but are usually created for some form of consumption that has to be negotiated, in that a person who has baked scones may ask other people to share them; a song writer usually presumes to write for an audience. They are premeditated activities that are quite complex, involving several stages of doing.

One might begin with the conceptualization of the scone. The occupation of scone making might be a spontaneous thought, a particular product amongst many alternative baking possibilities, but occurs because scones are part of the culinary cultural experience of the person who decides to make some. This scone baker is therefore able to anticipate the outcome of the action, having a concept of a scone to work towards. The baker may be able to assemble the necessary ingredients in the kitchen and produce scones there and then, but perhaps something is missing. Perhaps there is no dried fruit or margarine for baking. A visit to a corner shop or supermarket is necessary. The baker might go to the shop and collect the necessary items, at which the person on the till, eyeing the ingredients, might remark 'baking day, is it?' The baker might reply 'I'm going to bake some scones.' Now, the baker is already engaged in the occupation of making scones. Although the baker hasn't really started yet and is just stocking up on the ingredients, already the scones have progressed from being merely a concept towards becoming concrete. The baker has decided what is needed and organized a shopping trip for the ingredients. The other person in the conversation can see, simply from the ingredients going through the till, what kind of occupation is being engaged in. If they know the baker, perhaps because they live in the same community, they might respond with the parting comment, 'Great, well I'll be over for my afternoon break, get the kettle on and I'll have tea with mine.' It might be a joke, but the reading that has been made of the intended occupation of making scones is that they are to be shared. This short story concerning the occupation of making scones therefore has a number of dependent occupations relating to it which in part are related to the developing occupational narrative context.

Making scones (occupation 1)
Checking ingredients (occupation 2)
Shopping for ingredients (occupation 3)
Banter at the shop till (occupation 4)
Closing transaction (occupation 5)
Eating and sharing scones (occupation 6)

Breaking up and exposing different elements of occupation in this way illustrates the narrative stream in which occupation takes place. The narrative in which the baker might recount all these occupations arbitrarily starts with making scones and concludes with sharing them a little later. This is only one of many possibilities: it could potentially have started much earlier and in another occupational environment with, for example, the day in 1928 when as a little girl Grandma copied out her mother's scone recipe in a kitchen notebook, which forms the specific basis of the baker's conceptual scone.

In a broad respect, such as in this example of the occupation of baking, occupation can therefore be demonstrated to have a fairly stable structure. The scones may be very similar to the scones baked in 1928 two generations of cooks and several generations of cooking technology previously. Scones are a home baking product that many people will have prepared and eaten in similar ways. However, because occupation takes place in a social environment, the familiar elements of occupational context are intermixed with new ones. The story of the entry in the kitchen notebook is of an entirely different narrative stream to the present situation. The baker may have simply baked some scones for something to do, or because someone else was visiting, and scones might be a pleasant snack to offer them, but in 1928 the purpose of having a baking day in which several items were baked in the oven at the same time was to produce food economically within limited means. Grandma may have told the baker this story, and repeating to her in a phone call what happened today (because the baker used her recipe) might reconnect their narrative streams of doing, based around the similar occupational structure of 'baking scones'. Everything that people do has a connection with other events. Occupations form a continuous interweaving of narrative in which they can be interpreted as stable elements (perhaps that scones are baked traditionally on a Monday in a particular family), as well as moving elements (perhaps that scones are served at tea on a Monday by a later family generation, but no longer baked). Perhaps the regularity with which scones featured at tea time creates an aversion to scones in any form in one of Grandma's descendents, but there is still an occupational connection to be read.

Recognizing Occupation

In a profession that is centred on occupation, the professional needs to be capable of interpreting occupational events accurately in negotiation with the client. In many other contexts occupational therapists need only do this approximately because other people in the situation are also working to interpret roughly what is going on and continually make adjustments. These small changes enable people to accommodate others or come into conflict with them. Sometimes this approximation is not adequate because it works on assumptions and preferences based on our individual past experiences, and misunderstandings occur because other people, acting on the basis of their own experiences, act differently. Often we do not recognize the extent to which our experiences shape our preferences and biases in ways that are different from those of other people (Pronin, 2008). Usually we are able to recognize common experiences and actions but the way we attribute others may depend on individual interpretations based on the nuances of personal experience. Some situations are unfamiliar, almost as if they were described in another language, and people have to look for cues to work out the response they should make. Occupation, or the way that we understand 'doing', is heteroglossic and driven by different subjective experiences (Sakellariou and Pollard, 2008).

Occupation, or doing, may in some respects follow a structure rather like language. More often, it is not expressed in verbalized form. The term 'scone' may be applied to the thing a person makes out of flour, butter and some dried fruit, but it may be recognized as such by another person before its contents are actually discussed with anyone else. Scone recipes vary considerably: they may use grated cheese, preserved ginger, chocolate or toffee, different flours, cinnamon, saffron and other herbs and spices. The result of applying the recipes, many of them unwritten, but contained in the memories and experience of various cooks, will produce objects that correspond with the term 'scone' but exhibit a range of characteristics. They may vary considerably in colour, taste, shape, size, texture and content. Similar ingredients prepared in the same way but presented slightly differently might represent another culinary concept, to the extent that one might ask 'are these scones?' On the other hand, one person might recognize another's intention to produce scones even though the result bears little resemblance to the intended object. Here a 'minimalist program' allows people to make and present a variety of objects and to understand and interpret them within an occupational category of 'making scones'.

'Doingness'

Such a minimalist program seems to be important in determining how to arrive at a definition of 'occupation'. If there is a need to be engaged in purposeful doing, there seems to be a recognizable quality of 'doingness', which is the basis of determining whether a person is actively engaged in occupation, and yet allows them to be doing an infinite variety of activities. Generally occupational therapists have tended to qualify occupation with terms such as 'purposeful' (e.g. Golledge, 1998) and 'meaningful' (e.g. Salvatori, 1999). The suggestion is that the kinds of occupation with which a therapist should be concerned to promote should bring about positive outcomes. Thus the activities of Billy and Alex would not concern the therapist except where they form part of the reason for referral, and in Alex's case his activities do result in his selection for a new kind of aversion therapy. However, this is not to argue that their activities are not occupations, or do not express needs because they appear to be without any good purpose. The link between occupation and meaningfulness or purposefulness creates a problem. Both of these portrayals of young people present them as continuously engaged in doing something. Billy frantically covers over the problems created by one lie with yet further lies. He doesn't even understand why he tells some of them himself. Alex is always purposeful, unrelenting in his pursuit of violence for excitement.

Ordinarily, most people will be in the process of beginning or completing actions, doing things. They are all purposeful and meaningful, although the scale and interpretations of purpose and meaning may vary significantly (see Chapter 8). People may enter a room in their home without knowing why except perhaps to sit down in it. They may turn on the television and watch part of a programme with little more intention than to be entertained. These actions are banal but they are neither meaningless nor purposeless. A person with quadriplegia may have to engage in a considerable number of separate activities to be enabled to enter another room and require environmental controls that demand some effort to be able to turn on the television to achieve the same level of 'purposeless' occupation.

When can an action be identified as translating from passivity to the point of 'doing'? Is it possible that 'doing' is a constant state – that it is actually impossible to be doing 'nothing' because the presence of any person, or object, in the environment suggests that there must be a cause-and-effect relationship, which anticipates that presence. Is 'doingness' context dependent? A person 'John' may, as the euphemism to explain unemployment once said, be 'resting between engagements', but even this state is a state of 'doing'. If John is reading a book while resting between engagements it is still not clear that he is engaged in purposeful doing. He might be working for self improvement, or he might be procrastinating, putting off some more pressing occupational need. He could be 'doing nothing but reading a book'. Doing seems therefore to correspond to some notion of value. John's book reading could be of value to him, but not to someone else who might be expecting John to have prepared himself to go out for the day and look for work. John himself might find it hard to put the book down, despite his awareness that there are more significant tasks to engage in (see chapter 12 for further discussion of these issues).

This emergence of an act of 'doing' predates any distinctions of work, rest and play, whether a conceptualization of pleasure, productivity and restoration in the generative discourse of occupation identified by Doris Pierce (2001), negative actions, or, as we will discuss, a more complex interpretation of human needs and satisfiers. All such ideas are much further down the narrative stream of 'doing'. By the time productivity is identifiable there might already have been some indication of intent, a thought that might lead to an action, a thought that may not have become verbally articulated but which anticipates pleasure, productivity or restoration. Many human actions occur before the word to describe them can be formed; playing notes on a guitar, or the sensory responses needed to balance a bicycle, for example.

Physiologically there is no one centre of the brain in which 'doingness' is specifically conceived. Instead, the perception of social action appears to involve numerous areas of the brain according to the specific functions required for interaction (Hari and Kujala, 2009). The content of verbal expression is supplemented by other communicative signals that accompany what is being said. Facial expressions are very important in the development of early communication. Infants can be seen to imitate facial expressions although they have not seen the effect of movements in their own faces. Later on, this imitative impulse is less strong and parts of the brain inhibit and modify it (Hari and Kujala, 2009). Movements of the eyebrows, narrowing of the eyes and other facial gestures occur rapidly to form part of the content of communication. While these interactions are significant, words are also suggestive of behaviours and can generate changes in brain function, in some cases encouraging people to experience different sensations or perceptions (Hari and Kujala, 2009).

Morphemes

Even so, language does not determine thought and action. Much learning takes place through metacognitive processes without the need to verbalize it. Instead people learn to recognize situations that demand intentional, goal-directed responses, which are automatized, yet selective (Gollwitzer and Schaal, 1998). Thus the way that people experience and understand the phenomenon of doing is different to the unconscious interactions of synapses in the physical brain. While the interchange of neural impulses mirrors actions in the real world, individuals need a concept of 'doing' in order to be able to think about such functions in a way that corresponds with other aspects of their experience. For 'doing' to be analysed it may be supposed to have a structure that can be observed in some way. It may also be supposed that there is a minimal component of doing, in the same way that there is a minimal particle of meaning, particularly if doing and meaning are related aspects of human activity. Of course, no such particle literally exists, the morpheme we pursue here is metaphorical but some day-to-day conception is needed for us to think around the function of 'doing'. Is it useful for us to understand doing as intention and motivation combined with opportunity and resources form a molecular 'occupation', a systemic unit of components that might equate with the elements of a model of occupation? Or should the structure of 'doing' be more nebulous than that: the hazy distinction between instinct and drive, reaction and action in psychoanalytic theory?

Domains of Symbolic Logic

'Doing' can produce a state of 'flow' (Csikszentmihalyi, 1991), perhaps as a part of the spectrum of tension between doing and passivity. 'Doing' is done with other people and objects through humans being in a constant state of interaction with the world around them, an interaction that is anticipatory and active as well as reactive (Hari and Kujala, 2009). Hari and Kujala (2009) point out that some of these interactions concern the distribution of thinking tasks to others and to other objects in the environment – for example a notebook – to reduce the amount of cognitive effort required. Creative actions, as a form of 'doing', occur in domains that have a symbolic logic specific to them, such as art or mathematics (Csikszentmihalyi, 1997). Thus we might appeal to someone with expertise in the symbolic logic of specific domains to help us through a particular problem – such as assistance from someone who is good at maths with school mathematics homework.

This facility requires that art is recognized as 'art' and mathematics is recognized as 'mathematics'. The rate at which creative actions are admitted to a domain is determined by the nature of the field, and thus art may be a domain whose field allows a wide range of creative actions to be admitted to it because the domain has a loose identity. It is possible for an art domain object or 'doing' to use mathematical principles and be admitted into the field of art; it may be more difficult for an art domain object to be admitted into the field of mathematics because the principles of the mathematics domain may be less flexible: the object would clearly have to have a mathematical basis. Domains and fields represent forms of 'doing', ways in which 'occupation' can be categorized and classified. These may vary between cultures or as society changes, and so cannot necessarily be regarded as fixed. Activities such as coarse fishing may, for example, be regarded as part of the process of gathering food, a leisure activity, or a sport. Any of these can be regarded as specific but they may also overlap. A society of hunter gatherers, for example, may not need to make distinctions of this sort although the ability to fish well may be desirable both for meeting necessities of food supply and for social status.

If occupational speculation begins in a field of practices, of pleasure, productivity, and restoration, then the exploration of 'doing' will have already become ordered to a purpose. Of course, Pierce (2001) is talking about 'occupation', so some process of definition has already occurred that has elevated it from merely 'doing'. But by being, whether one is 'doing' something, or 'nothing', an individual is already occupying a space in the continuum of human society. Being and doing do not occur independently of each other. Though occupation may be broken theoretically into units, in medical, psychoanalytical, psychological or biological terms, it is actually perceived much of the time in flow between action and perception, both within people and between them as people interact (Csikszentmihalyi, 1991; Hari and Kujala, 2009). The intention to do something may or may not be followed with the action because other simultaneous events change the situation or alter the stimulus to action, or because there are insufficient resources to carry it out. Thus intention is continually informed and modified by the cues we receive from the environment and other people.

Although humans are physically distinct from each other and have individual experiences, sharing similar environments allows similar perceptions to arise from shared experiences. Language develops from these shared cues to allow terms to also be shared and it is learned through a process of simulation. As developing children we observe the actions of others and the sounds they make in response and try to emulate them for ourselves. Hari and Kujala (2009) point out that the development of cognitive processes in this order suggests that the development of the awareness of others predates the awareness of self. We seek cues from our environment to know how to act. These may be passive cues such as signs or features of the environment, or interactive. For example, we may seek reassurance that our behaviour is socially correct from the facial expressions of others.

References

Burgess, A. (1972) *A Clockwork Orange*. Harmondsworth, Penguin.

Chomsky, N. (1995) *The Minimalist Program*. (Current Studies in Linguistics 28.) Cambridge, MA, MIT Press.

Csikszentmihályi, M. (1991) *Flow: The Psychology of Optimal Experience*. New York, Harper & Row.

Csikszentmihályi, M. (1997) *Creativity: Flow and the Psychology of Discovery and Invention*. New York, HarperPerennial.

Golledge, J. (1998) Distinguishing between occupation, purposeful activity, and activity, part 1: review and explanation. *British Journal of Occupational Therapy* 61(3), 100–105.

Gollwitzer, P. M., Schaal, B. (1998) Metacognition in action: the importance of implementation intentions. *Personality and Social Psychology Review* 2(2), 124–136.

Hari, R., Kujala, M. V. (2009) Brain basis of human social interaction: From concepts to brain imaging *Physiological Review* 89(2), 453–479.

Kellett, A. (1994) *The Yorkshire Dictionary*. Otley, Smith Settle.

McLaren, J. (2009) African diaspora vernacular traditions and the dilemma of identity. *Research in African Literatures* 40(1), 97–111.

O Muirthe, D. (1977) *The English Language in Ireland*. Cork, Mercier.

Pierce, D. (2001) Occupation by design: dimensions, therapeutic power, and creative process. *American Journal of Occupational Therapy* 55(3), 249–259.

Pronin, E. (2008) How we see ourselves and how we see others. *Science* 320, 1177–1180.

Sakellariou, D., Pollard, N. (2008) Political challenges of holism: heteroglossia and the impossibility of holism. In N. Pollard, D. Sakellariou, F. Kronenberg (eds), *A Political Practice of Occupational Therapy*. Edinburgh, Elsevier Science, pp. 91–105.

Salvatori, P. (1999) Meaningful occupation for occupational therapy students: a student centered curriculum. *Occupational Therapy International* 6(3), 207–233.

Waterhouse, K. (1962) *Billy Liar*. Harmondsworth, Penguin.

5 Towards a Transformational Grammar of Occupation

Nick Pollard and Dikaios Sakellariou

Occupational literacy (Pollard, 2008; see Chapter 3) supposes the existence of synthetic blocks or components of doing that make access to occupation possible. These blocks refer to the elements into which a task can be broken down and understood and they can be described in linguistic terms as a 'transformational grammar', as opposed to a traditional or descriptive one. The overarching aim of any grammar is to be a tool that can lead to an understanding of language. A descriptive grammar does this by describing the observed elements and codifying these in rules. It provides regulation of the language, by establishing correct, 'normal' forms and irregularities. However, people communicate perfectly well without this set of rules. The first known descriptive grammar of the English language was the *Bref Grammar for English* by William Bullokar, published in 1586 (Bornstein, 1977). This did not stop people continuing to use the English language in ways that they had done before its publication. Being set in print, the rules described in this seminal work were not accessible to all English speakers and the language continued to develop through day-to-day oral usage. With the spread of print 'correct', or culturally dominant, ways to speak English emerged that reflected the values of a particular social class. Even within the range of English native speakers, there are considerable differences. As we have seen, Yorkshire dialects derive from earlier languages. They contain elements that are not elements of Received Pronunciation English (Kellett, 1994). Subsequent forms have developed from contact with many other cultures (Robson, 2008).

In contrast, a transformational grammar aims to provide knowledge on how a language functions. Instead of a set of rules, it might be more accurate to describe it as a platform from which to navigate the complexity of language. It facilitates an understanding of the heteroglossic context by providing conceptual tools to make sense of it (Bornstein, 1977). In effect the main aim of a transformational grammar is to understand the knowledge the native speakers have of their language.

Similarly, to understand the processes of occupation in all its complexity, it is not enough to codify it in sets of rules and categories. Although these might represent a necessary convention, primarily to facilitate communication, occupational therapists

Politics of Occupation-Centred Practice: Reflections on Occupational Engagement across Cultures,
First Edition. Edited by Nick Pollard and Dikaios Sakellariou.
© 2012 John Wiley & Sons, Ltd. Published 2012 by John Wiley & Sons, Ltd.

need to make sense of the knowledge that 'native speakers' of occupation have. They need to understand occupation as occurring in the context of the lives of people therapists are working with, valuing occupation as a diachronic concept (occurring within a historical continuity) and not only as a synchronic one (occurring here and now). A transformational grammar of occupation will not act as a handbook but as a tool for understanding, based on an open and dynamic process. Ikiugu (2004, 2010) developed his idea of instrumentality as a means to arrive at a pragmatic understanding of occupation and linked occupational actions to individual beliefs or cognitions about the world. Gramsci (1985) described how occupational actions and language are interlinked in his exploration of the development of Italian as the lingua franca of commerce in renaissance Italy. Such developments – especially in the relationship of language to the pervasive influence of activities such as commerce – have multiple layers as they permeate different arenas of human occupational functioning.

Human Scale Development Theory

Max-Neef (2010: 206) developed the human scale development theory as a matrix of constant human needs and variable satisfiers, which goes beyond the doing, being, becoming and belonging mantra. The listing of a need for 'idleness' in the matrix is significant for occupational therapists. 'Idleness' is a concept connected with purposefulness and meaningfulness. It is a quality of 'being' through 'imagination, curiosity, tranquillity, spontaneity', and may be obtained through 'having' 'games, parties, spectacles, clubs, peace of mind'. These opportunities involve actions such as to 'day-dream, play, remember, relax, have fun' and 'interacting' with 'landscapes, intimate places, places to be alone, free time.' The characteristics that Max-Neef describes here are positive aspects of idleness, although, returning to the narratives of Billy and Alex, it may be seen that they have resolved their need for idleness at the expense of other needs, such as affection, participation and understanding. The complexity of Max-Neef's matrix suggests that there is a balance operating across several dimensions of need at the same time.

Thus, in order to make sense of what occupation is, we need to move beyond the assumed and taken-for-granted nature of doing and being. Occupations appear to carry multiple meanings according to context: Ikiugu's (2010) modified instrumentalism in occupational therapy asks partners in a process to consider how their actions will be perceived by others, but this allows for different interpretations. Occupations occur in a flowing narrative context and they may often form a nexus in multiple narratives (because each action makes numerous other events possible in a chain of causality). People are able to make sense of occupation because they share an understanding of how actions and events are related, and can perceive motivations and interpret intentions (see, for example, Chapter 8). However, because of the influence of previous personal experience on individual understanding the objectives to which actions are intended are not always clear. The situation is rather like that of certain moves in chess that open multiple possibilities for the player. Although there may be a preferred strategy, a player may use moves to create several optional possibilities where advantage may be gained over the other player. In human action many choices are possible but they are not infinite. People are able to interact, correctly interpret intention and respond appropriately; human society is not chaotic.

However, as Chapters 12 and 14 demonstrate, there are points at which the intricate mechanisms of human interaction can break down. Kasnitz and Block (Chapter 14) give several examples where, because of disability, communication and other aspects of interaction operate at different speeds between individuals. The effort required to sustain communication over long periods can be exhausting, or the circumstances prove so difficult, that the participants run out of strategies. This can be frustrating, and sometimes events conspire against the best intentions.

Language and Occupation

Literacy is associated with reading and the written use of language. Due to the increasing complexity of information in human society, written forms of languages have become very important in reflecting and shaping culture. Whereas in certain historical periods people have, across parts of Europe, shared enough of the forms of their languages to make trade possible, they have evolved separately. The use of written language makes this very visible, even where similar alphabets are used. Where two groups of people with different linguistic traditions encounter each other there are inevitably exchanges about these differences. One of the features of these interactions is the acquisition of loan words from one language into another. The languages of cultures in which there has been much exchange with other people have many such words. English is rich in them: words like khaki, catamaran, caravan, tea, curry, all have origins in the colonial occupation of other cultures (Yule and Burnell, 1996). Many other words betray the influence of invading or migrant groups as we have already considered in the case of Yorkshire dialect (Kellett, 1994).

Burgess (1972: 91) chose to use Russian as the basis for nadsat to imply that it derived from Soviet propaganda, but perhaps also because of its unfamiliarity to most readers. English had few Slavonic loan words at the time he was writing. Alex's present-day peers might describe themselves by the word 'chav', which is currently used in the UK to describe an underclass of unemployed and uneducated youths (Hayward and Yar, 2006) and probably originated as a Romany word for 'youth' (Renouf, 2007). The extent to which such adoptions can be made is partly related to their affinity with the language into which they are adopted, which allows what Renouf (2007) calls 'lexical productivity'. Few of Burgess's terms, if any, found their way into English but there is a continuous process of assimilating and creating new words. Those that are more like English words, such as 'nimby' ('not in my backyard', a term that can be associated with territorial connotations of occupation) are perhaps more successful. Nimby can be developed into 'nimbyism' as an adjective, or 'nimbies' as a group noun.

This facility of linguistic development points to interesting effects in relation to grammar. The word 'nimby' has been accommodated to existing grammatical structures within English. On the other hand, as English has been exported to many countries, it is possible to see considerable differences between the variants spoken around the world. Thus some of the forms of English spoken in the Caribbean use a mainly English vocabulary but the grammatical structure has features derived from African languages. Exposure to the creative possibilities of patois and Caribbean forms of English through poets such as Linton Kwesi Johnson and Benjamin Zephaniah in the 1980s produced a phenomenon where white working-class poets would perform in patois themselves to give themselves a different voice.

Although this phenomenon was evident as a writing experiment, it did not extend to the spoken language these youths used off the performance stage, whereas many young white people have recently adopted 'Jafaican' terms into their 'multicultural London English' (Robson, 2008) speech, such as 'wazzup' and 'innit' but often incorporating elements with a global range of different cultural origins. Robson (2008) attributes this development to a social phenomenon of low-income lone-parent families. These are the same circumstances responsible for the 'chav' phenomenon identified by Hayward and Yar (2006), where many young people have developed their own cultural forms in situations of increasing independence from other elements of culture, much as Burgess foresaw in his novel. Because this manifestation seems to be a recent development it is not clear whether those who currently speak it will retain these features in their speech in future years. However, it is an illustration of how the use and form of language is linked to social status and occupation.

English is not the only language to experience such changes due to the influences to which it is open. French also has many phrases that derive from colonial cultural exchanges (Strutz 1999). The acquisition and use of these different terms is often a linguistic badging or identification, which in turn is linked with human occupations and their relationship with justice. Bonfim (2005) explains how, as a street child in Brazil, he learnt to use different forms of vernacular speech in order to survive in a socially marginalized existence. The ability to use the language of the street ensured his protection and also defined his occupational situation as a street child and a member of certain gangs.

This relationship between language and occupation is long established. Linebaugh (1991) explains how in the eighteenth century the language of the working and criminal classes was very distinct from that of the powerful and wealthy. Their 'cant' terms, which when used in defence statements sometimes had to be translated, originated in the cultural mix of itinerant labourers, workers in a range of trades, slaves, seamen, and prostitutes from anywhere with which Britain had commerce. Thus the relationship between language and a matrix of human development needs is something which can be explained and assessed through theoretical concepts, but is determined by human interaction. These linguistic changes are not a part of the forms of language that are taught in education systems and, if they are researched, they are usually explored by academics whose culture and social origins are removed from those who speak in them. They are not recognized as 'proper' forms of the language but as dialect. The forms of doing that are expressed through them are therefore also contained as external, even contaminating, to the dominant culture (McLaren, 2009; see also Chapter 11). Just as confusions over words such as 'baps' and 'fishcakes' mark out regional differences, the use of such terms may also be markers of class. The word 'bap' for example, is unlikely to feature on a high-class restaurant menu.

Conceptions such as purposeful and meaningful activity therefore have to be wielded with care. People may define themselves as belonging to society or a community through what they do, but they also define that becoming and belong-ingness in the way that they express that definition. The depiction of human occupations through changes in language, however, challenges some of the assump-tions about occupation. Linebaugh (1991) focuses on the eighteenth century as an era of particularly significant change, one that made the wealthy fabulously so in relation to the working classes, who struggled to survive. For the wealthy, there was no such concern as a general instrumentalism, which considered the opinions of others outside their own social class. The *purpose* and *meaning* of wealth *was* wealth, and it was dependent on maintaining social and economic differences that ensured poverty for others. Furthermore, even poverty, although necessary, was not enough, and those who stole to survive because they could not earn enough to eat were also to be hanged or transported to America or Australia. Stealing to survive appears to have been recognized as a meaningful and purposeful activity, although it was also recognized as a crime for which a person could be hanged or transported. It is perhaps hardly surprising that the gulf between the classes could be expressed in divergent forms of language just as is demonstrated in *A Clockwork Orange* and *Billy Liar*. Councillor Duxbury, having been subjected to Billy's Man O'Dales expressions, such as 'thraiped', points out to him that he need not try to talk as he does, a man who lacked educational opportunities, but should speak as he has been taught to do in school.

Alex's versions of doing, being, becoming and belonging have much more in common with those expressed by such traditional gallows ballads as *Sam Hall*: 'Oh my name it is Sam Hall, chimney sweep . . . and I've robbed both great and small/and my neck shall pay for all, when I die . . .' Such ballads have framed a continuous popular narrative of opposition to the status quo, from Robin Hood to the country and Western outlaw song, from Rebetika to the punk anthem or modern gangsta R + B. They represent a flamboyant end of the spectrum between criminal and legal occupations, and as Linebaugh (1991) suggests, present a form of criticism of dominant culture concerning the purpose and meaning of occupation, the understanding of doing and the language in which activities are expressed.

Territories of Words

Language itself is a convivial tool for the expression of ideas of change. The several uses of new forms of language, cant, patois, creoles and the assertion of regional dialect are ways in which language becomes a territory of words that can be occupied to articulate the needs of certain groups. Culture, the things people do and they way they do them, is framed in the languages they speak. In the UK this is not just about the languages that have arrived with migration but can be found in the variety of its native languages and connected identities, as expressed through the poetry of Nuala Ni Dhomnall, Sorley MacLean, Robert Burns (respectively Irish, Gaelic, Scots) or the Welsh *penillion* or folk verses (Jones, 1997).

The professional terminology that occupational therapists use is also a territory of words that frames ideas about doing. The word 'occupation' is used in specific ways. It has itself been 'occupied' to refer to certain areas of human activity with which occupational therapists are concerned as 'meaningful' and 'purposeful'. These linguistic actions in themselves give a moral force to certain kinds of doing and imply the proscription of other forms of doing. Other occupational therapists (e.g. Kronenberg and Pollard, 2005) have presumed the harnessing of 'meaningful' and 'purposeful' occupation to a transformational agenda in which the profession identifies itself with the pursuit of social and occupational justice issues.

The application of 'occupation' to a concept of justice, where meaningful occupation becomes a human right, is challenged by the possibility that if there is a minimal program concerning the understanding of doing, it breaks down at the junctures created by the language of property. Townsend and Wilcock (2004) remind us that occupation is much more than work but the meaningfulness of 'occupation' is confronted with notions of working, working for someone else who determines what the work is and what shall be paid for it, because somehow they have acquired a territorial claim to a place and resources through which work can be carried out. Furthermore, by setting a wage scale for remunerating that work, they can increase their territorial claims and the value of their property. Doing, being, becoming and *belonging*. Bloch (1965a, 1965b) traced how the modern notions of property emerged from the anarchic prefeudal society, to one that was governed by might. Property belonged to those with the power to assert their rights over others. This extended to land, so it also extended to those who inhabited the land and, whilst they may be subject to the depredations of their lord, in return their lord and his knights undertook to organize the defence of local inhabitants against the depredations of others.

The idea that occupation is connected with doing should not, then, be divorced from its connection with land rights and property ownership. The right to do something is connected with the space in which it is done. If the right to have ownership and control of a space, or a territory, is acknowledged, then the owner has the right to do and to allow others to do something in that territory. Those people who want to be occupied in that space, or who accept being given things to do for the right to occupy a portion of that space, acknowledgement of the right of the owner to exercise governance, or even to govern what else takes place in that space (see Chapter 1).

In most modern societies virtually all the geographical spaces are owned and controlled by people or organizations representing them. With the exception of their own homes, perhaps, every place to which people locate themselves is owned or controlled by others. They may move from a rented flat to a place of work, perhaps go to a restaurant or bar owned by yet another group of people, and return to their flats. Every space on this Monopoly board is owned by someone. The business of being occupied in all these spaces, whether eating, sleeping and bathing, working, or going out for the evening, is to some extent determined by all the owners of these spaces, and who set the price in terms of rent, wages and meal prices. Part of the price includes a charge for the space which is being occupied. Existence, the very right to exist, is itself determined by a concession to property rights; that is, to the physical occupation, ownership and control of space, which in turn determines the meaning of the occupations that are carried out in that space. The Monopoly player who runs out of money is, of course, out of the game.

This spatial control has become extensive, and further measures, such as the installation of closed-circuit television, electronic eyes and keycodes are increasingly taken to increase the surveillance and control of space, whether public or private (as in this conception of occupation and space many private functions take place in a space that is controlled and owned by others). Of course, there is also a counter narrative of resistance to these controls and, as Linebaugh (1991) suggested, many people contested the spatial regulation of occupation during the eighteenth century. De Certeau (1988) describes a process of resistance with his depiction of 'La perruque', a metaphorical wig that allows a person the exterior appearance of conforming to work expectations, while in fact using work facilities and space to do something for oneself, much as Billy Fisher seems to do in indulging his fantasy world while at his job at the undertakers. In Billy's case, this is not so much resistance as individual escapism, and one possible reading of *Billy Liar* is that resistance to conformity is futile; adulthood involves accepting and being satisfied with a far less grand counter narrative than the word 'resistance' suggests.

The application of occupation to the language of justice has to take account of these contextual issues. Elementary language-teaching systems usually involve the teaching of the present tense to enable the student to gain confidence in here-and-now situations. The more complicated concepts connected with past and future tenses, the history of the language and its dialects, are areas for advanced learning. To have a minimal program that recognizes different forms of doing, in order to admit the right to meaningful occupation, is perhaps to have a program that only deals with a superficial level of occupational 'parole' (or the discussion of doing). If meaningful occupation is a right, then it cannot be a right by itself without the right to a space in which to carry out that meaningful occupation.

The South African apartheid system allowed some forms of meaningful occupation to take place but operated its exclusions by determining the space in which occupation was to take place. People were accorded places to work and live and take their leisure according to their racial categorization, creating the rule of a place for everyone and everyone in their place. This meant that, because some places were denied to Black people, the occupations connected with those places were also denied (Luthuli, 1962). Acts of colonization and cultural dominance, from ancient times to the present, have been concerned with the denial of the right to practise occupations, such as religious or folk ritual, in particular places, often imposed through restrictions on the use of language, because to speak in one's own tongue is the 'language of struggle' (Ngugi, 1986: 3). These denials are repeated throughout the history of cultural dominance: Australian aboriginals were denied access to areas of spiritual significance, Native Americans were forced away from their traditional sources of food and sustenance and many peasant customs (which threatened the controls exercised by the state and Church) were suppressed. These exclusions served systems that valued the exploitation of people and their resources in terms of material wealth. It is for this reason that Max-Neef (2010) set out his matrix of human needs and satisfiers using terms that were qualities and did not lend themselves to being quantified. Max-Neef (2010) makes the point that qualities are the determinants of what is significant in human life, rather than economic formulae. Without people there would be no money, and therefore money, property, material things, have to serve life, rather than people having to serve social needs defined through dominant property relations.

Conviviality

If it is recognized that all humans define themselves as belonging to society or a community through what they do, then the concept of occupation as a human right is a logical development of this recognition. Terms such as 'occupational injustice', 'occupational deprivation', and even extremes that can be termed 'occupational apartheid' describe experiences where this human right is curtailed. This array of concepts depends on the reframing of elements of the social as occupational arenas or spaces, so that some aspects of social justice are viewed through an occupational lens. Max-Neef (2010) is one of a number of economists who refute the prevailing economic mantra of growth, which is linked to rising consumption. He argues that what people do has to be geared to self-sufficiency, sustainability and what Illich (1975) termed conviviality if the global population is to avoid consuming the resources available to it within a couple of generations. As Ikiugu (2008) points out, this has a clear occupational dimension that is expressed in the individual choices of everyone on the planet through everything that people choose to do. Such choices are means of working for development, rather than growth. Max-Neef (2010) argues against a number of myths that sustain progress only in terms defined by globalizing powers. Instead he argues for progress towards development, from the bottom up, at the level of human needs such as subsistence, protection, affection, understanding, participation, creation, idleness, identity, and freedom. This is a different language of economics and can be worked for through occupational forms other than those that privilege consumption and inequity. But it is not a task for a profession, such as occupational therapy, to attempt to take on as a mission for itself; it is an objective for the central idea of occupational therapy, which involves giving a key priority to the need to do.

This occupational lens also suggests a cultural lens. Doing and being are concepts that imply a narrative of action: 'this is what I/we did to be who I am/we are.' They are parts of a verb that is essential to the grammar of the depiction of action. If this is the client's narrative, the therapist making the assessment is writing the story in the second or third person: 'this is what you did . . .' '. . . to be who he or she is.' Each time the story is different, involving a different viewpoint and aspect of the same character. Each narrative is the nexus for a new set of grammatical constructions, new narratives, new understandings and further lenses with which to interpret other actions. A notional grammar of 'doing', which is flexible enough to accommodate all these variations in occupation, context and environment, allows each of them to be recognized and understood. It admits the formation of narratives that communicate more than the essential here and now of the what, but also the nuances contained in Kipling's (1987) other five 'serving men': who, why, when, where and how which are the essential components of any story.

Occupational therapy is one arena in which a language of doing can be articulated. A common complaint amongst occupational therapists (and other professional groups) concerns other professions or 'unqualified' people reinventing or 'poaching' their roles (Nancarrow and Borthwick, 2005: 902) or that due credit is often not given to the profession for its contributions (Wilding and Whiteford, 2007). The profession has yet to find the right language and use its grammatical skills to assert its terminology into the interprofessional lexicon. Perhaps this is merely jockeying for position amongst multidisciplinary rivals in professional boundary disputes, and usually the strategy which is then called for amongst professionals is the demand for more research but it is also necessary to argue effectively for the importance of occupational interventions (Wilding and Whiteford, 2007). Occupational science presents itself as a vehicle for the development of underpinning knowledge while other academics pursue the clinical evidence. These pursuits are necessary to the sustainability of occupational perspectives but practitioners are often dealing with events about which research evidence has not yet percolated and that are determined by policy, managerial and financial considerations, within which they have to manage the demand placed upon the services they offer. Occupational science might offer some perspectives to reach out further than the profession (do Rozario, 1997) but at the time of writing, it remains a narrow field that has yet to prove itself to be part of the curriculum in many professional education programmes or excite significant interest in other disciplines.

My Baby Took the Train . . .

Billy Fisher, having missed all his cues and used up all his alibis to the extent that he is thoroughly confused, dithers about at the station waiting for the last train to London to begin a life in show business as a scriptwriter. However, he does not get on it, seeming to recognize that he does not really have the resources to make that step and carry it through. His nineteen-year-old character, written in 1959, would now be in his seventies on a pension, which might be the reward for that decision to opt for the settled life of his home town. Perhaps he has managed to mature and develop a meaningful and purposeful life through his working years and up to retirement, achieving such social milestones as forming partnerships and raising children. As he walks past the infirmary where his Grandma died the night he had meant to go to

London, he might be contemplating his future needs in the light of his changing health, the reducing value of his income and the changing policy on healthcare. Perhaps, like many people, he has never heard of occupational therapy or really taken much notice of the term, even though it is possible that in the next few years his care needs may involve therapeutic interventions and assessments for aids and adaptations. Billy may be experiencing some arthritic pains, perhaps some loss of short-term memory. He grew up and lived through an era where access to healthcare was easily available but now his needs for subsistence, protection, affection, understanding, participation, creation, idleness, identity and freedom could be challenged. He might envisage himself in a few years attending a day centre, participating in activities such as crafts, music groups or reminiscence, or having to have social care input into his home. His existing relationships might be disrupted as he has to rely more on care facilities. Some of the changes may bring benefits and some of the opportunities offered to him may be enjoyable but these changes may not come out of choice but because this is what is available to him and they are the options to which he is directed by the health professionals he will encounter. The patterns and habits that he has established over his life may have to alter as a result. He may not be sure that this is the future he really desired or that will answer his wants. One of the questions he might be asking himself in response to considering these needs is 'what am I going to do?' Can an occupational grammar do more than help him to accept these solutions to his needs?

References

Bloch, M. (1965a) *Feudal Society. The Growth of Ties of Dependence*. L. A. Manyon (trans.). London, Routledge.

Bloch, M. (1965b) *Feudal Society. Social Classes and Political Organisation*. L. A. Manyon (trans.) London, Routledge.

Bonfim, V. (2005) Once a street child, now a citizen of the world. In. F. Kronenberg, S. Simo Algado, N. Pollard (eds) *Occupational Therapy without Borders – Learning from the Spirit of Survivors*. Edinburgh, Elsevier Science, pp. 19–30.

Bornstein, D. D. (1977) *An Introduction to Transformational Grammar*. Cambridge, MA, Winthrop.

Burgess, A. (1972) *A Clockwork Orange*. Harmondsworth, Penguin.

De Certeau, M. (1988) *The Practice of Everyday Life*. S. Rendall (trans.) Berkley, CA, University of California.

do Rozario, L. (1997) Shifting paradigms: the transpersonal dimensions of ecology and occupation. *Journal of Occupational Science* 4(3), 112–118.

Gramsci, A. (1985) *Selections from Cultural Writings*. D. Forgacs, G. Nowell-Smith (eds), W. Boelhower (trans.). London, Lawrence & Wishart.

Hayward, K., Yar, M. (2006) The 'chav' phenomenon: consumption, media and the construction of a new underclass. *Crime Media Culture* 2(1), 9–28.

Ikiugu, M. (2004) Instrumentalism in occupational therapy: An argument for a pragmatic conceptual model of practice. *International Journal of Psychosocial Rehabilitation.* 8, 109–117.

Ikiugu, M. (2008) *Occupational Science in the Service of Gaia*. Baltimore, PublishAmerica.

Ikiugu, M. (2010) Influencing social challenges through occupational performance. In F. Kronenberg, N. Pollard, D. Sakellariou (eds) *Occupational Therapies without Borders*, Vol. 2. Edinburgh, Elsevier Science, pp. 113–122.

Illich, I. (1975) *Tools for Conviviality*. London, Fontana.

Jones, G. (1997) *A People's Poetry: Hen Benillion*. Bridgend, Seren.

Kellett, A. (1994) *The Yorkshire Dictionary*. Otley, Smith Settle.

Kipling, R (1987) *Just So Stories*. London, Penguin.

Kronenberg, F., Pollard, N. (2005) Overcoming occupational apartheid: a preliminary exploration of a political nature of occupational therapy. In F. Kronenberg, S. Algado, N. Pollard (eds) *Occupational Therapy without Borders: Learning from the Spirit of Survivors*. Edinburgh, Elsevier/Churchill Livingstone, pp. 58–86.

Linebaugh, P. (1991) *The London Hanged. Crime and Civil Society in the Eighteenth Century*. Harmondsworth, Penguin.

Luthuli, A. (1962) *Let My People Go*. London, Fontana.

Max-Neef, M. (2010) The world on a collision course. *AMBIO* 39, 200–210.

McLaren, J. (2009) African diaspora vernacular traditions and the dilemma of identity. *Research in African Literatures* 40(1), 97–111.

Nancarrow, S. A., Borthwick, A. M. (2005) Dynamic professional boundaries in the healthcare workforce. *Sociology of Health and Illness* 27(7), 897–919.

Ngugi wa Thiong'o, (1986) *Decolonising the Mind: The Politics of Language in African Literature*. Oxford, Heinemann.

Pollard, N. (2008) When Adam delf and Eve span: occupational literacy and democracy. In N. Pollard, D. Sakellariou, F. Kronenberg (eds) *A Political Practice of Occupational Therapy*. Edinburgh, Elsevier Science, pp. 39–51.

Renouf, A. (2007) Tracing lexical production and creativity in the British Media. In J. Munat (ed.) *Lexical Creativity, Texts and Contexts*. Amsterdam, John Benjamins, pp. 61–89.

Robson, G. (2008) Social change and the challenge to RP: approaching the British cultural revolution through accents and dialects. In I. Ramos, A. J. M. Guijarro, J. I. A. Hernandez (eds) *New Trends in English Teacher Education*. La Mancha, Universidad de Castilla, pp. 199–211.

Strutz, H. (1999) *Dictionary of French Slang and Colloquial Expressions*. Hauppauge, NY, Barrons Educational Series.

Townsend, E., Wilcock, A. A. (2004) Occupational justice and client centred practice. *Canadian Journal of Occupational Therapy* 71(2), 75–87.

Wilding, C., Whiteford, G. (2007) Occupation and occupational therapy: knowledge paradigms and everyday practice. *Australian Occupational Therapy Journal* 54, 185–193.

Yule, H., Burnell, A. C. (1996) *Hobson-Jobson, the Anglo Indian Dictionary*. London, Wordsworth.

6 Narratives of Recognition

Dikaios Sakellariou and Nick Pollard

In Chapter 1 we concluded that occupational therapy positions itself as an advocate of doing, being, becoming and belonging. As these terms are very similar to those used to describe quality of life (Phillips, 2006) and human development needs (Max-Neef, 2010), this position is not unique. Indeed, it looks as if many professional groups such as nursing, social work, education and youth workers have a claim to a place in the complex shield wall facing the greedy barons of William the Conqueror in the defence of the ancient virtues of individual freedoms. Harold, King of England only represented those freedoms in myth, having many connections with the feudal world William was about to impose which were instrumental in the reasons for the conflict, and himself representing a similar form of property relations (Loyn, 1962; Miles, 2006). This has subsequently formed a key element of legends such as Robin Hood or has been reinterpreted in practices such as poaching (see Chapter 1). There are no clear goodies and baddies in this story and the negotiation of language extends into a narrative of the negotiation of best fit. The claim that any group may make to the defence of occupational rights is complex (Hammell, 2008; Galheigo, 2011). The occupational therapist fits the client into their practice and fits their practice around the client. At the same time the therapist has to negotiate practice in a multidimensional team, managerial and policy environment (Hammell, 2007, 2008, 2010). The therapist and the client may also have to take account of the communities around them so that outcomes can be sustained (Iwama, 2006). Their stories embody different standpoints and multiple viewpoints.

Occupational Therapy Stories

As a result there are several stories in occupational therapy that are dialogical in nature. One is the story of its client-centred practice (Sumsion, 1999) and the healing plot (Mattingly, 1998). Another story is that of professional practices, motivations, and responsibilities versus practical experiences (Detweiler and Peyton, 1999; Wilding and Whiteford, 2007). This, while being a cycle of stories in itself, has a new subset related to the emerging concept of occupational justice, which is starting

Politics of Occupation-Centred Practice: Reflections on Occupational Engagement across Cultures, First Edition. Edited by Nick Pollard and Dikaios Sakellariou.
© 2012 John Wiley & Sons, Ltd. Published 2012 by John Wiley & Sons, Ltd.

to be hailed as one of the *raisons d'être* of the profession through a claim to an origin in social reform. Yet further stories concern the people occupational therapists work with: stories of illness, stories of life with an illness, stories of occupation and stories about occupational therapists (Mattingly, 1998). While some storylines are often written, or at least directed, within professionals' discourses and to some extent owned by healthcare professionals, the last storyline is one that occupational therapists may or may not fit into and it is authored by people who live with an illness or disability. Of course, there can be a co-constructed storyline too, where professionals and service users develop a common horizon of understanding and develop intersecting or joint stories (Mattingly, 1998), perhaps through the use of the Kawa model (Iwama, 2006).

Each has its dialectical tensions: social justice versus a disabling society that poses a limitation on what the therapist can effectively work out with the service user; the narrative of the 'client' (i.e. as interpreted by the therapist), or the narrative of disability (the disabled person's *own* meanings of occupation, function, purpose, etc. – see discussions in Chapters 12 and 14) versus the hegemonic medical discourse, which determines the scope for the action of the therapist. This is often an informal narrative, constructed by the service user and carers based on their interpretations and geared toward an audience of friends and relatives, based in forms of tacit knowledge and vernacular expression.

Even though one may be a health professional, when *we* have a relative in care or are in care ourselves we narrate the plot from *our* perspective, privileging our story over that constructed with the therapist. We then do not necessarily respect the hegemonic dominance of medicine or science – because very often our knowledge of the world is informed by our experience, even where this differs from the norm (see for example, Rippere and Williams, 1985). It is, as I (NP) discovered for myself even with a mild episode of mental distress, bewildering. During this period, while in the town centre market, I met a client who recognized me and with concern asked 'are you alright, lad?' 'Fine,' I replied, not, 'no, I feel bloody dreadful.' I could not explain my story as this would have breached professional boundaries, and yet I had crossed them through my episode of illness. While I was fortunate enough to be able to return to practice, this was a useful lesson in how mental distress is part of normal experience and yet pushes the individual into a zone of marginalization.

The clinical process disrupts our narrative, curtailing this to the essentials demanded by the doctor (Frank, 1995), or by the technical process of adaptation suggested by the therapist (Mattingly, 1998). The person with a disability is rendered silent and invisible, objectified, less than a person, although Mattingly found that occupational therapists tended to interact well with their clients because their role involved forms of engagement that were more than physical care interventions but concerned task-related activities.

All these narratives can be read in multiple ways, or multiple glossias, each dependent on the viewpoint and expression of the person who is speaking in the narrative, like the changes of position in a metanarrative such as Tolstoy's *War and Peace* (1978). Tolstoy combines multiple plots, which intersect with each other at various points to weave a complex embroidery or tapestry from different stories.

It can be seen, therefore, 'that other narrative accounts are possible, based around subplots in these stories, just as Jean Rhys' (1968) novel *The Wide Sargasso Sea* tells the tale of the first Mrs Rochester, who is the mad woman in the attic of Charlotte Bronte's (2003) earlier novel *Jane Eyre*. Within and around the central plot of the client and professional that may be privileged by an occupational-therapy-based presentation there are several subplots. Each of these subplots may also represent an intersecting major narrative to which the story of client and therapist may be yet another sub plot:

- client and professional and carer;
- employer and institution;
- institution sets conditions for care to client and carer;
- interaction between professional groups;
- external contextual plots: the home and social circumstances surrounding each character which influence their participation in other plot elements.

Consequently, multiple interpretations can exist of the *same* phenomena (see also Latour, 1996). The stories around a person who lives with a progressive paralytical condition and needs to use a wheelchair for mobility can include many possible scenarios, such as:

1. A wheelchair is desired by all involved, perceived as good, and is also easily accessible and usable.
2. A wheelchair is desired by all involved, perceived as good and is available, but cannot be easily used outdoors.
3. A wheelchair is desired by all involved, perceived as good and usable but is too expensive.
4. A wheelchair is desired by all involved, perceived as good, and is also easily accessible and usable, but the waiting time is too long.
5. A wheelchair is perceived as good by the partner of the person who needs it, but to the disabled person it acts as a reminder of the paralysis.
6. A wheelchair is desired as good by all involved but it has some negative points.
7. Despite the wheelchair being perceived as good by all involved, the partner of the person who needs it cannot push it.

The possibilities are many, and several of them co-exist. All of them are equally plausible and they depend upon the standpoints of the participating actors. Possible scenarios range from the one extreme that everyone is in consensus about the goodness that a wheelchair, or any other technology, represents, in the knowledge that one is both accessible and usable, to the other end where the question about the potential use of a wheelchair is not even raised.

These narratives and subplots can be said to have a grammatical structure because generally they have replicable beginnings and ends according to the treatment process or cycle. This can be observed at the linguistic level in the emergence of the professional cant, which can be exemplified through the use of such terms as 'referral', 'assessment to establish aims', 'treatment', 'reassessment to establish outcomes', 'discharge'. The language of health professionals requires a range of dictionaries and formularies to define the terms employed in the subplots of interaction between professional groups. Just as in a television hospital drama serial, but depending on the treatment context, the subplots may deal with many different issues. Examples might be the plot line of individual interactions between occupational therapist and support worker, or nurse; managerial subplots concerning the processing of clients through the treatment environment and the staffing issues; or different aspects of team interaction. Peck and Norman (1999), for example, reveal many such narrative plots operating concurrently in multidisciplinary community psychiatric teams. A drama serial may, for example, play on the tensions between Goffman's (1990) 'front of house' and 'back of house' dramatic presentations, the professional face versus the relaxed office environment where personal relationships between staff might be more clearly exposed; contrasted with a similar difference in the way relationships between client and carer are presented to professionals and when in private (see discussion of occupational effect in Chapter 1). In actuality the intersection of such subplots is more complicated than a 60-minute soap opera episode, which has to be tied up neatly for the viewer. There may be several clinical subplots because team members possess different perspectives but, in each, the specific use of professional language offers one plane of narrative. In other dimensions different uses of language are used to describe the experiential autobiographical narrative of the client, carers, and possibly also in professional critical reflective diaries.

These elements correspond to the notions of high literature or professional discourse, and an oral lay discourse (sometimes a community published version may also be developed – see Chapter 11), in which the same events are described in vernacular form. 'I went into hospital and this is what happened to me.' Just as in the discourses surrounding literature, the professional discourse (often supported by differences in social class, education and economic status and the access all these give to the means of expression through professional authority and avenues for dissemination as knowledge) is often privileged over the lay version of the same events.

High literature frequently contains inconsistencies and variations between different editions of the text. Part of the interest such books may have for us is not only in the story being told, but the background to the production of the text, the influences on the author and the relationship between what is depicted in the writing and the experiences of the writer. There is always more to be discovered in what may be a series of subtexts that frame the circumstances of the main narratives. In this sense no narrative is ever complete, just as many treatment episodes remain incomplete. People discharge themselves and the rest of their story is not known to the professional. An intervention may occur once a week or once a month but the therapist may have little idea of what might have happened in the meantime. The healing narrative of the professional and the client is a small part of the autobiographical narrative of either and, as we have discussed, the space is maintained by professional boundaries. However, how it is told can also be determined by the client's ability to express their story as well as a frequent anticipation that the professional understands and can speak for the service user who has difficulty in verbalizing their experiences (Jackson and Stevenson, 2000). Perhaps in a psychiatric review meeting the professional is trying to tell a healing narrative of interactions with the client and what the client has reported of life between interventions. This represents the professional's story of the client but it may prove to be unreliable. Sometimes other professional team members or clients themselves give quite different explanations, perhaps because relations in other treatment milieux have allowed a more familiar and informal interaction, producing deeper exploration of key issues, for example where a professional works with clients in their own home (Jackson and Stevenson, 2000).

In other situations the professional returns to the office after having seen the client and indulges in what Goffman (1990) terms 'back of house' conversations with colleagues. While there is a professional discourse concerning the client there is also a private professional discourse between professional intimates. This may be at least as significant as the 'front of house' discourse because it may differ considerably both from the information formally recorded in notes or used in professional meetings and in terms of the presentation of self. Professional intimates may use different language to signify that they are talking informally, and may use these situations to explore or second guess at aspects of their observations that they may be struggling to make sense of. They may also discuss issues such as how their work or interactions with clients affect them personally, perhaps exploring the distinction between their use of self when maintaining a boundaried familiarity with the client and the self they reveal to colleagues (Jackson and Stevenson, 2000).

These 'dramatic' scenes present a further possibility. A professional arrives at the home of a client, or a client arrives in the department. The door opens, the scene begins, as if the curtains are raised on a stage. The ensuing scene is improvised by what both people find when they meet. What happens next may make sense to the participants, but then again it may not. If the client's narrative and the professional's narrative do not meet, the narrative of client-centred practice may be interrupted. It is also possible that there are other needs being supported by the engagement. For example, users of mental health services do not always articulate their needs directly but show signs and symptoms. What is being intended or communicated by one person is not necessarily correctly interpreted by the other. The previous narrative understood by each of them may be of use, but it may not. In effect, this can be viewed in the same way as an absurdist dramatic scene, like a play by Harold Pinter, or the music of Luigi Nono; the story has started before the spectator/occupational therapist arrives and will go one after she leaves the stage. What is perceived as the beginning of the story is not a 'beginning' in the literal sense of the word. It is merely the phase in which observation of a process commences. Once the curtain goes up, anything can happen and anything can make sense because the previous scene may not be available to us. As Jean Rhys's novel *The Wide Sargasso Sea* may suggest, narrative is actually interrupted in order to make a beginning, an end and to allow interpretation; the biography of the first Mrs Rochester offers a different reading of the sense we may have made of *Jane Eyre's* story. History is not bounded within convenient dates, to begin in 1066 with the conquest of England and end in 1992 (see Fukuyama, 1992).

The professional dealing with such loose ends uses structural concepts such as the cycle of assessment, treatment, review, assessment to develop a narrative and make sense of phenomena such as symptoms. These concepts offer a language, or a set of rules that occupational therapists, for example, can employ to act in congruence with others and facilitate the perception of continuity and coherence in the progress of treatment. However, the use of these rules within the storied account of action also disguises the truths that it represents. They are made to conform to a professional subtext or perhaps a personal subtext, a narrative of the experience of working with a client. Possibly clients may feel similar constraints in the way that working with a therapist may imply obligations to them for the interventions they have received; the tale told might represent a path to independence but the meaning might be one of interdependence, where the therapist refines her practice in the light of the experience given by the client while the client gains by the interaction with the therapist. Such stories have many dimensions and authors (Mattingly, 2010) so the appropriateness of any intervention ultimately needs to be negotiated within a context of heteroglossia.

Heteroglossia

Heteroglossia refers to the presence of 'another's speech in another's language', for example, the presence of multiple perspectives around disease: those of the service user and those of the healthcare providers, but also those of close and extended family, friends, work colleagues and other social actors. These multiple discourses are interconnected and are grounded in the diverse cultural discourses operative in every society, which in turn are termed social heteroglossia (Kroeger, 2005). In an analogy with the textual construction of a novel where heroes are situated in interactions initiated by the author and act within preset boundaries, social actors operate within an inescapable dominant cultural discourse. These multiple 'languages', the diverse perspectives of the various actors together with the scripts, beliefs and attitudes present in society comprise the social whole that is the setting of human action. The various vantage points from which people view the world, their different perspectives and the different languages they speak are intertwined in relationships of power.

Some languages do not need any translation to make people understand them as they express experiences that are widely recognized as representative of society as a whole. Some others have been marginalized and the realities they communicate need to be reframed according to the rules of the dominant discourse (Beetham, 2002). The construction of a common language does not eradicate the possibility of misinterpretation, as it both perpetuates power differentials (communications take place according to the norms and experiences of a dominant group) and also excludes people whose experience cannot be understood according to these conventions (Beetham, 2002). In the context of health and illness, the biomedical, scientific knowledge demonstrated by healthcare professionals has been legitimized and gained power of authority over the narrative knowledge developed by people living with an illness.

As Bakhtin (1981/1994) reminds us, language can never be neutral, but it is always rich with meanings, constituting an operational means for discourse. The way people talk, and through their speech, represent the world around them, expresses their perception of reality and the way they live in the world. Consequently multiple discourses co-exist, including: official and vernacular, personal and political, explicit and implicit, scientific and narrative. These occur in the context of illness, as much as they may do in every other aspect of life, but when they enter formal relationships such as that between health service client and clinician these discourses form an arena for the negotiation of power and choices.

The transcript that follows is an excerpt from a study on how people make sense of living with motor neurone disease (MND). In the following excerpt, Dikaios discusses with Cerys, who has been living with MND for 15 years, and her husband Glyn, about a procedure called percutaneous endoscopic gastrostomy (PEG). This procedure is used to ensure that people get enough nutrition despite being unable to chew and/or swallow due to progressive paralysis of the bulbar musculature:

Dikaios: I remember you telling me last time that you know when they told you about the PEG at the hospital you didn't want it.
Glyn: no, Cerys didn't want it, no.
D: why not?
G: Because it is another step down the road, you see. Each step you lose you going further down under. As I said before, today she could do ... today, not now but years ago, next week she couldn't do it so it was another step further down the road. [Cerys: starts synthesizing answer on her lightwriter.] So having the PEG was another step down the road, She didn't want that, she wanted to stay as she was. I felt that she didn't need it, I said don't do it, she don't need it. She is OK as she is, right. He [neurologist] says, he insisted that she should have it.

Glyn moves on to describe how a decision was finally taken, and why.

G: Because when she was in the hospital for a couple of days, she didn't have anything to eat, because it wasn't mashed or anything. And of course they weren't feeding her either. You can't take it out as such, like. So the doctor said, well, she will starve to death, you got to have a PEG like. For she blamed me for having had the PEG put in but it wasn't my fault, I didn't want it in the first place.

Up to this point the story suggests that the decision to have a PEG was one taken unilaterally by healthcare professionals. Food was not mashed like at home, and there was no time to feed Cerys. Not only this, but healthcare professionals could know with a certain degree of certainty that Cerys's bulbar musculature would progressively get so weak that she would not be able to swallow even mashed food. Still, Cerys blamed Glyn for not protecting her against a decision taken despite her. But also despite Glyn. Ten years after the procedure, when this interview was taken, Glyn comments:

G: But best thing that ever happened to her.
C: I felt it was too life changing
G: Too life changing, you see. So . . . everything . . . awkward. cleaning the teeth in the morning is awkward. Before she could do it alright, now it's very difficult, now we get to fight [she laughs] to clean her teeth in the morning like, you know. I want to do it for her, she wants to do it herself. If I do it for her, it's another step down the road, isn't it. So, I'm putting toothbrush, toothpaste in her hand and she can't get it up there, in her mouth like, around [Cerys smiles] and of course she is fighting me because she wants to do it herself, and I am fighting her because let's get on with it for Chrissake. We can't have all day on it.

More than against a single procedure like the PEG, the fight is against change that signifies a lost skill – an ability that may not be regained. It is also a fight against changes in how daily life, or occupation, is being experienced. From receiving food *normally* and *normatively* through the mouth, to washing her teeth alone, Cerys knows what she wants. But other people's wishes are important as well and their perceptions of what is the *good* do not always meet. At least not immediately. These different languages can be explored through the use of stories, or narratives, as discussed in the following chapter.

References

Bakhtin, M. (1981/1994) The heteroglot novel. In P. Morris (ed.) *The Bakhtin Reader; Selected Writings of Bakhtin, Medvedev, Voloshinov*. London, Arnold, pp. 112–122.

Beetham, M. (2002) Speaking together; heteroglossia, translation and the (im)possibility of the just society. *Women's Studies International Forum* 25(2), 175–184.

Bronte, C. (2003) *Jane Eyre*. London, Penguin.

Detweiler, J., Peyton, C. (1999) Defining occupations: a chronotypic study of narrative genres in a health discipline's emergence. *Written Communication* 16, 412–468.

Frank, A. W. (1995) *The Wounded Storyteller. Body, Illness and Ethics*. Chicago, University of Chicago Press.

Fukuyama, F. (1992) *The End of History and the Last Man*. New York, Free Press.

Galheigo. S. M. (2011) What needs to be done? Occupational therapy responsibilities and challenges regarding human rights. *Australian Occupational Therapy Journal* 58, 60–66.

Goffman, E. (1990 [1959]) *The Presentation of Self in Everyday Life*. London, Penguin.

Hammell, K. W. (2007) Client-centred practice: Ethical obligation or professional obfuscation? *British Journal of Occupational Therapy* 70(6), 264–266.

Hammell, K. W. (2008) Reflections on . . . well-being and occupational rights. *Canadian Journal of Occupational Therapy* 75, 61–64.

Hammell, K. W. (2010) Contesting assumptions in occupational therapy. In M. Curtin, M. Molineaux, J. Supyk-Mellson (eds) *Occupational Therapy and Physical Dysfunction*. Edinburgh, Churchill Livingstone/Elsevier, pp. 39–54.

Iwama, M. (2006) *The Kawa Model: Culturally Relevant Occupational Therapy*. Edinburgh, Churchill Livingstone/Elsevier.

Jackson, S., Stevenson, C. (2000) What do people need psychiatric and mental health nurses for? *Journal of Advanced Nursing* 31(2), 378–388.

Kroeger, J. (2005) Social heteroglossia: the contentious practice or potential place of middle-class parents in home-school relations. *The Urban Review* 37(1), 1–30.

Latour, B. (1996) *Aramis, or the Love of Technology*. C. Porter (trans.). Cambridge, MA, Harvard University Press.

Loyn, H. R. (1962) *Anglo-Saxon England and the Norman Conquest*. London, Longman.

Mattingly, C. (1998) *Healing Dramas and Clinical Plots: The Narrative Structure of Experience*. Cambridge, Cambridge University Press.

Mattingly, C. (2010) *The Paradox of Hope: Journeys through a Clinical Borderland*. Berkley, CA, University of California.

Max-Neef, M. (2010) The world on a collision course. *AMBIO* 39, 200–210.

Miles, D. (2006) *The Tribes of Britain*. London, Phoenix.

Peck, E., Norman, I. J. (1999) working together in adult community mental health services: exploring interprofessional role relations. *Journal of Mental Health* 8(3), 231–242.

Phillips, D. (2006) *Quality of Life: Concept, Policy and Practice*. London, Routledge.

Rhys, J. (1968) *Wide Sargasso Sea*. Harmondsworth, Penguin.

Rippere, V., Williams, R. (eds) (1985) *Wounded Healers. Mental Health Workers' Experiences of Depression*. Chichester, John Wiley & Sons, Ltd.

Rowles, G. D. (1991) Beyond performance: being in place as a component of occupational therapy. *American Journal of Occupational Therapy* 45(3), 265–271.

Sumsion, T. (1999) *Client-centred Practice in Occupational Therapy: A Guide to Implementation*. Edinburgh, Elsevier/Churchill Livingstone.

Tolstoy, L. (1978) *War and Peace. Rosemary* Edmonds (trans.). Harmondsworth, Penguin.

Wilding, C., Whiteford, G. (2007) Occupation and occupational therapy: knowledge paradigms and everyday practice. *Australian Occupational Therapy Journal* 54, 185–193.

7 Narratives and Truths

Dikaios Sakellariou and Nick Pollard

The *Merriam Webster* dictionary (www.merriam-webster.com/dictionary/narrative, accessed 2 September 2011) gives three definitions for narrative: something that is narrated, a story, or an account; the art or practice of narration; the representation in art of an event or story. For Chase (2005) a narrative can be written or oral and can be short and topical, it can take the form of an extended analysis of an aspect of one's life, or it can be presented as a story of one's whole life. In essence, narrative refers to the stories people say (or embody) about aspects of their life.

Narratives, in the form of written or oral stories, have been used throughout human history to record, convey, explain and essentially make sense of information, experience and life itself. The long narrative poem, the epic, for example, is a format encountered in many parts of the world, blending facts and fiction and demonstrating a specific linguistic structure as described by Bakhtin (1941/1981). The epic was used not only as a form of information recording and communication, but also as a way to make sense of the recorded information (Bakhtin, 1941/1981).

Labov (Labov and Waletzky, 1967; Labov, 1997) introduced the importance of stories in social sciences and sought to offer a working definition of the term 'narrative'. For Labov a narrative refers to a speech event that is told in natural situations and which has a structure that includes the following elements: abstract, orientation, complicating action, evaluation, resolution and coda, or lesson learnt. Labov viewed narrative from a linguistic perspective, and understood it as organized speech, structured both thematically and temporally, which represents reality and relays events that have happened.

People make sense of their lives in different ways, finding ways to connect the past with the present, and to project their sense of self into the future. Mace (1998) and Chodorow (1978), for example, relate different ways in which the replication and narration of domestic activities represents a contiguity, a sense of continuity through the generations between mothers and daughters. Bull (2009) suggests that (at least for anglers) the same might be true for the handing on of male experience between generations. The construction of stories that look backwards and forwards

Politics of Occupation-Centred Practice: Reflections on Occupational Engagement across Cultures, First Edition. Edited by Nick Pollard and Dikaios Sakellariou.

give meaning to a person's life, so that life is experienced as a connected whole rather than as a multitude of fragments in time and space (Ricoeur, 1984). These stories can be relayed through different means; they can be enacted, written, narrated in their entirety, or in snippets, or in any other way that is available and resonates with a person's life.

Rather than emphasizing overarching qualities, such as courage, wisdom, or loyalty as exemplified in the literature of Arthurian romances or satirized in picaresque novels such as Fielding's *Tom Jones*, in our times narratives, or stories, are more attuned to the personal experience as conveyed and also constructed through the process of narration. In other words, we live in postmodern times and ours are postmodern stories. If modernity as an ontological framework was based on the existence of permeating stories, the grand narratives (or theories about the world and the way it works), then postmodernity has argued for attention to the personal (Lyotard, 1984). Discourses of race, ethnicity, illness and disability are constructed, lived and talked about in ways that depend on the standpoint of the narrator. This does not negate the existence of common experiential elements across narratives but the usefulness of creating an all-explaining story that can be *true* to every person's experience is doubtful. In this context 'true' refers to a story that can resonate with an individual's experience and recognized as doing so by that individual.

Features of Narratives

The testimonio, or first-hand witness account (Beverley, 2005), the autobiography (Oakley, 1993), the memoir and the manifesto are some of the things that people have constructed in order to narrate life experiences. In the late twentieth century, Kura Sunazawa (1983) told the story of her life and her peoples, the Ainu, in northern Japan, giving it the title 'memories from my century'. Moving between languages, Ainu and Japanese, across geographic regions as the Japanese occupied Ainu land, and experiencing two World Wars with significant impact on the country, Sunazawa manages to find a connecting thread that gives meaning to these experiences; despite all the changes and interruptions her life makes sense.

According to Mattingly (1998) narratives have three distinctive features. They are event centred, experience centred and they create new experiences. Sunazawa not only narrated events as they unfolded in time (occupation of land, the wars, and legislative changes) but also discussed the interaction between the social and political contexts and herself. Or as Mattingly would say (1998), she not only wrote about what she did to the world but also about what the world did to her. The story invites further interpretation and exploration of possibilities and alternative scenarios. Narrating the experience means transforming the experience as events are put in some order and meaning is sought.

Events and experience form the basis of narrative (see Chapter 11). This becomes strikingly obvious when the memory of events is taken away. In *The Lost Mariner*, Sacks (1985) tells the story of Jimmie, a man who had retrograde amnesia and a short-term memory of a few minutes as a result of Korsakov syndrome. While he could remember very clearly events in the distant past, the present appeared to be disconnected from that past as the thematic continuum had been ruptured due to the amnesia. While Jimmie enacted and embodied many stories, he could not narrate them simply because he could not remember the events and how they made him feel. Somebody else had to do the narrating (i.e. produce a story).

Narratives also have a temporal aspect, in that they are about events that have happened in time and sometimes follow one from the other. Aristotle, in Poetics, said that a narrative has a beginning, a middle and an end, and many scholars agree that narratives have a temporal structure that calls for start and end points, with events unfolding in between. Polkinghorne (1994) argues that these events are organized thematically, through the plot. A plot is the organizing theme that structures the story and makes it function as a unified whole rather than as a series of disjointed events. Plot, for Ricoeur (1984: 171) is 'the intelligible whole that governs a succession of events in any story.' The existence of a plot is a vital difference between lives as lived and lives as narrated. From the perspective of the individual who is going through it, lived experience lacks plot as events and their effects are not known and so cannot be organized either thematically or temporally. It is only after the events have been lived that the individual or someone else acting as a narrator has an overview of events and discerns a plot.

Mattingly (1994) described the process whereby a clinician produces a plot explaining the course of an intervention as therapeutic emplotment. This distinction between plot and emplotment is useful because it reminds us that plot is not given but produced by the narrator, or by the audience. The existence of a plot does not imply that narratives run smoothly in a cause-effect way, neither does it assume the existence of an end beyond which further stories are no more possible. Narratives can be fragmented and disconnected, and the plot may be hard to detect.

Narratives presuppose the existence of a narrator and an audience who will partake in the sharing of the story, interpret and shape it accordingly. Narrator and audience give the story its meaning and construct its plot. Chase (2005) referred to narratives as interactive performances, whereas Good (1994: 143) stated that 'in order to constitute narrative, the story must be appropriated by a reader or an audience'. For Riessman (2008) storytelling is a relational activity. Not only does the narrator transform an experience and construct new experiences through telling a story but the audience gives its own interpretations to the events narrated and draws its own conclusions. In other words they develop their own plots. Narratives are posited on the premise that they are dynamic rather than concerning a truth, or a grand narrative; their remit and focus is with individuals and their own interpretation of events (Rodriquez, 2002).

According to Chase, narratives are socially situated events, 'produced in this particular setting, for this particular audience, for these particular purposes' (2005: 657). Gelya Frank (2000) chose to tell the story of DeVries, a woman born with tetra-amelia, in a particular way; both women were situated in space, time and culture; several events from both women's lives were mentioned and all this was complemented by Frank's analysis and interpretations. Writing for an academic journal would require a different structure and focus, with events being put in the background and Frank's interpretations being foregrounded (see, for example, Frank 1984 for a different telling of the story). Had DeVries told the story it would have had yet another focus as the standpoint of the narrator would have been different (see Chapters 12 and 14). The Federation of Worker Writers and Community Publishers was formed in the UK in 1976 in order to represent marginalized experiences directly through the narratives of those who were excluded from the dominant cultural forms. Through the organization of community publications, working-class people, people from a wide range of cultural minorities and those with disabilities disseminated their narratives to their local communities (see Chapter 11).

This constant refocusing of stories depending on the standpoint of the narrator becomes even more obvious when a story is narrated by many different people. Seeking to understand why a particular technology failed (an innovative transportation system) Latour (1996) studied the stories that people related to this technology had to share; his informants included a long list of engineers, bureaucrats, politicians, representatives of the public and scientists and the data consisted of oral and written accounts on this transportation system and on individuals' and organizations' relation to it. The product of the study was a book that is half a novel and half a scientific report. Halfway through it Norbert, a young sociologist, is exasperated by the multitude of the different stories that each informant gives, despite all starting from the same externally observable and verifiable facts. It was not only the existence of a multitude of voices that was so challenging for Norbert. It was the fact that these voices were not hierarchical and none took precedence over the other that made it impossible to find one 'true' answer to why the technology failed, as all answers were plausible and true in their own right. All narrators were telling a story that made sense to them.

This multitude of voices that Latour (1996) observed points to another feature of narratives: they are concerned about individuals as the protagonists in stories, not about the events narrated. That is not to mean that the events themselves are not important but their significance lies in how they are interpreted and experienced by the narrators, as similar events can mean different things to different people. Arthur Frank (1995), writing about his experience of being diagnosed and treated for testicular cancer, narrates how, after the treatment was concluded, he ran into a colleague who as it turned out had also been treated for testicular cancer in the past. In contrast to Frank's experience, however, his colleague's cancer was diagnosed early, operated soon after and testicular cancer as an event never gained prominence in his life. While from a medical point of view both men presented with the same diagnosis, testicular cancer, their experience and interpretation of this and the role it played in their lives was vastly different (Frank, 1995).

Narrative and Illness

The postmodern notion of a fragmented, yet interconnected world, where stories can illuminate people's perspectives and create meaning, has been taken up by social scientists such as Annemarie Mol, Arthur Frank, Arthur Kleinman and Laurence Kirmayer, all of them exploring stories of living with illness. Some of them are narrating their own personal stories of living with illness (for example Murphy, 1990; Frank, 1991; Wikan, 2000). Others are co-constructing stories with other people who live with illness or disability (for example Kleinman, 1998; Robinson and Hunter, 1998; Shakespeare *et al.*, 1996; Charmaz, 1991; Cole, 2004; Kirmayer, 2000) and yet some others are exploring these stories, which happen in the space in-between healthcare professionals and people living with illness (for example Good, 1995; Mattingly, 1998, 2010; Park, 2008).

In the opening paragraph of Gareth Williams' (1984) classic article on the genesis of chronic illness, Bill, one of the study participants, breaks out asking: 'how the *hell* have I come to be like this' (p. 175, emphasis in the original). Williams (1984) was one of the first researchers who explicitly referred to narratives in the context of health and illness. In the context of a fieldwork study with people living with rheumatoid arthritis, Williams conducted semi-structured interviews with 30 people diagnosed with the disease, looking for illness-explanatory models that would answer the question 'why do you think you got arthritis?' Data pointed to a process whereby participants discussed their changing relationship to the world and constructed pasts that could lead to their lived presents, so as to make it possible for the disease to emerge. Williams defined this process as *narrative reconstruction*.

Williams' statement that '[disease] assaults the taken for granted world and demands explanation' (1984: 197) reminds us of the fundamental human need for meaning. Stories of illness are effectively stories about life. Sometimes, and for some time, they can be dominated by illness, while some other times illness is just in the background, as a possibility or as a lived normality.

In his story about living with a benign tumour wrapped around his vertebrae, gradually leading to total paralysis, Murphy (1990) describes the loss of meaning brought about by disability, the loss of social standing and the loss of identity. However, rather than being a narrative of hopelessness and lost meaning, Murphy's is a narrative that presents disability as another way of being in the world, one way among so many others.

Drawing from personal experience and from empirical material, Frank (1995) presented three storylines of illness narratives. Rather than being thought of as fixed categories, they can be more accurately conceptualized as points between which stories of illness constantly gravitate. These storylines are restitution, chaos and quest.

Restitution stems from the human needs for safety and also control that lead to a desire to know that 'all will be fine'. Life-threatening disease or disability ruptures life in a fundamental way, creating a schism between an experienced past and an uncertain future. When a fundamental point of reference – the body and its health – is modified, the sense of identity is threatened. The first reaction the person has is to believe that things will go back to normal and their sense of identity will not be threatened. The emergence of what Mol (1990) refers to as the logic of choice, has led to the dominant construction of the patient-consumer who views healthcare as a product. In that context, disease is but a disruption of the normal rhythm of life and the main problem lies in finding the right way/product to deal with it so that health can be restituted. Sometimes this is possible. Sometimes it is not and other stories need to be told.

Chaos narratives refer to these stories where restitution is not conceivable (irrespective of whether it is possible or not) and the sense of identity has been affected in such a deep way that meaning making is not possible. The thread that was connecting one's story from the past, to the present and on to a projected future has been sheared and the person is lost in the present. According to Frank (1995), a chaos storyline is a non-narrative as a person living it cannot engage in a process of narration. In Chapter 6 we discussed briefly how narrative and interpretation may become disconnected and one has to make sense of events in the present. A person whose thoughts have become very disordered might perhaps experience a phase of having the past, present, and the anticipated future jumbled up, but whereas the example of Jimmie represents a permanent condition, in the experience of psychosis there is a possibility that the episode can be recalled later and given an interpretation, the chaos reintegrated into a story, as related in Peter Mackie's *The Madhouse of Love* (Mackie, 2010).

The final storyline described by Frank refers to quest narratives. In these narratives, the narrator engages in a dialogical relationship with disease, which is seen neither as an external element (as in the restitution storyline) nor as an all-destructive force (as in the chaos storyline). Instead, in quest narratives, disease is viewed as part of the person's sense of identity, and emphasis is placed on learning to live with disease. As Frank (1995: 117) put it, 'quest stories tell of searching for alternative ways of being ill', placing emphasis on personal transformation. Frank draws parallels between quest narratives and the heroic journey as described by Joseph Campbell (1968) in his study on the construction of the 'hero'. Campbell described the hero's journey as unfolding in three main stages: departure, initiation and return. All of these can have their equivalent in stories of illness, with departure being the stage where the person first notices symptoms or consults a specialist; initiation the stage where it becomes clear that the prospect of restitution and a return to previous normality is not likely; and return could refer to the stage where a person is transformed through living with an illness. There is a crucial difference however between the 'hero's journey' as described by Campbell and stories of illness; ill people do not choose to embark on a life with illness. Illness is presented to them, leaving them no choice. They can, however, try to live with illness, making those choices that seem more sensible in the context of their lives (Frank, 1995).

The role of stories becomes even more prominent when a projected or desired future never comes, due to unforeseen developments such as serious illness or disability. This process whereby one's life story is disrupted, and the lived past does not lead any more to a previously envisaged future, has been defined by Bury (1982) as biographical disruption. The thematic thread that was leading from the past, to an unfolding present and through to a projected future is ruptured and new meanings and links need to be established so that people can once again make sense of their lives (Charmaz, 1991). This sense making has been described as biographical repair

(Locock *et al.*, 2009: 1043), whereby people can re-establish a notion of continuity between a good past, a difficult present and a desired future.

Other typologies of illness narratives have also been proposed, for example Hydén (1997). Rather than focusing on storylines as Frank (1995) did, Hydén bases his discussion of illness narratives on the relationship between narrator, narrative and illness. What most authors agree on however is that people living with an illness repair their biographies and re-establish meaning in their lives by engaging in storytelling. In Frank's (2002: 5) words 'stories give lives legibility; when shaped as narratives, lives come from somewhere and are going somewhere.' A life that makes sense is not necessarily a desired life. Making sense of life does not mean that interruptions are sutured and fractures repaired, allowing the protagonist of the story to resume life as normal. For Mattingly, making sense refers to constructing a plot, which links elements of a person's story to a thematic whole. Narratives can thus contribute towards developing an explanation, understanding one's life in context (Frank, 1995).

Postmodernism has debated widely against the notion of one explanation, or one *truth* or one *reality* (see, for example, Lyotard, 1998 and Latour, 2007) and instead understands the world as a nexus of unique, intersecting meanings and stories. According to Said (1979: 272–273) 'the real issue is whether there can be a true representation of anything, or whether any and all representations, because they are representations, are embedded first in the language and then in the culture, institutions, and political ambience of the representor.' To put it in other words, life as lived is different to life as narrated for the two reasons mentioned earlier in the chapter; plot and authoritative voice are present in narratives. Experience is transformed by the very nature of being told, as the narrator decides where to put emphasis, how to present certain characters and what to leave untold. Rather than mimesis, it is construction of meaning then that occurs when a story is narrated.

Whose Narrative and Whose Language?

In going about their daily life, people interact with other people. They each perceive life in a unique way, depending on their standpoint. And they have access to different languages through which they not only make sense, but also articulate their experiences. A moving viewpoint would be required to sample all the different perspectives, as argued by Good (1994). As Lyotard (1994) reminds us all these perspectives are equally valid, although some may exercise more power than others, for example, as we have discussed, the health professional may have the position of interpreter for a client who has difficulty expressing their story (Jackson and Stevenson, 2000). The elements of a narrative are at some point actually constructed, told and sometimes written by one individual, for example, a healthcare professional, a researcher, a journalist. This implies that, by virtue of being a narrator, one person's voice assumes authority to select, present and explain lived life in a particular way.

There can be as many stories as there are listeners, narrators and narrative contexts. The therapist tells the version that meets professional needs, the client tells the narrative that relates to the experience of disability. Each may tell more than one version of the narrative according to context. Certain details may be omitted, for example, in deferment to the listener's sensitivities, or matters of confidentiality; others may be exaggerated, perhaps to accentuate humorous aspects. Language will change to suit the audience and the situation, and is used to stress some points, foregrounding certain aspects of the experience, while putting in the background elements that are not as central to what the narrator wants to communicate.

References

Bakhtin, M. (1941 /1981) Epic and novel: towards a methodology for the study of the novel. In M. Holquist (ed.) *The Dialogic Imagination*. Austin, University of Texas Press.

Beverley, J. (2005) Testimonio, subalternity, and narrative authority. In N. Denzin, Y. Lincoln (eds.) *Handbook of qualitative research* (3rd ed). Thousand Oaks, CA, Sage, pp 547–558.

Bronte, C. (2003) *Jane Eyre*. London, Penguin.

Bull, J. (2009) Watery masculinities: fly-fishing and the angling male in the South West of England. *Gender, Place and Culture: A Journal of Feminist Geography* 16(4), 445–465.

Bury, M. (1982) Chronic illness as biographical disruption. *Sociology of Health and Illness* 4(2), 167–182.

Bynner, J. (2009) *Life-long Learning and Crime: A Life-course Perspective*. London, Institute of Education.

Campbell, J. (1968) *The Hero with a Thousand Faces*. Princeton, Princeton University Press.

Charmaz, K. (1991) *Good Days, Bad Days: The Self in Chronic Illness and Time*. New Brunswick, NJ, Rutgers University Press.

Chase, S. E. (2005) Narrative inquiry: multiple lenses, approaches, voices. In N. K. Denzin, Y. S. Lincoln (eds) *The Sage Handbook of Qualitative Research*, 3rd edn, Thousand Oaks, CA, Sage Publications, pp. 651–679.

Chodorow, N. (1978) *The Reproduction of Mothering*. Berkeley, CA, University of California Press.

Cole, J. (2004) *Still Lives*. Cambridge, Harvard University Press.

College of Occupational Therapists (2010), *Code of Ethics and Professional Conduct*. London: College of Occupational Therapists.

Cook-Gumperz, J. (1986) Literacy and schooling: An unchanging equation? In J. Cook-Gumperz (ed.) *The Social Construction of Literacy*. Cambridge, Cambridge University Press, pp 16–44.

Council of Occupational Therapists' Registration Boards (Australia and New, Zealand)/OT, Australia, (2010) *Towards a National Safe System for Occupational Therapy Practice*. Mile End, SA, Council of Occupational Therapists' Registration Boards (Australia and New Zealand/Fitzroy, Vic: OT Australia.

Denshire, S. (2002) Reflections on the confluence of personal and professional. *Australian Occupational Therapy Journal* 49, 212–216.

Detweiler, J., Peyton, C. (1999) Defining occupations: a chronotypic study of narrative genres in a health discipline's emergence. *Written Communication* 16, 412–468.

Frank, A. (1991) *At the Will of the Body: Reflections on Illness*. Boston, Houghton Mifflin.

Frank, A. (1995) *The Wounded Storyteller. Body, Illness and Ethics*. Chicago, University of Chicago.

Frank, A. (2002) Why study people's stories? The dialogical ethics of narrative analysis. *International Journal of Qualitative Methods*, 1(1), http://ejournals.library.ualberta.ca/index.php/IJQM/article/viewArticle/4616, accessed 10 September 2011.

Frank, G. (1984) Life history model of adaptation to disability: the case of a congenital amputee. *Social Science and Medicine* 19, 639–645.

Frank, G. (2000) *Venus on Wheels: Two Decades of Dialogue on Disability, Biography, and Being Female in America*. Berkeley, CA, University of California Press.

Gesler. W. M. (1992) Therapeutic landscapes: medical issues in light of the new cultural geography. *Social Science and Medicine* 34(7), 735–746.

Goffman, E. (1990 [1959]) *The Presentation of Self in Everyday Life*. London, Penguin.

Good, B. (1994) *Medicine, Rationality and Experience: An Anthropological Perspective*. Cambridge, Cambridge University Press.

Hagedorn, R. (2001) *Foundations for Practice in Occupational Therapy*, 3rd edn. Edinburgh, Churchill Livingstone/Elsevier.

Hammell, K. W. (2007) Client-centred practice: ethical obligation or professional obfuscation? *British Journal of Occupational Therapy* 70(6), 264–266.

Hammell, K. W. (2008) Reflections on.. *well-being and occupational rights. Canadian Journal of Occupational Therapy* 75, 61–64.

Hocking, C. (2007) The romance of occupational therapy. In J. Creek, A. Lawson-Porter (eds) *Contemporary Issues in Occupational Therapy: Reasoning and Reflection*. Chichester, John Wiley & Sons, Ltd, pp. 23–40.

Hydén, L. C. (1997) Ilness and narrative. *Sociology of Health and Illness* 19(1), 48–69.

Iwama, M. (2006) *The Kawa Model: Culturally Relevant Occupational Therapy*. Edinburgh, Churchill Livingstone/Elsevier.

Jackson, S., Stevenson, C. (2000) What do people need psychiatric and mental health nurses for? *Journal of Advanced Nursing* 31(2), 378–388.

Kinsella, A. (2006) Poetic resistance: Juxtaposing personal and professional discursive constructions in a practice context. *Journal for the Canadian Association for Curriculum Studies* 4(1), 35–59.

Kirmayer, L. (2000) Broken narratives: clinical encounters and the poetics of illness experience. In C. Mattingly, L. Garro (eds) *Narrative and the Cultural Construction of Illness*. Berkeley, CA, University of California Press.

Kleinman, A. (1988) *The Illness Narratives: Suffering, Healing, and the Human Condition*. New York, Basic Books.

Labov, W. (1997) Some further steps in narrative analysis. *Journal of Narrative and Life History* 7, 395–415.

Labov, W., Waletzky, J. (1967) Narrative analysis. In J. Helm (ed.), *Essays on the Verbal and Visual Arts*. Seattle, University of Washington Press, pp. 12–44. Reprinted in *Journal of Narrative and Life History* 7, 1–38.

Latour, B. (1996) *Aramis, or the Love of Technology*. C. Porter (trans.). Cambridge, MA, Harvard University Press.

Latour, B. (2007) A textbook case revisited; knowledge as a mode of existence. In E. Hackett, O. Amsterdamska, M. Lynch, J. Wajcman (eds) *The Handbook of Science and Technology Series*. Cambridge, MIT Press, pp. 83–112.

Locock, L., Ziebland, S., Dumelow, C. (2009) Biographical disruption, abruption and repair in the context of motor neurone disease. *Sociology of Health and Illness* 31(7), 1043–1058.

Loyn, H. R. (1962) *Anglo-Saxon England and the Norman Conquest*. London, Longman.

Lyotard, J. F. (1984) *The Postmodern Condition; A Report on Knowledge*. G. Bennington, B. Massumi (trans.). Manchester, Manchester University Press.

Mace, J. (1998) *Playing with Time: Mothers and the Meaning of Literacy*. London, UCL Press.

Mackie, P. G. (2010) *The Madhouse of Love*. Brentwood, Chipamunka.

Mattingly, C. (1994) The concept of therapeutic 'emplotment'. *Social Science and Medicine* 38(6), 811–822.

Mattingly, C. (1998) *Healing Dramas and Clinical Plots: The Narrative Structure of Experience*. Cambridge, Cambridge University Press.

Mattingly, C. (2010) *The Paradox of Hope: Journeys through a Clinical Borderland*. Berkley and Los Angeles, University of California.

Miles, D. (2006) *The Tribes of Britain*. London: Phoenix.

Mol, A. (2008) *The Logic of Care; Health and the Problem of Patient Choice*. New York, NY, Routledge.

Murphy, R. (1990) *The Body Silent*. New York, Norton.

Oakley, A. (1993) Telling stories: auto/biography and the sociology of health and illness. *Sociology of Health and Illness* 15, 414–418.

Office for National Statistics, (2011) *Earnings: 2010 Survey of Hours and Earnings*, www. statistics.gov.uk/cci/nugget.asp?id=285, accessed 3 May 2011.

Park, M. (2008) Making scenes: imaginative practices for a child with autism in an occupational therapy session. *Medical Anthropology Quarterly* 22(3), 234–256.

Peck, E., Norman, I. J. (1999) working together in adult community mental health services: exploring inter-professional role relations. *Journal of Mental Health* 8(3), 231–242.

Perrin, T., May, H., Anderson, E. (2008) *Wellbeing in Dementia: An Occupational Approach for Therapists and Carers*, 2nd edn. Edinburgh, Churchill Livingstone/Elsevier.

Pollard, N., Walsh, S. (2000) Occupational therapy, gender and mental health: an inclusive perspective? *British Journal of Occupational Therapy* 63(9), 425–431.

Prospects (2011) *Occupational Therapist Salaries and Conditions*, http://ww2.prospects.ac. uk/p/types_of_job/occupational_therapist_salary.jsp, accessed 3 May 2011.

Rhys, J. (1968) *Wide Sargasso Sea*. Harmondsworth, Penguin.

Riessman, C. (2008) *Narrative Methods for the Human Sciences*. Los Angeles, Sage Publications.

Rippere, V., Williams, R. (eds) (1985) *Wounded Healers. Mental Health Workers' Experiences of Depression*. Chichester, John Wiley & Sons, Ltd.

Robinson, I., Hunter, M. (1998) *Motor Neurone Disease*. London, Routledge.

Rodriguez, A. (2002) *Redefining our Understanding of Narrative. The Qualitative Report*, Volume 7(1), www.nova.edu/ssss/QR/QR7-1/rodriguez.html, accessed 10 September 2011.

Rowles, G.D. (1991) Beyond performance: being in place as a component of occupational therapy. *American Journal of Occupational Therapy* 45(3), 265–271.

Sacks, O. (1985) *The man who mistook his wife for a hat and other clinical tales*. New York, Summit.

Said, E. (1979) *Orientalism*. New York, Vintage.

Schon, D.A. (1987) *Educating the Reflective Practitioner*. San Franciso, Jossey Bass.

Shakespeare, T., Gillespie-Sells, K., Davies, D. (1996) *The Sexual Politics of Disability.* London, Cassell.

Sunazawa, K. (1983) *Watashi no ichidai no hanashi* (the story of my life) Sapporo, Hokkaido, Shinbunsha.

Wikan, U. (2000) With life in one's lap: the story of an eye/I (or two). In C. Mattingly, L. Garro (eds) *Narrative and the Cultural Construction of Illness.* Berkeley, CA, University of California Press, pp. 212–236.

Williams, G. (1984) The genesis of chronic illness: narrative re-construction. *Sociology of Health and Illness* 6(2), 175–200.

8 Occupation in a Greek Town: Flowing, Emergent, Flexible across Time and Space

Sarah Kantartzis, Matthew Molineux and Sally Foster

Introduction

Occupation, understood to be 'all the things that people need, want, or have to do' (Wilcock, 2006: xiv) has historically been explored within occupational therapy and occupational science from an individual perspective, where the individual emerges as a conscious actor engaging with and influencing his or her environment through occupation, reflecting Western individualism and neoliberal politics (Kantartzis and Molineux, 2011). Recent work on occupation and place (Hamilton, 2011; Townsend *et al.*, 2009) and the proposal for an occupational theory of landscape with the concept 'occupationscape' (Hudson *et al.*, 2011) suggest the importance of a more dynamic and critical exploration of occupation and context. An alternative to the focus on the individual is to explore occupation as emerging from a dialectical interaction between economic, social and political structures and individuals, across time and space (Giddens, 1984; Dear, 1988; Lefebvre, 1991). This approach may be particularly useful for occupational therapists and occupational scientists who wish to move beyond the hegemony of contemporary Anglophone theoretical discourse (Frank and Zemke, 2008) to understand occupation in other contexts.

In developing understandings of occupation it is important to recognize that 'daily life, like language, contains manifest forms and deep structures that are implicit in its operations, yet concealed in and through them' (Lefebvre, 1981: 2). These forms and deep structures become the conditions of possibility within which individuals construct their daily lives.

Politics of Occupation-Centred Practice: Reflections on Occupational Engagement across Cultures, First Edition. Edited by Nick Pollard and Dikaios Sakellariou.
© 2012 John Wiley & Sons, Ltd. Published 2012 by John Wiley & Sons, Ltd.

Only recently has the socially constructed nature of space and time, and how they are integrally bound up with the everyday activities of individuals, been recognized in social theory, particularly through the work of Lefebvre and later Foucault, Bourdieu and in the structuration theories of Giddens and others (Pred, 1984). The spatial, temporal and social form a triad and together structure and are structured by daily life in an ongoing dialectical process (Soja, 1989). Occupation, usually referred to as action or practice in these theories, does not occur in a vacuum but is situated in a particular time and space, within particular social institutions (Giddens, 1984). The daily path of the individual (Pred, 1984) takes him or her through a particular series of places or locales at particular times, according to the structuring features of these locales and their temporal frameworks. The routinization of such daily activities leads to the ongoing reconstitution of these institutions, locales and temporal frameworks (Giddens, 1984).

Exploring the spatial and temporal fabric (Dear, 1988) upon which occupation is woven therefore provides a rich and lens that is an alternative to that which focuses directly on the individual. This is not to propose a structural approach to understanding the emergence of occupation, but rather to observe that there is an iterative relationship between space, time and the occupation of the individual; each is affected and in some ways made possible by the other (Kaiser, 2008).

The following discussion focuses particularly on space and time in a small Greek town and on the occupations of which they form an embodied and integral part (Crabtree, 2000). An ethnographic study is in progress that is exploring the occupation of the inhabitants of the town through participant observation and interviews. The study is ongoing and this discussion is based on the unfolding analysis and emerging understandings.

Following a brief introduction to Melissa (Melissa is a pseudonym), the town within which this study is being undertaken, focus will turn to the temporal and spatial framework within which occupation arises and is performed. Giddens (1984) pointed out that daily life emerges in an ongoing flow in time and space. An ongoing flow and flexibility is particularly characteristic of occupation in this town. There are flexible boundaries between and around concepts such as work and leisure, public and private, individual and social. These flexible boundaries of occupation would seem to be facilitated and partially constituted by the flexible boundaries between and within the spatial and temporal organization evident in the town. The discussion will aim to explore these issues as illustrated by the daily life in this town.

Introduction to Melissa

The town of Melissa with 3500 inhabitants (Panepistimio Thessalias, 2009) is located in central, mainland Greece, at the base of a range of mountains rising to 2,500 metres behind the town. Archaeological excavations and documentary evidence indicate that the town was thriving from Mycenaean times (1600–1100 BC) (Enisleidi, 1978). The contemporary town rises up the lower slopes of the mountain and is built mainly of stone with red tiled roofs. The wide valley spreads out in front of it with fertile land for farming. The river runs through the centre of the valley, along with the main train line from Athens (the capital city) to northern Greece, and the town's station is located here, approximately 2 km from the town. The main road links the neighbouring villages and the two nearest large towns, forty minutes drive away, also accessed by the thrice-daily bus. Athens is reached in approximately two hours by car or train.

Historically the town was, and continues to be, a farming community and *kefaloxori* (head town), the centre of the municipality. There are a small number of locally owned businesses and some development of tourist services together with shops, bars, *tavernes* (restaurants) and *kafeneion* (cafés).

The places of everyday life

Daily life in the town of Melissa takes place in the land around the town, in the homes, in the streets and squares with their *kafeneion* and *tavernes*, in the businesses and shops, and in the buildings housing the public services. These are the primary locales in which the majority of time of the inhabitants is spent (Soja, 1989).

All these locales provide opportunities for a variety of occupations to be undertaken within them, with a variety of purposes. Some examples will illustrate this variety and the difficulties of defining occupations according to categories of purpose such as for work and leisure, as is common practice in occupational therapy (Christiansen, 1994; Molineux, 2010). Also evident are the social networks that are (re-)constructed through these occupations, both an influence on, and an outcome of, occupation.

Ta xorafia (the fields)

Land around Melissa (commonly referred to as *ta xorafia* – the fields) is used in multiple ways. Melissa is traditionally, and currently, a predominantly farming community, with one-third of the working population engaged in farming (Panepis-timio Thessalias, 2009). Farming takes place on the land that extends up to 20 km in either direction from the town. Part of the land has been cultivated and mainly wheat, corn, cotton and olives are grown. Almost 5000 sheep and goats are grazed in the rough land around the fields (Panepistimio Thessalias, 2009). Dotted amongst the fields and within the town, are smaller areas, *perivolia* (kitchen gardens) where chickens are kept and vegetables, fruit and nuts are grown for mainly private consumption. At certain times of the year, dead trees are cut for fire wood, and *pournari* (a small holly bush), which covers much of the uncultivated land, is collected and used in the town for communal bonfires during carnival celebrations and for cooking the Easter Sunday lamb. Many families have olive groves to supply them with olive oil for the year. The land is also used for hunting, mainly of small birds, and for gathering *xorta* (greens), which is popular both as an occupation and as a food.

Occupations on the land therefore fulfil a variety of purposes. The land is used for profit through cultivation and animal husbandry, to provide direct food supplies to family members and *gnostous* (acquaintances, friends), as a source of heating fuel, and in social activities, either as a location or as a supplier of necessary materials.

These occupations vary from being intensely individual, for example shepherding, to the intensely social, for example harvesting of olives, which is carried out in family groups and is a highlight of the year for many, with its combination of hard work, singing and *kalabouri* (jokes and banter). Husband and wife traditionally worked together on their land, while today many farmers employ foreign labourers. Family and friendship networks are maintained through regular supplies of freshly slaughtered lamb and other produce. *Xorta* that is gathered is often shared. Men hunt together, while the *pournaria* brought to the town for carnival enables an all-night bonfire and party attended by the whole town.

To spiti (home)

Traditionally land and home are intricately interrelated in farming communities (Giddens, 1984). The oldest houses in this town are built with storerooms on the ground floor for animals, grain and farming supplies, while the family home is on the first floor. Many new homes continue to be built in this style and although animals are no longer kept within the town, farming machinery and supplies are often kept under or next door to the home, or the ground floor used for an office or shop.

The house is the location of a variety of occupations. The household tasks and care of children and elderly relatives are considered the responsibility of the *noikokura* (housewoman). The *noikokuris* (houseman) is responsible for providing the necessary income or raw materials to enable his wife to look after the family, while he also undertakes repairs and community-based occupations such as heavy shopping or paying bills. Together the couple ensure the quality of the *noikokurio* (the household), a central element in Greek daily life (Salamone and Stanton, 1986). Extended family members and neighbours may help, when necessary, with heavy or particularly tiring occupations – usually men helping men and women helping women. For all family members the house is a place for rest and restorative occupations. For women it is also the place where they meet their female neighbours and relatives, who may drop by in the late morning or early evening for a coffee and a chat.

Occupations in the house, therefore, also serve a variety of purposes. Primarily they transform the house into a home (Rowles, 2008); they maintain the *noikokurio* and sustain the family, practically, emotionally and symbolically. The home is a place for rest and sleep but also for maintaining relationships with extended family and neighbours, particularly for women, on a daily basis. On special occasions, the house becomes the centre for celebration. For example when a family member has their name day (Saint's day), the house is opened and all pass by to wish the person well. Food and wine is offered and dancing and singing may go on until early morning.

Oi plateies (the squares)

The three public squares, surrounded by *kafeneion* and *taverns,* are the third important location of daily life in the town, providing the focal point for most social activities, as in other Greek towns (Friedl, 1962). Many adults, particularly the men, will spend part of each day in one of the squares, perhaps for the first coffee of the morning or a last drink at night. People usually sit with their *parea* (companions) and most *pareas* have their own *steki* (favourite haunt).

As well as these regular occupations, the lower square, in particular, is used throughout the year for festivals and celebrations and has space for 2000 to 3000 people. Carnival, Independence Day celebrations and occasional cultural events with traditional songs and dancing are organized by the municipality and the Women's and Folklore Associations. These involve a considerable amount of preparation as men build stalls or put up a stage, put up loudspeakers or cut *pournaria* from the fields for the bonfire. Women cook food that will be offered to all participants and passers by. The intense work in preparing for these events is followed by several hours of dancing, music, eating and drinking, with *kefi* (intense heightened emotion), enabling people to *ksespasoun* (burst or break out), a perceived necessary release from the pressures and tensions of daily life.

Occupations in the square therefore have a variety of purposes. For men, in particular, being in the square would seem to be an essential part of their lives, an embodiment of their place in the town. Through their daily presence, through seeing others and being seen, they maintain their membership in the community (Cowan, 1990). Going to the *kafeneion* is a physically relaxing occupation, a time for winding down and coming in tune with oneself. It is also a time to learn all the news and plans of the other men, to discuss local and national politics, to create alliances and partnerships, and to arrange business deals. The *kafeneion* thereby plays an important role in the maintenance and development of male social relationships (Cowan, 1991; Papataxiarchis, 2006).

Traditionally the *kafeneion* was the site of sexual regionalization (Giddens, 1984) having been a strictly male institution. Although there is no longer a taboo against women, they continue to use the square and the *kafeneion* in a different way from the men. They enjoy going to the square to 'go out', irregularly, as a special event, to relax and meet their friends.

Finally the public celebrations and events held mainly in the lower square, serve to re-establish the bonds of community and a common identity as inhabitants of Melissa. They are also important in providing a break from the daily routines, by requiring a change in occupations, temporal rhythms and the way places are used.

Magazia kai ipiresies (shops, businesses and public services)

The commercial shops, businesses and public services are primarily a location where a customer goes to buy a service or item, or to arrange a particular administrative procedure. Alongside this, in a town where most inhabitants are interrelated or known to each other, these places also provide opportunities for social interaction. Therefore, apart from those occupations directly related to their function, occupations taking place include popping in (or out) to greet an acquaintance, sitting and having coffee or a drink with them, or just chatting. Shopkeepers may also spend a considerable amount of time alone in their businesses with very few customers. Occupations related to these locations may also be carried out in other places, for example a shopkeeper may be asked to order a particular pair of work boots over a coffee in the square in the evening.

For shop owners and employees the primary purpose of occupations in these locales is economic, to gain an income. A secondary but equally important purpose is the maintenance of a public role in community life and in their social networks.

Independence and interdependence

Greece has been described as a society with collectivistic features, particularly in its more rural regions (Triandis, 1989; Hofstede and Hofstede, 2005). The places of the town and the temporal rhythms can be seen to have emerged from and to support an intertwining of independence and interdependence in the ways in which people organize and undertake their occupations.

In this community, as already mentioned, the majority of people are landowners and self-employed. Farmers, although owning tracts of land many kilometres from the town, have not built homes on their land, but instead within the town. They built stone barns close to their fields where they kept their tools, but also where the family would live at harvesting time, and these have also been built close to others, forming two small hamlets, one north and one south of the town.

Organization of occupations on the land has traditionally been a combination of the demands of the particular season or crop and the personal preference and needs of the individual and family. For example some farmers are seen to work harder than others; certain families keep sheep and goats, other do not; some men cut their own firewood, others buy it; farming equipment may be shared within family groups. However, a growing financial interdependence with the state and with the European Union is evident. From 1982 the European Common Agricultural Policy (CAP) provided considerable financial support, with a significant increase in the production of certain crops (Baltas, 2010). Recent CAP policy changes for the 2007 to 2013 period have aimed to discourage such intensive farming with direct subsidies to farmers, focusing on quality and rural development (Euromed sustainable connections, 2008), increasing the economic dependency of the local farmers. The Greek government is strongly supporting investments by farmers in renewable energy schemes, particularly solar panel systems on their land, with favourable, guaranteed return on investment for twenty years. Thus a long-lasting financial interdependence between state and land owner is being maintained.

The inter-relationship between the land and ancestors is very deep for some inhabitants, affecting the occupations they choose to undertake. Some families have been land owners for generations, farming the same land as ancestors named as local *arxontes* (lords) from the time when Greece formed part of the Ottoman empire (Enisleidi, 1978). Some people working in public services continue to keep sheep and goats in memory of and in respect for their fathers. This is comparable to women's descriptions of the deep meaning linked to cooking for their families (Primeau, 1996b). Identity is closely linked both to the town and to one's family name, and this creates responsibilities and expectations for behaviour. People's memories, stories and shared histories around places, including feuds, sales and dowries, create an additional focus to the occupations of the present, as past debts and favours are taken into account in today's negotiations.

Most inhabitants also own their own homes, and women, who have the main responsibility for running the home, have considerable independence in how they do this. However the son who inherits the *patriko* (family home), usually also takes responsibility for the ongoing care of the parents. The daughter-in-law, who frequently is a *kseni nifi* (foreign bride/wife – from other villages), therefore faces particular demands for sharing household tasks and responsibilities with her mother in law, into whose house she has moved, and with other female relatives of her husband. In other cases, families will live in close proximity, on different floors of the same house or within a short walking distance of each other. Young people living in the village will usually continue to live at home until they marry. On marrying, and particularly with the birth of grandchildren, the young couple will continue to receive considerable practical support from the grandparents, which will be returned as the grandparents' needs increase, arrangements practically facilitated by the physical proximity of homes.

Interdependence is also illustrated in the particular importance given to the *geitonia* (the neighbourhood). The *geitonia* consists of the five or six homes in the immediate vicinity of one's house. Women talk to their neighbours across the balconies of their homes, meet for coffee in each other's homes, help each other with heavy household tasks and share food. Men cook the Easter lamb, together with the *geitonia*, in one pit in the street between the houses. Not quite family, neighbours are, however, an essential resource and support, and may provide a relief from more demanding family relationships. As the population of the town declines and new houses are built on the lower levels of the town, several *geitonies* have only one or two elderly people living in them, isolated and fearful now that their *geitonia* is almost deserted.

Shopkeepers also maintain an intricate network of obligations with the wider community. Commonly they have chosen the type of shop they will open, or have retained their father's shop, and are responsible for its day-to-day running. However, they develop their trade, including not only the general items but also the specific items they sell, in response to the immediate needs of the community, vulnerable to the increasing competition from the nearby large towns. They are also vulnerable to their personal and family characterization by the other families within the town, who are aware of, and use, their power to promote and support a local business, or to fail to support it. However, in turn, customers are also careful of their obligations, shopping from relatives or neighbours, or consistently from a certain supplier, from whom in return they expect good service. Such interdependence is also characteristic of the occupations of the *kafeneion, taverna* and bar owners, whose opening and closing times depend on the customers rather than institutionalized regulations, and who also display flexibility in the spatial arrangements of their business according to customers' wishes. The importance of mutual obligations is evident in the commonly heard description of someone, that *tous exo ipoxreosi* (I am obliged/indebted to them); a debt that should be repaid according to the value prescribed to it.

Public and private places

Public and private places can refer to the ownership of the place but also frequently discussed in the literature is the idea of front and back regions, originally discussed by Goffman (1959). Referring to the position of the body in encounters, the front, the public, is where ritualized public behaviour occurs and where supervisory power is present, and the back is where one can speak one's mind and engage in more regressive behaviour (Tuan, 1977; Giddens, 1984). In this town, with its extensive kinship-based social networks and publicly owned spaces, the boundaries between public and private display flexibility.

The majority of inhabitants, while often living as a nuclear family, are nevertheless part of an extended network of *soi* (relations). Special rights and obligations exist with *soi*, which are extended to *koumparoi* (best man/woman, often also godparent to one's child). Practically, these relationships permit almost free access to one's home, advice about and involvement with day-to-day occupations and participation in major decision-making and family celebrations. This network demands an ongoing balance of obligations and debts and flow of information, which provide not only social capital (Coleman, 1988) but also a good deal of intimate knowledge of a wide group of fellow citizens (relations).

Regarding the public spaces, for example the squares, these are not privately owned but belong to the municipality and by extension the inhabitants. Inhabitants perceive themselves to have a right to be involved in the decision-making, if not the actual practice, regarding the way these public spaces will be used and developed. A similar close relationship exists with one's *steki*, which may be a café that one has sat in with one's *parea,* once or twice a day for over 30 years.

Therefore, in this town where the majority of the inhabitants can trace a family relationship with each other and families have lived for generations, there is an intimate knowledge of the daily lives of many others, of the ways of the town, its activities and services. Many inhabitants therefore experience as back regions, as places where they can be themselves, not only their own home but also those of family members, together with the squares, *kafeneion* and other public locales. However, at the same time, they are visible with high levels of surveillance of their occupations (Giddens, 1984), even within their own homes. This conflict between the private and the public is evident in the practice of, and complaints around, gossiping.

Temporal rhythms

Time is multiple and heterogeneous, varying between individuals, societies and spaces (Dodgshon, 2008). In Melissa, various forms of time influence daily occupations: seasonal, biological, institutional and social, including the common sense of when certain events should occur in the lifecycle and the rhythm of daily routines (Bash, 2000; Mills, 2000). The various forms of time are nested within each other and draw meaning from each other (Bender, 2002).

The cyclical rhythms of nature influence the working patterns of farmers and others who use the land. Daylight, seasonal weather conditions, growing seasons and rates, all affect when and for how long certain occupations may take place. This both enables and demands flexibility in occupations throughout the year. Shepherds are required to follow a more rigid daily and seasonal pattern, as herds need milking twice each day and are herded daily through the fields of the valley. The changing seasons also affect when occupations take place for all the population. For example, the heat of summer days leads to night time becoming a time for occupations, particularly socializing and play. Poor weather, snow and rain, keep many people indoors – also due, in part, to the absence of covered shopping streets and malls and the steep inclines of the streets.

Other important rhythms are biological, circadian rhythms, which have led to the ongoing tradition of the mid-afternoon rest (Green, 2008). Between 15.00 and 17.30 is *mesimeri* (middle day), almost a nontime, when it is illegal to disturb the public peace and many people will rest. In the full heat of summer, this time may be extended, while farmers and shepherds working far from the town will rest in shade. The underlying temporal synchronies, and in particular the physical pace of movement (Larson and Zemke, 2003) is slow; people take their time and rarely hurry. Biological rhythms, as in a sense of what the body needs, are carefully monitored. People place much importance on avoiding *agxos* (anxiety), which can cause people to work too hard physically or be too upset emotionally, leading to health problems. Although people may work very hard, they say that they are careful to do this within their body's capacities.

The cyclical rhythms of nature have been incorporated in the linear rhythms of the educational and administrative institutions (Lefebvre, 1992/2004). Working hours for public service employees are 07.00 or 07.30 to 15.00, and schools start at 08.00, finishing at the latest at 14.00. Shops and offices also follow these opening times but open again in the *apoyevma* (aftermeal/afternoon) – that is from approximately 17.30 to 20.00 except for Monday and Saturday. These institutional times are those most rigidly kept, although even these may be overridden by social rhythms.

Social rhythms are important and may take priority over the other temporal forms. For example, one may celebrate one's name day with a day off work (a semi-official holiday for public servants). Births and deaths will lead to the closure of an office or shop for one or more days. Strikes and poor weather will usually close public services and schools at least once each year.

The self–employed, whether professionals with offices or shop keepers, while largely complying with official opening times will, from time to time and dependent on other obligations, open later, close earlier and put up 'back soon' signs during the course of the day. The opening hours of *tavernes*, bars and *kafeneion* respond to the flexible needs of the inhabitants and will usually serve throughout the day, closing when the last customer leaves at night.

Social rhythms also illustrate considerable flexibility; school classes may finish early and children may hang out before going home, and men may drop by for a quick drink on the way home for work. Social time places the midday meal between 14.00 and 15.00 but it can be flexible. The type of meals prepared, which rarely need to be 'eaten immediately', enables this flexibility. In addition, food is usually cooked in quantity to ensure sufficient for the unexpected visitor. Appointments are often flexible, for example, meeting for a coffee in the afternoon will take place between six and eight, an exact time is neither made nor expected. Finally, the institutional temporal rhythms of the Church take priority for all inhabitants at certain times of the year, for example Easter, Christmas and saints' day celebrations, while many follow its timetable regarding weekly and special periods of *nisteia* (fasting).

Spatio-temporal rhythms

The 'Time-Geography' work of Hägerstrand and his colleagues illustrates the importance of the boundaries limiting behaviour across time and space – boundaries set by the physical context interacting with the capabilities of the individual within a certain time budget (Giddens, 1984; Hallin, 1991; Dodgshon, 2008). In this town, the physical boundaries of most occupations, the principal locations, are within about 20 minutes walking distance of each other (apart from the land). Many people live above or close to their work place and children live close to their schools and afterschool occupations. The absence of violent crime and people's familiarity with both the places and the people of the town also facilitate movement through the town.

Therefore people can quickly and easily (and independently, even in the case of school-age children) traverse the town, and this is regarded as a key feature of quality of life in the town. The short travelling times enable people to 'pop out' of their workplaces to attend to other occupations. Some women go home to put on the lunch, to check on a sick child or elderly relative, or to go to the street market before work. Other people go to pay a bill or post a letter, and if a shop is closed the customer will return later presuming that the shopkeeper is out for a short time. The short travelling times and the high presence availability – that is the close physical proximity – of the inhabitants to each other (Giddens, 1984), also facilitate ongoing social relationships as people drop in on relatives' homes or the *kafeneion* or pass each other in the street.

Discussion

Emerging from this traditional farming community with a large percentage of autonomous self-employed and a largely stable, small population of interrelated families, daily occupations have a flowing quality as people move recursively through the various locations and within an interlinking network of temporal frameworks and social relationships.

In this context, the difficulties of categorizing the purpose and nature of occupations in ways commonly found in the literature, such as for work and leisure, are apparent. The dichotomy of work and leisure is generally regarded as having emerged as a result of industrialization (Giddens, 1984; Lefebvre, 1958/2008; Carrasco and Mayordomo, 2005). This led to work taking place in specific places for a specific length of time, usually regulated by the employer and involving the payment of a salary (Primeau, 1996a). Leisure, defined as an activity freely chosen and with value or positive outcomes to the individual (Neumayer and Wilding, 2005) is difficult to identify as a separate, bounded occupation.

Institutionally organized, serious leisure occupations (Suto, 1998; Stebbins, 2004) or hobbies for adults are restricted to the folk-dancing group and choir. Some people cycle, walk, or ski, for example, but at the time and in the place that suits the individual and the *parea,* so there has not been the routinization (Giddens, 1984) of these practices that may lead to the emergence of related social institutions (for example, the rambling groups in the United Kingdom). The absence of theatres, cinemas and sports centres with prebookable facilities has enabled an ongoing flexibility to temporal rhythms. Opportunities for relaxation and meeting friends, taking place in the public spaces of the town, are available at almost any time and with a flexible time frame.

There are specific temporal frameworks for occupations but these frequently do not require tight temporal coordination (Larson and Zemke, 2003) between participants. This temporal 'looseness' enables and is maintained by the performance of occupations according to the subjective experience of the person, the occupation's form, and the social context. Satisfactory completion of a previous occupation may require one to be 'late' for the next. Additionally frequent changes of, or breaks in, the routine across the days and weeks are enjoyed and anticipated.

Attitudes to time are also significant. Time has not come to be seen as money, as a commodity to be wasted or spent sensibly, in the way described in industrialized nations (Carrasco and Mayordomo, 2005). Many people, when required, work extended hours, beyond the prescribed eight hours of employment; farmers may work throughout the night in the summer and the owners of the *kafeneion* and *tavernes* work 364 days of the year. However, such intensive working times are seen as a necessity and there is an ongoing awareness of the need to avoid *agxos* (anxiety) and 'doing too much'. Time is associated with the duration of life and with the maintenance of friendships and so as something not to be wasted in a broad sense. Also important and sought after is time to enjoy oneself and to relax.

The way work is enfolded (Bateson, 1996) into other occupations, particularly social occupations, is also evident. For example, a business deal is completed over ouzo in the square, a friend drops into the office for a chat and a woman pops home from her shop to put on the lunch. In the absence of fixed working hours and breaks and preset production targets, people have greater flexibility to work at their own pace or in accordance with the demands of the job, a relational construction of temporal events (Dodgshon, 2008), rather than clock regulated.

Although not specifically discussed here, also important to this emergent, flexible, flowing of occupation are other factors. For example, it is unusual to find self-identification with a particular occupation (job) as a lifetime career (O'Halloran and Innes, 2005), and people retire easily as they maintain their central social identity and occupations. One may be asked 'whose are you?' referring to one's kinship line, rather than 'what do you do?' illustrating the centrality of social identity.

Some of the beliefs and values around daily life are also important. Many people support the idea of being *metrimenos* (moderate, prudent), to not overdo things (physically or emotionally), which requires moments for rest and relaxation. This concept is also present in the need to avoid *agxos*, previously discussed. It is believed that, overall, life is largely in the hands of God. Plans for the future are always expressed together with the phrase 'God willing'. Working hard, providing for one's family, taking care of one's children are all important and believed to be within one's own responsibility but beyond that it is difficult to know what '*h moira*' (fate) will bring. The compulsive drive towards new experiences and activities which Abraham's (1986) described to be characteristic of Western societies, is not evident.

Conclusion

This discussion has focused on the spatio-temporal framework within which occupation emerges in this Greek town, providing an alternative viewpoint to studies that focus on the individual. The importance of understanding occupation as a complex phenomenon emerging within specific contexts, connected to the community (Whiteford *et al.*, 2005), was emphasized.

The spatio-temporal organization of the town supports flexible and fluid occupational boundaries (Zemke, 2004) between productive and leisure occupations and between concepts such as independence and interdependence, the private and the public. The characteristics of family run shops and businesses, the nature of agricultural occupations, combined with the importance of family life, and an awareness of one's own physical and mental needs, lead to occupations emerging as an ongoing flow without fixed and static boundaries in time and space. Lives are composed as the elements are combined and harmonized (Bateson, 1996).

Spatial, temporal and social structures can be seen to be in a dialectical relationship with the individual, from within which daily occupation emerges. Occupation is indivisible from the person and their context as the individual engages in the world through their occupations in an ongoing, intricately constructed performance.

References

Abrahams, R. D. (1986) Ordinary and extraordinary experience. In V. W. Turner, E. Bruner (eds) *An Anthropology of Experience*. Chicago: University of Illinois Press, pp. 45–72.

Baltas, N. (2010) *The Convergence of Agricultural Policy of Greece towards the Common Agricultural Policy: Lessons for New EU member States*. Paper presented at the Workshop 'Public administration in the Balkans – from Weberian bureaucracy to new public management', www.balcannet.eu/papers_grecia/Baltas_Nicholas.pdf.

Bash, H. H. (2000) A sense of time: Temporality and historicity in sociological inquiry. *Time & Society* 9 (2/3) 187–204.

Bateson, M. C. (1996) Enfolded activity and the concept of occupation. In R. Zemke, F. Clark (eds), *Occupational Science. The Evolving Discipline*. Philadelphia, PA, F. A. Davis Company, pp. 5–12.

Bender, B. (2002) Time and landscape. *Current Anthropology* 43 (Suppl.) S103–S112.

Carrasco, C., Mayordomo, M. (2005) Beyond employment. Working time and living time. *Time and Society* 14 (2/3) 231–259.

Christiansen, C. H. (1994) Classification and study in occupation. A review and discussion of taxonomies. *Journal of Occupational Science: Australia* 1(3), 3–20.

Coleman, J. S. (1988) Social capital in the creation of human capital. *American Journal of Sociology* 94, S95–S120.

Cowan, J. K. (1990) *Dance and the Body Politic in Northern Greece*. Princeton, NJ, Princeton.

Cowan, J. K. (1991) Going out for coffee? In P. Loizos, E. Papataxiarchis (eds) *Contested Identities. Gender and Kinship in Modern Greece*. Princeton, NJ, Princeton University Press, pp. 180–202.

Crabtree, A. (2000) Remarks on the social organisation of space and place. *Journal of Mundane Behaviour* 1(1), 25–44.

Dear, M. (1988) The postmodern challenge: reconstructing human geography. *Transactions of the Institute of British Geographers* 13(3), 262–274.

Dodgshon, R., A. (2008) Geography's place in time. *Geografiska Annaler Series B*, 90(1), 1–15.

Enisleidi, C. (1978) *H A. (To polisma kai i peri ton Parnason xora)* (in Greek) Athina, Ellenikos Oreivatikos Sullogos A.

Euromed Sustainable Connections (2008) 2.1 *EU Agricultural Policy Analysis*, www.awish-hellas.org/images/2.1-%20EU%20agric%20policy%20analysis.pdf accessed 3 May 2011.

Frank, G., Zemke, R. (2008) Occupational therapy foundations for political engagement and social transformation. In N. Pollard, D. Sakellariou, F. Kronenberg (eds) *A Political Practice of Occupational Therapy*. Edinburgh, Churchill Livingstone Elsevier, pp. 111–136.

Friedl, E. (1962) *Vasilika. A Village in Modern Greece*. New York, Holt, Rinehart & Winston.

Giddens, A. (1984) *The Constitution of Society*. Cambridge, Polity Press.

Goffman, E. (1959) *The Presentation of Self in Everyday Life*. London, Penguin Books.

Green, A. (2008) Sleep, occupation and the passage of time. *British Journal of Occupational Therapy* 71(8), 339–347.

Hallin, P. O. (1991) New paths for Time-Geography? *Geografiska Annaler. Series B, Human Geography* 73(3), 199–207.

Hamilton, T. B. (2011) Occupations and places. In C. Christiansen, E. Townsend (eds), *Introduction to Occupation. The Art and Science of Living*, 2nd edn, Upper Saddle River, NJ, Pearson, pp. 251–279.

Hofstede, G., Hofstede, G. J. (2005) *Cultures and Organizations. Software of the Mind*. New York, McGraw-Hill.

Hudson, M. J., Aoyama, M., Diab, M. C., Aoyama, H. (2011) The South Tyrol as occupationscape: occupation, landscape, and ethnicity in a European border zone. *Journal of Occupational Science* 18(1), 21–35.

Kaiser, T. (2008) Social and ritual activity in and out of place: the 'negotiation of locality' in a Sudanese refugee settlement. *Mobilities* 3(3), 375–395.

Kantartzis, S., Molineux, M. (2011) The influence of Western society's construction of a healthy daily life on the conceptualisation of occupation. *Journal of Occupational Science* 18(1), 62–80.

Larson, E., Zemke, R. (2003) Shaping the temporal patterns of our lives: the social coordination of occupation. *Journal of Occupational Science* 10(2), 80–89.

Lefebvre, H. (1958 /2008) *Critique of Everyday Life*. Volume I (J. Moore trans.) London, Verso.

Lefebvre, H. (1981/2008) *Critique of Everyday Life*, Volume 3 (G. Elliott, trans.) London, Verso.

Lefebvre, H. (1991) *The Production of Space* (D. Nicholson-Smith, trans.) Oxford, Blackwell.

Lefebvre, H. (1992/2004) *Rythmanalysis: Space, Time and Everyday Life*. London, Continuum.

Mills, M. (2000) Providing space for time: The impact of temporality on life course research. Time & Society 9(1), 91–127.

Molineux, M. (2010) The nature of occupation. In M. Curtin, M. Molineux, J. Supyk (eds) *Occupational Therapy and Physical Dysfunction: Enabling Occupation*, 6th edn. Edinburgh, Elsevier, pp. 17–26.

Neumayer, B., Wilding, C. (2005) Leisure as commodity. In G. Whiteford, V. Wright-St Clair (eds) *Occupation and Practice in Context*. Sydney, Elsevier Churchill Livingstone, pp. 317–331.

O'Halloran, D., Innes, E. (2005) Understanding work in society. In G. Whiteford, V. Wright-St Clair (eds) *Occupation and Practice in Context*. Sydney: Elsevier Churchill Livingstone, pp. 299–316.

Panepistimio Thessalias. (2009) *Epixeirisiako programma, Dimou A. 2007–2010*. Volos: Panepistimio Thessalias.

Papataxiarchis, E. (2006) O kosmos tou kafeneiou. Tautotita kai antallagi ston andriko sumposiasmo. In E. Papataxiarchis, T. Paradellis (eds), *Tautotites kai fulo sti sugxroni Ellada*, 3rd edn. Athina, Aleksandreia, pp. 209–250.

Pred, A. (1984) Place as historically contingent process: Structuration and the time-geography of becoming places. *Annals of the Association of American Geographers*, 74(2), 279–297.

Primeau, L. (1996a) Work and leisure: transcending the dichotomy. *American Journal of Occupational Therapy*, 50(7), 569–577.

Primeau, L. (1996b) Work versus nonwork: the case of household work. In R. C. Zemke, F. (ed.), *Occupational Science: The Evolving Discipline*. Philadelphia, PA, F. A. Davis Company, pp. 57–70.

Rowles, G. (2008) Place in occupational science: a life course perspective on the role of environmental context in the quest for meaning. *Journal of Occupational Science* 15(3), 127–135.

Salamone, S. D., Stanton, J. B. (1986) Introducing the Nikokyra: ideality and reality in social process. In J. Dubisch (ed.) *Gender and Power in Rural Greece*. Princeton, NJ, Princeton University Press, pp. 97–120.

Soja, E. W. (1989) *Postmodern Geographies: The Reassertion of Space in Critical Social Theory*. London, Verso.

Stebbins, R. A. (2004) *Erasing the Line between Work and Leisure in North America*. Paper presented at the 'Leisure and liberty in North America' conference, http://people.ucalgary.ca/~stebbins/leisurelibertyinnpap.pdf, accessed 23 December 2011.

Suto, M. (1998) Leisure in occupational therapy. *Canadian Journal of Occupational Therapy* 65(5), 271–278.

Townsend, E., Stone, S. D., Angelucci, T., Howey, M., Johnston, D., Lawlor, S. (2009) Linking occupation and place in community health. *Journal of Occupational Science* 16(1), 50–55.

Triandis, H. C. (1989) The self and social behaviour in differing cultural contexts. *Psychological Review* 96(3), 506–520.

Tuan, Y.-F. (1977) *Space and Place: The Perspective of Experience*. Minneapolis, MN: University of Minnesota Press.

Whiteford, G., Klomp, N., Wright-St. Clair, V. (2005) Complexity theory: understanding occupation, practice and context. In G. Whiteford, V. Wright-St. Clair (eds), *Occupation and Practice in Context*. Sydney, Elsevier Churchill Livingstone.

Wilcock, A. (2006) *An Occupational Perspective of Health*. Thorofare, Slack Incorporated.

Zemke, R. (2004) The 2004 Eleanor Clarke Slagle lecture – time, space, and the kaleidoscopes of occupation. *American Journal of Occupational Therapy* 58(6), 608–620.

9 Indigenous Ainu Occupational Identities and the Natural Environment in Hokkaido

Mami Aoyama[1]

Modernity has brought convenience and an abundance of commodities as a result of unprecedented development achieved by the use of fossil fuels and resulting economic efficiency. The same system has, however, weakened identities and increased stress due to changes in the length, location, organization and form of work, weakened communities due to hyperindividualism, brought about environmental destruction on a global level, led to a crisis in the sustainability of life forms and human societies, and reduced human wellbeing. Rebuilding community-based cultures has recently been proposed as a solution to these problems of modernity and as a way to achieve sustainable societies as well as human health and wellbeing (McKibben, 2007).

Occupational science and occupational therapy aim to support the occupational dimensions of human health and wellbeing and to this end have developed growing research on the meanings of occupation, on occupational potential, on occupation and place, on occupational identities and on transactional approaches to occupation. It is now recognized that the performance of meaningful occupations is closely connected to an individual's health and wellbeing (Wilcock, 1998, 2006). Inability to perform meaningful occupations, in contrast, has an adverse effect on health but it is becoming increasingly accepted that such inability is not simply an individual problem but also has significant social causes. In 1986, the Ottawa Charter for Health Promotion proposed eight prerequisites for health: 'peace, shelter, education, food, income, a stable eco-system, sustainable resources, social justice and equity' (World Health Organization, 1986). The Public Health Agency of Canada similarly lists 12 key determinants of health: income and social status, social support networks, education and literacy, employment/working conditions, social environments, physical environments, personal health practices and coping skills, healthy child development, biology and genetic endowment,

[1] Translated by Mark Hudson.

Politics of Occupation-Centred Practice: Reflections on Occupational Engagement across Cultures, First Edition. Edited by Nick Pollard and Dikaios Sakellariou.

health services, gender and culture (Public Health Agency of Canada, 2010). Reflecting these changing social views of health, research on the social determinants of occupation and health has been increasing in occupational science and occupational therapy.

At the same time there have been changing views of how humans relate to the natural environment. The fourth report of the Intergovernmental Panel on Climate Change (IPCC) concluded that it is 'very likely' (meaning a 90–99% probability) that current global warming is caused by anthropogenic greenhouse gas concentrations, i.e., by human activity (Solomon *et al.*, 2007). The Millennium Ecosystem Assessment (2005) conducted for the United Nations has discussed the connections between ecosystems services and health and wellbeing and between human activity and declining biodiversity. In recent years, occupational science and occupational therapy have begun to stress the importance of research linking the natural environment, occupation and health and the necessity of approaches to environmental change using occupational dimensions (Wilcock, 1998, 2010; Hudson and Aoyama, 2008; Ikiugu, 2008; Aoyama, 2009; Aoyama *et al.*, in press). There are, however, still few studies that examine concrete connections between occupation and the natural environment (Aoyama and Hudson, 2005; Blakeney and Marshall, 2009).

In order to further our understanding of the relationships between the natural environment, occupation and health, in previous research the author has analysed and compared occupations of the Okhotsk culture of cold-temperate Hokkaido (ca. AD 550–1200) and the Late Prehistoric culture of the subtropical Sakishima Islands (ca. 500 BC–AD 1200) (Aoyama and Hudson 2005, 2009). I have also investigated the traditional occupations and worldview of Ainu hunter-gatherers (Aoyama, 2011). Building on the results of this Ainu research, in this chapter I describe the effects of social changes on Ainu health and occupations.

Ainu are an indigenous people who traditionally lived in Hokkaido and the surrounding regions of northern Honshu, Sakhalin and the Kuril Islands (Figure 9.1). Until the late nineteenth century, hunter-gathering formed the main subsistence base of Ainu people, although some Ainu were also involved in long-distance trading with Japan and the Amur region (Hudson, in press). 'Subsistence' here refers to the many occupations that comprised Ainu lifeways. A historically recognizable Ainu culture began in the medieval era around the twelfth century AD, when a rich culture with a separate Ainu language was developed as a result of complex interactions between Japan and Northeast Asia (Hudson, 1999a). During the early modern Tokugawa period (1600–1868), Japan was ruled by military leaders known as *shōgun*, although power was held in a delicate balance with the great barons of regional feudal domains. In this period Ainu gradually came under the control of the Matsumae domain that ruled part of the southern end of Hokkaido. From the mid-nineteenth century, Ainu territories were directly colonized by Japan and Russia. In Hokkaido, Japanese assimilation policies resulted in laws that banned many aspects of Ainu culture and occupation, forcing huge occupational transformations in the name of modernization. In this chapter I

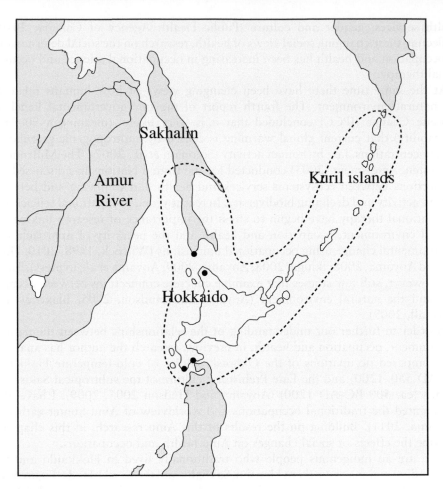

Figure 9.1 Map of Hokkaido and surrounding regions. Dotted line shows main area of Ainu settlement.

divide Ainu history into two periods, the first prior to the Tokugawa era when Ainu possessed a more or less autonomous life as hunter-gatherers and the second from the Tokugawa period onwards when Ainu came under the growing influence of the Japanese state. The first part of the chapter summarizes the Ainu worldview and traditional occupations in the premodern period, while the second part goes on to discuss the occupational changes brought about by outside pressure from the early modern era. The chapter concludes with a discussion of the connections between occupation and the natural environment and presents some suggestions as to how the study of Ainu occupations may aid in developing an occupational dimensions-based approach to current environmental problems.

Ainu Worldview and Traditional Occupations in the Pre-Tokugawa Period: Occupations and Worldview Linked with Nature's Cycles

I begin by describing the traditional Ainu worldview as found in rituals such as the *iyomante* (bear festival) and in *yukar* epic poems and other oral literature. I then analyse Ainu occupations associated with the main subsistence activity of hunter-gathering and discuss connections between Ainu worldview and subsistence occupations.

Ainu worldview

Ainu believed that spirits reside in all things that surround humans, including in animals, plants and tools. Things over which humans had no control were deified as *kamuy*. There were nature *kamuy* of fire, water and the sun, animal *kamuy* such as those of bears and owls, tool *kamuy* such as pots and boats, and *kamuy* of the ancestors. These were good spirits that protected humans, bringing food and many other blessings. Furthermore, these *kamuy* were not absolute but possessed the same spiritual existence as humans with whom they were mutually interdependent. Dreaded diseases such as smallpox and famines were also considered as *kamuy*. *Kamuy-nomi* were prayers that Ainu offered to the spirits to give thanks or to ask for protection. These *kamuy-nomi* ranged from ordinary prayers as part of everyday life to special ceremonies such as the *iyomante* or 'bear festival'. The *iyomante* is a ceremony in which bears and other animals were killed and their spirits sent back to the land of the *kamuy*. Ordinary *kamuy-nomi* were performed on a regular basis to the spirits of the house and fire and to the mountain spirits before entering the mountain space. Larger ceremonies such as *iyomante* were conducted by the *kotan* (village community) and were held over several days with people from other communities also being invited.

The author conducted an analysis of the structure, process, objective occupations and occupational meanings for Ainu of *iyomante* based on reports from the Ainu Museum published in 1989, 1990, and 1994, on *Ainu-e* genre paintings, and on published *yukar* tales (Aoyama, 2010). From this process analysis it was shown that these occupations were part of a culture with particular meanings for Ainu that were quite different from the objective, etic interpretations of Ainu occupations. Box 9.1 provides a summary of a *yukar* tale of a bear festival, which demonstrates both the occupational meanings of Ainu bear hunting and the Ainu worldview.

Using this example of the bear ceremony, it can be seen that the Ainu worldview was based on feelings of gratitude respect and fear of the spirits and, at the same time, relations of mutual interdependence between humans and *kamuy* in which both needed each other. On this basis, the Ainu worldview also emphasized symbiosis and reproduction. In a comment on Minamata disease[2] reported in the Record of

---

[2] Minamata disease was the name given to methylmercury poisoning caused by pollution from a factory in Minamata City, Kumamoto Prefecture, Japan in the 1950s to 1960s. The mercury moved up the food chain to fish and then to people that consumed those fish.

BOX 9.1

SUMMARY: 'I am a Mountain God... [I respected my wife, but] one day... I thought to myself:... 'I want to go and visit the god ruling the Lower Heavens...' [While there, one day a crow appeared and said]: '... your wedded wife, decided that she wanted to visit the humans. She left behind your little baby.' [Returning home and] picking up my little baby,... I went outside, intending to go down... to ravage the human village. [Attacked by humans] the God of Aconite Poison came dashing out [and said]: 'The Fire Goddess has sent me to bear this message: "O weighty deity, please come to pay me a peaceable visit"... After sleeping for a while, I [saw] I was sitting on a tree branch,... Underneath me a big old he-bear was lying outstretched.... [The men] began to prepare the he-bear and worshipped him. [The next morning] a large crowd of people came [and] began to skin that bear. When they had finished, [they] went down the mountain bearing the meat on their backs. [In a house at] the center of the village... I... was seated under the sacred window. My wedded wife was already there before me... crowds of young men [and] women [were busy] making dumplings [and] whittling *inaw* (sacred shaved sticks) [to send me off]. I was given [*inaw* and dumplings and] went on my way until I came back to my own home. After... two or three days... my wedded wife, came along after me... loaded down with much wine, many *inaw*, and dumplings too. [Then we invited the gods to a] delightful banquet... Afterward, all of the gods left for home, expressing their thanks... After some time... our dear little child came back from the humans... Once again we invited the gods [to a] peerless feast...' (Translation by Philippi, 1979.)

INTERPRETATION: The bear changes into black clothing (wears fur) to visit the human world. He chooses an honest human who removes the bear's disguise so that he can return to the world of the gods. In thanks he leaves his fur, meat, gall bladder, etc and only his spirit returns to the mountain. Humans are happy to entertain this distinguished god, to receive his gifts, to remove his disguise, and to send off his spirit with many gifts back to the world of the gods. If the humans treat him badly, the bear gets angry and will not come again to the village. The *kamuy* go back to the world of the gods (*kamuy-moshir*) and tell the other gods about the affluent and enjoyable world of the humans (Ainu *moshir*). When the other *kamuy* hear such stories, they also want to visit the land of the Ainu. *Kamuy* who have often visited the Ainu *moshir* and been ceremonially sent back were also thought to gain extra status in the *kamuy-moshir*. The sending back ceremony worked through mutual interaction to maintain good relations between the gods and the Ainu.

the Environment Special Committee, National Diet House of Councillors for 9 November 1994, Ainu elder Shigeru Kayano argued that this feeling of coexistence was much stronger than perhaps most of us living in industrial societies can imagine:

> Minamata disease first made fish sick.... In other words, humans caught Minamata disease by eating fish and shellfish that had been polluted with mercury.... Humans could confirm each other's feelings and made some explanations to each other. But how difficult must have been the feelings of the fish and shellfish who could not talk like humans and could not conduct *charanke* (ritual negotiations).... How many humans really apologized from the heart to the fish? If the fish stood with fists raised facing

humans, I, an Ainu named Shigeru Kayano, would stand together with the fish in anger. (Cited in Matsuna, 2007.)

Until at least the later nineteenth century, most Ainu possessed a worldview that emphasized *kamuy* and co-existence with 'nature' and it can be said that their occupations and lifestyles were based upon this worldview. In the next section, I will describe Ainu occupations of the premodern period.

Traditional Ainu occupations and the occupational cycle

Ainu traditional occupations were intimately connected with place. According to Mashiho Chiri (1984), the *iwor* is the world where the Ainu spirits reside, the places in the mountains or on the sea for hunting and fishing and the places where the materials for daily life (clothes, foods, fuel and building materials) were obtained. Matsuna (2007) saw the *iwor* as the place where the spirits reside and where the hunting and gathering necessary for life was conducted. If the *iwor* was the place of the spirits (*kamuy*), the *kotan* was the place of the human beings (Ainu). Ainu built up to about a dozen houses along rivers or coasts that were resilient to natural disasters to form *kotan* villages. The village was protected by many *kamuy*, including the spirit of the Blakiston's owl, the spirit of the fire, and the spirit of the house. In this way, the *iwor* and *kotan* were strictly differentiated concepts (Matsuna, 2007). For this analysis, I examined published reports of the traditional Ainu occupations of 'subsistence' in the *iwor* and *kotan*. Depending on where they were conducted, 'subsistence' occupations were classified into (1) occupations of the mountains, sea and rivers (*iwor*), (2) occupations of the living place (*kotan*), and (3) occupations that straddled or went beyond the *kotan* and *iwor*. Further classification was based on (1) type of occupation, (2) resources obtained from occupations, (3) tools used in occupations, (4) sexual division of labour of the occupation, (5) raw materials obtained from resources, and (6) products made from raw materials (Table 9.1).

Ainu entered the *iwor* of the mountain, river or sea and obtained animals and plants such as deer, bears, salmon, seals, reeds and bamboo grass as resources. From these resources they acquired raw materials such as meat, furs and bone that they used to produce objects and tools for everyday life such as houses, storehouses, boats, foodstuffs, clothing, fuel, harpoons, arrows, knives, needles, toys and other items for children, and ritual objects.

Based on these results, Figure 9.2 shows the occupational cycle that provided the catalyst for the material cycle in Ainu society. Through this cycle, resources were obtained from the ecosystem and transformed into foods or goods necessary for life or else absorbed by the body. Things that were no longer needed were returned to nature, sometimes in 'sending back' ceremonies that were performed in the hope that these things would once again visit the land of humans. The 'occupational cycle' is defined here as the chain of occupations that provide the mechanism by which resources move through the social-ecological system. 'Occupational cycle processes' (OCP) are clusters of particular occupations by which resources are transformed into the next stage. 'Supplemental occupations' (SO) are those that impact the

Table 9.1 A classification of early modern Ainu occupations related to 'subsistence'.

Occupation and location	Resources	Tools used	Division of labour	Raw materials	Products	Miscellaneous comments
Mountain hunting	Deer, bear, otter, hare, marten, fox, raccoon dog, white tailed eagle, Steller's sea eagle, raven; reindeer and musk deer (Sakhalin only)	Bow, poison arrow, traps, small knife (makiri), large knife	Mainly males	Meat, internal organs, fur, bone, sinew, antler	Food, medicine, clothing (animal furs, bird feathers), shoes, cord, decorations, bone and antler tools	Deer were the most important land animals used for food
Marine hunting	Whales, dolphins, Steller sea lion, sea otter, seals, fur seal, sea lion	Boats, harpoons (kite), fish hooks	Mainly males	Meat, skins, bone, cartilage, fat	Food and oil, clothing (gloves, etc), bone tools (knives, harpoons, fish hooks, etc), materials for boats, fat for lighting and heating	Redistributed (partly used for trade)
Fishing (sea and rivers)	Salmon, trout, char, herring, sardine, cod, flounder, sculpin, smelt, Crucian carp, swordfish, ocean sunfish, turtles	Marek (spear), nets, dogs (for salmon and trout fishing), hooks, weirs	Mainly males	Meat, skins	Food, clothing (fish skins), shoes	Redistributed and stored (partly used for trade). Salmon was the staple
Marine gathering	Abalone, sea urchin, konbu and other seaweeds	Baskets	Males and females	Meat and shell	Food, tools (shell reaping knives, lamps, dishes, etc)	Partly used for trade
Plant collecting	Japanese tree lilac, Manchurian ash, Japanese elm, Katsura tree, nettles, Phragmites grass,	Axes, baskets	Mainly females	Leaves, stems and bulbs, bark, plant fibres, dried grasses	Houses, storage buildings, weirs, boats, wooden tools (handles for knives, containers,	Clothing included work and ceremonial clothes. Embroidery and

Activity	Natural resources	Tools/equipment	Division of labour	Food/medicine	Products
	kaya yew, lilies, nuts, berries, bark, syrup			Food, medicine	bows, traps, combs, musical instruments, toys, ceremonial artefacts, grave markers, etc), clothing (tree bark and plant fibres), foods, flavourings, medicine, decorations, mats, baskets, cradles, roof post twine, rope, nets; other designs were applied. Cotton was imported
Plant cultivation	Foxtail millet, common millet, barnyard grass, turnip, buckwheat, beans, potatoes	Axes, spades, shell reaping knives	Mainly females	Food, medicine	
Processing and storing foods	Salmon, lily bulbs, nuts, cultivated plants	Drying equipment, casks for sake, raised floor storage buildings, baskets	Mainly females		Food (preserved)
Collecting water and firewood	Water for drinking and cooking, firewood for cooking and heating	Baskets			Fuel, drinking water
Trade	Marine products, animal furs, bear gall bladders	Boats	Mainly males		Rice, sake, lacquerware, iron, clothing, ornaments

No shading: occupations of the mountains, seas and rivers (*iwor*)
Light shading: occupations performed in the *kotan* (village)
Dark shading: occupations performed beyond the *iwor* and *kotan*

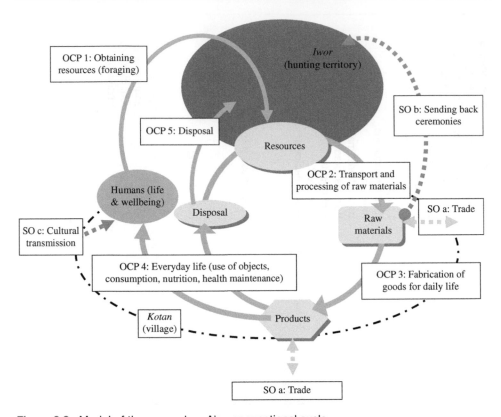

Figure 9.2 Model of the premodern Ainu occupational cycle.

occupational cycle, even though they do not directly contribute to the resource cycle. Five occupational cycle processes and three supplemental occupations were identified in Ainu society.

The occupational cycle processes (OCP) included foraging (OCP 1), which involved travelling to the *iwor* to obtain resources, initial processing (OCP 2), comprising the transport of materials, butchering animals, removing fibres from trees or plants, and so on, final processing and fabrication (OCP 3), including cooking, weaving, basket making, woodworking and building, the practice of daily life (OCP 4), the actual use or consumption of goods, including eating foods, wearing clothes, living in houses, praying with sacred objects, and playing with toys, and finally disposal (OCP 5), the discard of things that had been used in daily life and were no longer needed or serviceable. In addition to these occupations that formed the catalyst to the material cycle, Ainu society was also reproduced through a number of supplemental occupations (SO) including the trade and exchange of goods and materials (SO a), the sending back of spirits to the land of the *kamuy* (SO b), and the transmission of folklore about creation and the lessons of the past (SO c).

Through this occupational cycle, Ainu made the foods, clothing, houses and other necessities for everyday life out of resources obtained from the natural environment and lived through utilizing these foods and objects. The practice of everyday life (OCP 4) served to maintain Ainu health and survival, to store energy, and to provide a source for the next occupational activities. In other words, we can say that the practice of everyday life in premodern Ainu society depended on resources obtained from the natural environment in order to maintain life and health and to create the capability for future occupations.

In Ainu society, winter was called the 'men's season' and summer the 'women's season' (Keira and Keira, 1999), symbolizing a seasonal division of occupations by sex. Occupations were also performed through the cooperative efforts of the *kotan* community. Men were primarily engaged in hunting and trapping, fishing, and the production of tools related to these activities. Women gathered and cultivated plants, processed foods and prepared meals, made clothes, baskets and mats, and cared for children and families. Women would process salmon that men caught in the autumn, putting up the fish by smoking or salting. Religious ceremonies were held by the *kotan* with men making altars and ritual objects and women preparing food and wine. After prayers by male elders, women would perform songs and dances. Gender is important in Ainu society but age is also significant and it is thought that the older one gets the closer one becomes to the spirits. Male elders played an important role during ceremonies while female elders cared for the bear cubs that were thought to be *kamuy*.

When it came time to build a house, other members of the *kotan* cooperated in collecting building materials and in construction. Salmon was a food indispensable to everyday life and a gift from the *kamuy* and, when the time approached for salmon to swim upstream to spawn, the *kotan* community began to observe strict taboos to preserve the water quality of the rivers. Bushes growing along the banks of rivers were quickly removed and, one of the main causes of river pollution, washing clothes in rivers where salmon swim upstream was prohibited. When the salmon arrived, men would refrain from speaking in loud voices near the river (Matsuna, 2007), displaying respect for the spirit of the fish as well as avoiding disturbing those same fish. Traditional Ainu occupations were performed through a division of labour within the household and through the cooperation of the *kotan* community.

Hokkaido is in a cold, temperate zone where winter monsoon winds from Siberia bring heavy snows to the western part of the island. Sea ice blocks the eastern Sea of Okhotsk coastline from January to March. In order to survive in this environment it can be said that Ainu reproduced occupations through which they collaborated with other participants in Ainu society to obtain resources, fabricated various products needed for everyday life, and attempted to maintain their health and wellbeing. However, this chain of occupational performances related to nature was not confined to occupations designed to satisfy needs necessary for survival. Collecting resources (OCP 1) involved not just physical movements but psychological healing from being in nature (cf. Morita *et al.*, 2007), feelings of competitiveness and chance, and aspects of play. These occupations can also be said to have met psychological needs through feelings of social belonging and social ethics derived from cooperative work and role performance as well as from feelings of self-esteem, respect for others, and the sense of achievement from solving problems

(Aoyama, 2011). The occupations involved in initial processing (OCP 2) and final processing and fabrication (OCP 3) can also be argued to have contributed to supporting psychological desires for creativity and self-efficacy (cf. Thompson, 1976). Maslow (1943) proposed that physiological requirements, safety, love/ belonging, esteem and self-actualization comprise a hierarchy of needs. The linked chains of occupational performance directly connected to nature in which premodern Ainu participated can be said to have contributed to all of these needs. In short, the traditional Ainu occupational cycle not only produced foods and objects that were essential to everyday life, but also contributed to the promotion of physical and spiritual health and to occupational satisfaction.

Traditional occupations and worldview

This section first used *yukar* to explain the Ainu worldview of co-existence with *kamuy* – with what we would call 'nature'. An analysis of traditional Ainu occupations was then used to propose a model of the occupational cycle in Ainu society. As well as demonstrating that Ainu livelihoods were dependent on nature, it was argued that participation in the occupational cycle led to occupational satisfaction and contributed to basic survival and to the maintenance of physical and mental health. If we consider this occupational cycle from a different perspective, it can also be said that Ainu possessed the knowledge and technology to make good use of nature. The products used for the practice of everyday life and to maintain life and health (OCP 4) required the knowledge and technology to make objects necessary for daily life (OCP 3), as well as the knowledge and processing technology to prepare raw materials for these objects (OCP 2) and the knowledge and technology of foraging needed to obtain a diverse range of resources (OCP 1). For this reason, Ainu had a rich vocabulary and an extensive body of knowledge relating to humans-in-nature. The *kotan* community can be assumed to have possessed all of the technology and knowledge about nature, processing and fabrication needed for the occupational cycle.

Objects made through the application of knowledge and technology to materials obtained by the *kotan* were made in different ways in different communities, a process that led to the formation of Ainu art as well as to supporting everyday life. Furthermore, Ainu participating in the occupational cycle could physically experience how Ainu life depended on nature, experiences that can be said to have resulted in the development of particular occupations such as giving thanks to the *kamuy* and sending back ceremonies (supplemental occupation a). Through close connections with the natural environment during the occupational cycle, Ainu society came to recognize the laws of that environment, giving birth to a system of knowledge by which the community and individuals understood how best to relate to nature. This system of knowledge was transmitted between the generations by *yukar* and other folklore practices such as the *iyomante* and other *kamuy-nomi* and became what we can call a worldview. This worldview provided models by which Ainu society reproduced itself. The resulting accumulation of occupational experiences related to nature was transformed into rich knowledge and technology as well as into a worldview – elements that can be said to have formed Ainu culture.

The worldview of Canadian Inuit, who are hunter-gatherers like Ainu, is described by Svenson and Lafontaine (1999) as a concentric circle with the creator on the outside surrounding nature, community, family and individuals. This is a worldview based on what we might call 'humans-in-nature'. These hunter-gatherers constructed community norms based on the 'laws' or cycles of their gods and of nature, and families and individuals can be said to have lived their lives guided by these norms. Native Americans such as the Iroquois nation are said to have considered the effects of their actions on seven future generations before making major decisions. This shows that, in order to continue survival with nature over the generations, the performance of community, family and individual occupations that followed the cycles of nature were thought to be necessary by these Native peoples. Through traditional occupations following such cycles of nature in Hokkaido, Ainu also built a rich worldview and Ainu culture continued to develop over a period of more than 600 years prior to colonization. This interaction between nature and occupation can be said to have formed the basis of Ainu culture and identity.

Wilcock (2006) argued that survival and health are made possible by doing, being, belonging, and becoming, a relationship that she expresses by the formula $d + b^3 = sh$. She also proposes that for this relationship to be possible, one has to be free to participate in meaningful occupations and also that eco-sustainable community development is necessary. While limited to the small social unit of the *kotan*, until the early modern era Ainu society followed a worldview as part of the cycles of nature and the members of the society found their roles by participating in the associated occupational cycle and thus maintaining the health and survival of the community in a society that can be said to have preserved occupational justice.

Ainu Occupational Changes from the Early Modern Period: Domination by Japanese Social Norms and Contempt of the Cycles of Nature

In this section, I summarize the history of Ainu occupational changes that resulted from the forced imposition of norms from Japanese society. This Ainu example is used to consider occupational deprivation and occupational injustice resulting from social pressure.

Ainu history and occupational changes from the early modern period

The formation of Ainu society in the twelfth to the thirteenth centuries AD was linked with the expansion of long-distance trade stimulated by the so-called 'medieval economic revolution' in China (Hudson, 1999a,b). This period saw major transformations in the practices of everyday life. The design and construction of Ainu houses changed and imported iron and, later, porcelain vessels replaced local earthenwares. From around the mid-fourteenth century, Japanese settlers began to move into southern Hokkaido (or Ezo as it was then known) and in the fifteenth to early sixteenth centuries Japanese incursions into *iwor* hunting territories began to destroy the economic base of Ainu society. Disputes over taxes for trading ships led to the outbreak of conflict between Ainu and Japanese. As noted above, however, the medieval Ainu were still able to maintain an autonomous lifestyle through free trade and an occupational cycle that followed the cycles of nature. In the early modern Tokugawa period, however, the peripheral border regions were reorganized as parts of the Tokugawa state. The Matsumae domain of southern Hokkaido was given monopolistic control over the Ainu trade. Matsumae cut off free trade and cultural contacts between Ainu and other peoples except for Matsumae retainers. This system was called the trading post fief system (*akinaiba chigyōsei*). Under this system, Ainu became passive participants in trade and gradually lost their economic autonomy, being forced to accept prices and conditions offered by Matsumae. Ainu were forced to supply more and more goods to meet the price increases, thus damaging their resource base. Furthermore, since only chiefs were now allowed to trade, the system increased social divisions in Ainu society. As a result, large regional groupings were formed within Ainu society leading to new conflicts both between Ainu groups and also with the Japanese, most notably during the Shakushain War of 1669.[3]

In the first half of the eighteenth century, Matsumae retainers began to rent trading rights to merchants, giving rise to the contract fishery (*basho ukeoi*) system. In order to pay back these rents, the merchants began to force Ainu to work for wages in fishing stations that were established across Hokkaido. Ainu were forced from their villages into these fishing stations where conditions were terrible and wages meagre. Ainu gradually became wage labourers, building roads and performing other tasks as well as fishing. For this work Ainu were paid about two *ryō* a year, a salary that was much lower than Japanese workers doing similar work who could expect to earn seven or eight *ryō* a year (Howell, 1995; Walker, 2001; Emori, 2007).

The Japanese explorer Takeshirō Matsu'ura left many records of deteriorating conditions in Ainu settlements at this time. One example is the fishing station at Kudō on the Japan Sea coast of Hokkaido. According to Matsu'ura (2002), in the period from 1764 to 1788, the population of this settlement was about 87 people with 13 houses, but by 1821 this had declined to 25 people and only five houses. Ainu were made to work very hard and most males only lived to their 30s or 40s. Old people and children had nothing to eat and no clothes to wear and many died of starvation and cold. Matsu'ura's descriptions reflect harsh conditions even by the standards of the time and Ainu living standards were probably much worse than those of many Japanese people during a time when historians such as Hanley (1997) have argued that population and physical wellbeing were both increasing in Japan.

In 1804 the Hokkaido Ainu population was reported to be 21,697, but by 1854 this had dropped to 15,171. The main causes of this population decline were forced labour, violence, especially toward women by the heads of the fishing stations, forced

---

[3] The largest Ainu uprising in the early modern era, caused by opposition to the injustices of the trading system of the Matsumae domain.

abortions, an increase in the number of unmarried Ainu, and the spread of smallpox, syphilis and other epidemic diseases through contact with Japanese (Yoshida, 2007, 2008). At the same time, Japanese traders and settlers began to damage the natural environments that supported Ainu livelihoods. This destruction can be said to have begun as early as the seventeenth century with the expansion of placer mining for gold in many rivers in Hokkaido. This mining diverted stream flows and deposited sediments that seem to have adversely affected many salmon runs. Both Japanese merchants and Ainu themselves associated this mining with starvation from poor salmon runs (see Walker 2001: 84). By the early eighteenth century, Japanese officials and merchants were noting major declines in deer populations in Hokkaido resulting from overhunting for the trade in deerskins; these declines also frequently led to the starvation of Ainu communities (Walker, 2001: 118–123). For these reasons, Ainu forced into heavy labour in the fishing stations became unable to maintain their own lives and those of their families. At this stage, however, Ainu as a whole still retained their own traditional beliefs and lifestyles.

In the nineteenth century, as Russian expansion began to be perceived as a threat, Japan's Ainu policy changed from one that emphasized the differences of the Ainu people to an assimilation policy that denied Ainu ethnicity. Meanwhile, in 1868 the military control of the Tokugawa shoguns came to an end and the emperor was returned to power in the Meiji Restoration. Japan began to develop a modern, industrial nation-state that followed the Western powers in imperial expansion overseas. In 1869, the Meiji authorities established a colonial government and sent growing numbers of soldiers and settlers to Hokkaido. From 58,467 in 1869, the population of Hokkaido increased to more than 1,738,000 by 1912. The name of the island was changed from Ezo-chi (meaning 'land of the barbarians') to Hokkaido (the 'Northern Sea Circuit') and in 1872 the homeland of the Ainu people was legally erased when Hokkaido was made the territory of Japan. Ainu hunting grounds, the *iwor* where the *kamuy* resided, were subdivided and sold to Japanese immigrants. In this way, Japanese settlers gained private ownership of lands and then proceeded to cut down the forests and make fields, destroying the places that had supported Ainu subsistence. In 1871, Ainu were forced to adopt Japanese-style names and were made citizens of Japan. Following this, in 1878, Ainu were designated 'former aborigines' to distinguish them from the ethnic Japanese. Ainu customs were banned, with violators severely punished. Such bans included those on women's tattoos and men's earrings (1871), bans on deer hunting and the use of traps and poisoned arrows (1876), and bans on salmon fishing (1879). Kayano (1994) relates how his father was arrested for poaching salmon in the early 1930s. A report produced in 1884 by the Banseisha colonial company noted that, removed from their traditional sources of subsistence, famine stalked Ainu who were 'just sitting waiting for death'. Losing both their lands and their traditional occupations, Ainu experienced great hardships in their everyday lives.

The Hokkaido Former Aborigines Protection Law was passed in 1889 with the aim of saving Ainu from the sad plight into which they had fallen. This law, however, ignored traditional Ainu occupational experiences and was designed to assimilate Ainu to Japanese culture and to force them into agriculture. An example of this agriculturalization policy was the forcible movement of large groups of Ainu from Sakhalin to Hokkaido and from the northern Kuril Islands to Shikotan in the south of the Kuril archipelago. These movements aimed to turn Ainu into farmers but the traditional livelihood of these people had been fishing and the Japanese policy resulted in great suffering with almost half of the 841 Ainu who had been brought from Sakhalin dying within just over a decade. Miyajima (1998: 98) comments that, 'The high death rate was the inevitable result of the forced relocation and the changes in daily life that it forced upon the people.' Ainu were forcibly resettled for a range of reasons, including perceived security threats in border zones, but the link with the policy of occupational change, especially agriculturalization, is clear in many cases (Siddle, 1996: 65).

As part of the Former Aborigines Protection Law, schooling for Ainu children was begun, but this schooling was primarily in the so-called 'imperial education' and in Japanese language. As a rule there were separate schools for Ainu and Japanese children and education was promoted based on the discriminatory assumption that Ainu culture was inferior to Japanese culture and that Ainu should be happy to assimilate to Japanese culture. Hirata (2009: 38) notes that

> The increase in Ainu children attending school, from around 9.2% in 1886 to 92.2% some 15 years later in 1910, was not due to the effectiveness of educational policies but to the fact that the increase in *shamo* [Japanese settlers] had destroyed Ainu livelihoods and, for their very survival, Ainu had no choice but to decide to discard their own culture.

Hirata goes on to write that, 'In the following generation of Ainu that were educated by *shamo*, there grew a trend toward "detesting Ainu". In order to dilute Ainu blood, this generation did not hesitate to produce mixed blood children with *shamo*, consciously ceased from teaching the Ainu language and folklore to their children, and themselves extinguished Ainu customs and culture' (Hirata 2009: 38).

Kiyotaka Kuroda, the first director of the Hokkaido colonization office, was typical of most Japanese of the nineteenth century when he described Ainu as retaining 'inferior customs' and 'repugnant practices' in an official report in 1872 (cited in Miyajima, 1998: 77). Concepts of biological race and social Darwinism, introduced from the West, supported the idea that the Ainu were a 'dying race', doomed to extinction in the modern world of Meiji Japan. Siddle (1996: 75) cites a Hokkaido newspaper making the following comment in 1886: 'According to the principle of the survival of the fittest, as civilisation advances superior races succeed while inferior races die out... This can clearly be seen in the case of the Aino [i.e., Ainu], that is to say, the natives.'

Such examples show that Ainu were treated as a 'dying race' doomed to extinction, that their social position was low, and that Ainu culture was dismissed. The performance and transmission of traditional Ainu occupations became difficult and, in the midst of a very harsh situation, Ainu found themselves in a situation where they could not but throw away Ainu culture and assimilate themselves with the Japanese. Some Ainu found this too hard and committed suicide.

The invasion of Japanese society and occupational injustice

In the previous section I summarized the history by which Ainu society was coerced to fit the norms of Japanese society with its values of wealth and power. Seen from an occupational perspective, this is clearly a history in which Ainu occupations were transformed by outside pressure from the Japanese. This occupational transformation was not uniform but can be divided into three phases based on the historical background. The first transformation was the loss of occupational autonomy as a result of changes in the objective and quality of work (occupation). The early modern Ainu continued their traditional occupations but their trading activities were limited by labour in the Japanese trading stations and Ainu livelihoods were transformed from those in which their occupations maintained their own lives to becoming wage labourers. Through this change in the form of labour, Ainu lost their occupational autonomy and their occupations became those coerced by their employers.

The second phase was occupational deprivation resulting from legal prohibitions against traditional occupations. These legal restrictions were the immediate cause of the occupational deprivation but more basic causal factors included forced migrations and removal from the land and environmental destruction due to overhunting, overfishing and unrestrained land development by the growing population of Japanese settlers. Such factors destroyed the lands where Ainu had carried out their traditional occupations of hunting, fishing and gathering.

The final transformation was the coercion – by Japanese who ignored Ainu culture – away from traditional occupations, which held value for Ainu people, into new, unfamiliar occupations, notably agriculture. This change resulted from the state policy of assimilation (which was influenced by foreign relations with Russia and the West) and from educational policies emphasizing the 'survival of the fittest'.

Ainu occupational changes resulting from outside pressure can thus be summarized as follows: (1) loss of occupational autonomy and the coercion of occupations; (2) deprivation of traditional occupations; and (3) coercion of occupations that differed from those having value for Ainu people. The outside pressure forcing these occupational changes included legal measures instituted by the state but the effect of such measures was worsened by land removals, interventions by merchants with their market principles, forced migrations, environmental destruction and discriminatory educational policies.

As a result of these occupational changes forced upon Ainu people by the Japanese, Ainu became destitute. Due also to the spread of epidemic diseases by the Japanese, Ainu health was impaired and there was a dramatic decline in population. Ainu society began to weaken and the *kotan* started to collapse.

Kronenberg and Pollard (2005) use the term 'occupational apartheid' to describe restrictions to occupation that are part of systematic and deliberate political policies based on discriminatory frames of reference such as race, class, gender or disability. Pollard, Kronenberg and Sakellariou (2008: 56) have already mentioned Ainu as an example of occupational apartheid. Townsend and Wilcock (2004) proposed that all people have the right to occupation and that there is occupational injustice when that right is damaged. Through an examination of the history of Ainu occupations, this chapter has shown that the performance of traditional Ainu occupations was damaged by the pressure of the Japanese state and society and that Ainu health and well-being deteriorated to a dangerous condition as a result. It can thus be concluded that the occupational changes experienced by Ainu correspond to what Townsend calls occupational injustice or what Kronenberg and colleagues call occupational apartheid.

For the Ainu nation, their history of injustice through the deprivation of traditional, meaningful occupational experiences and their treatment as a 'dying race' meant that 'Ainu were themselves embarrassed and felt ashamed of anything Ainu' (Fujimoto, 1973). Such feelings played an important role in the weakening of Ainu pride and identity.

It was argued above that the performance of an occupational cycle connected with nature contributed to the satisfaction of Maslow's hierarchy of needs not only through the maintenance of physical health but also by psychological satisfaction. Prior to the Early Modern period, it was also argued that Ainu possessed a worldview of humans-in-nature in which members of the *kotan* participated and fulfilled their roles in the occupational cycle, protecting the survival, health, and occupational justice of Ainu society. From the Tokugawa period, however, as a result of the priority given to the economy and development within Japanese society, social norms that scorned nature and life came to dominate the Ainu world. The only way for Ainu to survive was to accept the social norms of the more powerful Japanese society but this resulted in the collapse of the *kotan* community and a growing destruction of nature, which threatened Ainu health and survival. Social norms that ignored the cycles of humans-in-nature not only brought about occupational injustices but also threatened the health of communities, families and individuals.

Ainu today

In 1997 the Former Aborigines Protection Act was replaced by the Ainu Cultural Promotion Law and legal discrimination was officially ended. However, education about Ainu is still insufficient and Shirō Kayano (2009) notes that many Japanese continue to think Ainu are still wandering around the mountains, hunting bears and deer and catching salmon like in traditional times. More explicit discrimination against Ainu people still exists in Japan. According to the 2006 survey conducted by the Hokkaido government, there are 23 782 Ainu living in 72 cities, towns and villages in Hokkaido (Hokkaido Prefecture, 2006). However, this survey was limited to Hokkaido and only includes people who identify themselves as Ainu. It is said that there might be 50 000 Ainu today in Japan as a whole. The 2006 Hokkaido survey found that 38.3% of Ainu were receiving social welfare benefits as compared to a total average of 24.6% for the same communities. Only 17.4% of Ainu entered university as compared with an overall total of 38.5%. The percentage of Ainu who reported having experienced some form of discrimination in the past was 16.8%; experiences of discrimination over the previous six or seven years were recorded as 13.9% when searching for work, 39.1% at work, 21.7% at school, 13.0% in respect to marriage, and 9.5% from government agencies. These figures show that discrimination still continues against Ainu people.

In 2009, the author met Ainu artist and activist Kōji Yūki at a *kamuy-nomi* ceremony in Shiretoko, eastern Hokkaido. During this ceremony, Yūki apologized to the *kamuy* in Japanese: 'I am very sorry not to speak Ainu.' Later he said, 'I came out as Ainu because my son had pride in being Ainu. But I had no confidence because I grew up without learning about Ainu culture.' These words demonstrated to me that even if discriminatory laws were removed, the long history of prejudice and occupational deprivation had stopped the functional transmission of everyday life. For contemporary Ainu, the acquisition of the Ainu language and meaningful Ainu occupations is not easy. The inability to speak Ainu and to perform occupations meaningful to Ainu can be said to affect the pride and identity of Ainu people.

At the same time, however, a movement to restore pride in Ainu culture began in the 1920s during the time of assimilation policies. Yukie Chiri was one example of an Ainu who began to translate and publish *yukar*. The publication of these texts meant that the rich worldview of the Ainu could now be transmitted to Japanese and other peoples. *Yukar* are now highly regarded as one of the great world traditions of epic poetry. Furthermore, in recent years there has been a growing interest in indigenous peoples. In 2007, the United Nations passed a Declaration on the Rights of Indigenous Peoples. The following year an indigenous peoples' summit was held in Hokkaido and the World Indigenous peoples Network AINU was established. An indigenous peoples' summit was also held in Aichi Prefecture to coincide with the 2010 COP10 meting of the Convention on Biological Diversity. Events here included a forum on 'Biological diversity and indigenous peoples' wisdom of coexistence' and a music festival on the theme of 'Links between nature and humans and links between humans and humans.' As global environmental problems become ever more serious, the values and wisdom of indigenous peoples who lived closely with nature are invaluable. Through participating in this global community and debating their indigenousness, Ainu are presently attempting to restore the worldview, ethnic identity, pride and cultural occupations that they had lost.

Conclusions

In this chapter I have used a historical analysis of Ainu occupations to discuss the occupational cycle and occupational injustices resulting from Japanese social norms. The first part of the chapter proposed a model of the dynamics of the material cycle based on an 'occupational cycle' and demonstrated that Ainu everyday life was dependent on the resources of the natural environment. Prior to the Early Modern period, Ainu developed a 'humans-in-nature' worldview that co-existed with nature and developed and reproduced Ainu culture through a traditional occupational cycle that was directly linked with the cycles of nature. It was also argued that through their participation in traditional occupational cycles, Ainu maintained their survival and health as well as obtaining occupational satisfaction. The second part of the chapter then discussed Ainu occupational changes from the Early Modern period onwards. As a result of the arrival of Japanese in Hokkaido, Ainu people were subjected to (1) loss of occupational autonomy and the coercion of occupations; (2) deprivation of traditional occupations; and (3) coercion into occupations that differed from those having value for Ainu people. It was also shown that these occupational changes led to problems such as environmental destruction, the collapse of communities and families, increased mortality and morbidity, and weakened identities. It was concluded that these occupational injustices resulted from the norms of a modern society that valued wealth and power and ignored the cycles of humans-in-nature.

Based on the above analysis of the history of Ainu occupations, I want to conclude with some suggestions relating to contemporary occupations and the natural environment. In contemporary society the resources for human life, including food, freshwater, wood, fibres and fuel, are provided by ecosystem services. However, many people are now unaware of their most basic ecological dependencies (Cornell, Costanza, Sörlin and van der Leeuw, 2010). The chain of occupational cycles that formed the catalyst for the material cycle in traditional Ainu communities is separated by industrialization into primary, secondary and tertiary sectors of industry in contemporary societies in the global north. This can be said to have resulted in a decline in people whose occupations connect them directly with nature and a loss of opportunities to learn about the links between nature and everyday life through occupational cycles. Furthermore, the norms and mechanisms of contemporary society place value on the efficient mass production and consumption of commodities and the accumulation of money through economic growth. Thoughts of giving thanks to nature have been shunned from everyday life. These processes have encouraged occupations that ignore natural cycles, communities and families and which can be assumed to have provoked many contemporary social problems.

As mentioned in the introduction to this chapter, contemporary society is plagued by many social problems deriving from the norms of modernity, such as those relating to health, the collapse of communities and families, and environmental pollution. I suggest that the main reason that little progress is being made in resolving these problems is that we ourselves live within these social norms, even though our time left to reach a solution is clearly running out. The 'World Scientists' Warning to Humanity' signed by many Nobel prize laureates in 1992 describes the dangers to the environment in the following terms: 'Human activities inflict harsh and often irreversible damage on the environment and on critical resources. … No more than one or a few decades remain before the chance to avert the threats we now confront will be lost and the prospects for humanity immeasurably diminished' (Union of Concerned Scientists, 1992).

What sort of occupations should we choose and perform in order to avoid such a crisis of human survival and to develop sustainable societies? What needs to be done to produce new, sustainable social norms? There are no easy answers to these questions, but in aiming for human health and wellbeing we have to find lifestyles that balance nature, scientific technology and human beings. In our attempts to reconstruct new social norms that recall worldviews based on humans-in-nature, we have much to learn from the worldviews and traditional occupations of Ainu and other indigenous peoples.

References

Aoyama, M. (2009) *The Natural Environment and Human Health in Occupational Therapy and Occupational Science*. Paper presented at the 50th annual meeting of the Society for Medical Anthropology, Yale University, New Haven, CT.

Aoyama, M. (2010) *Nature and Occupation in Narratives of Ainu Bear Ceremonialism*. Poster session presented at the Fifteenth World Congress of the World Federation of Occupational Therapists, Santiago, Chile.

Aoyama, M. (2011) Nichijō seikatsu to shizen kankyō no kankei: Ainu no 'seigyō' o tōshite manabu [Relationship between everyday life and the natural environment: Learning from Ainu 'subsistence']. *West Kyushu Journal of Rehabilitation Sciences*, 4, 23–28.

Aoyama, M., Hudson, M. J. (2005) Occupation and lifestyle in a hunter-gatherer society: the Okhotsk culture of Hokkaido. *Hokkaido Journal of Occupational Therapy* 22, 68–83.

Aoyama, M., Hudson, M. J., Aoyama, H. (2009) *Sakishima shotō ni okeru shūryōsaishūmin no sagyō to seikatsu* [Occupations and lifestyles of hunter-gatherers in the Sakishima Islands]. Poster session presented at the forty-third Annual Congress of the Japanese Association of Occupational Therapists, Fukushima, Japan.

Aoyama, M., Hudson, M. J., Hoover, K. C. (in press) *Occupation Mediates Ecosystem Services with Human Wellbeing*. Journal of Occupational Science.

Blakeney, A. Marshall, A. (2009) Water quality, health, and human occupations. *American Journal of Occupational Therapy* 63, 46–57.

Chiri, M. (1984) *Chimei Ainugo shojiten* [Ainu place name dictionary]. Sapporo, Hokkaido Shuppan Kikaku Sentā.

Cornell, S., Costanza, R., Sörlin, S., Van der Leeuw, S. (2010) Developing a systematic 'science of the past' to create our future. *Global Environmental Change* 20, 426–427.

Emori, S. (2007) *Ainu minzoku no rekishi* [History of the Ainu nation]. Urayasu, Sōfūkan.

Fujimoto, H. (1973) *Gin no shizuku furufuru* [Silver droplets falling]. Tokyo, Shinchō Sensho.

Hanley, S. B. (1997) *Everyday Things in Premodern Japan: The Hidden Legacy of Material Culture*. Berkeley, CA, University of California Press.

Hirata, M. (2009) Kaitakushi kari-gakkō fuzoku 'Hokkaidō dojin kyōikujo' ni okeru Ainu kyōiku no jittai: kyōkasho kara miru Meiji shoki no Ainu kyōiku seisaku [The actual state of Ainu education at the temporary 'Hokkaido Aborigines School' attached to the Hokkaido Colonial Office: Early Meiji Ainu education policy as seen from textbooks]. *Sauvage* (Graduate Students Bulletin, Graduate School of International Media, Communication and Tourism Studies, Hokkaido University) 5, 29–42.

Hokkaido Prefecture (2006) *Ainu seikatsu jittai chosa hokokusho*, www.pref.hokkaido.lg.jp/ks/ass/grp/H18houkokusyo.pdf, accessed 22 June 2011.

Howell, D. L. (1995) *Capitalism from With in: Economy, Society, and the State in a Japanese Fishery*. Princeton, Princeton University Press.

Hudson, M. J. (1999a) *Ruins of Identity: Ethnogenesis in the Japanese Islands*. Honolulu, University of Hawai'i Press.

Hudson, M. J. (1999b) Ainu ethnogenesis and the Northern Fujiwara. Arctic Anthropology, 36, 73–83.

Hudson, M. J. (in press) Ainu and hunter-gatherer studies. In M. J. Hudson, A. E. Lewallen, M. W. Watson (eds), *Beyond Ainu Studies: Changing Academic and Public Perspectives*. Honolulu: University of Hawai'i Press.

Hudson, M. J., Aoyama, M. (2008) Occupational therapy and the current ecological crisis. *British Journal of Occupational Therapy* 71, 545–548.

Ikiugu, M. N. (2008) *Occupational Science in the Service of Gaia*. Baltimore, MD, PublishAmerica.

Kayano, Shigeru (1994) *Our Land was a Forest: An Ainu Memoir*. Boulder, CO, Westview.

Kayano, Shirō (2009) Senjūmin samitto no seika oyobi Ainu minzoku no genjō to kongō [The results of the Indigenous Peoples' Summit and the present and future of the Ainu people]. *Journal of Cultural Symbiosis Research* 2, 97–107.

Keira, M., Keira, T. (1999) Village work: gender roles and seasonal work. In W. W. Fitzhugh, C. O. Dubreuil (eds) *Ainu: Spirit of a Northern People*. Washington, DC, Arctic Studies Center, Smithsonian Institution, pp. 234–239.

Kronenberg, F., Pollard, N. (2005) Overcoming occupational apartheid: a preliminary exploration of the political nature of occupational therapy. In F. Kronenberg, S. Simó Algado, N. Pollard (eds) *Occupational Therapy without Borders: Learning from the Spirits of Survivors*. Edinburgh, Churchill Livingstone/Elsevier, pp. 58–86.

Maslow, A. H. (1943) A theory of human motivation. *Psychological Review* 50(4), 370–396.

Matsuna, T. (2007) Iwor-kō [An essay on 'iwor']. *Ninchi Kagaku Kenkyū* 5, 11–29.

Matsu'ura, T. (2002) *Ainu jinbutsushi* [Ainu biographies]. Tokyo, Heibonsha.

McKibben, B. (2007) *Deep Economy: The Wealth of Communities and the Durable Future*. New York, Times Books.

Millennium Ecosystem Assessment (2005) *Ecosystems and Human Well-being: Synthesis*. Washington, DC, Island Press.

Miyajima, T. (1998) *Land of Elms: The History, Culture, and Present Day Situation of the Ainu People*. Etobicoke, Ontario, United Church Publishing House.

Morita, E., Fukuda, S., Nagano, J., Hamajima, N., Yamamoto, H., Iwai, Y., Nakashima, T., Ohira, H., Shirakawa, T. (2007) Psychological effects of forest environment on healthy adults: Shinrin-yoku (forest-air bathing, walking) as a possible method of stress reduction. *Public Health* 121, 54–63.

Philippi, D. L. (1979) *Songs of Gods, Songs of Humans: The Epic Tradition of the Ainu*. Princeton, Princeton University Press.

Pollard, N., Kronenberg, F., Sakellariou, D. (2008) Occupational apartheid. In N. Pollard, D. Sakellariou, F. Kronenberg (eds) *A Political Practice of Occupational Therapy*. Edinburgh, Churchill Livingstone/Elsevier, pp. 55–67.

Public Health Agency of Canada (2010) *Key Determinants of Health*, www.phac-aspc.gc.ca/ph-sp/determinants/index-eng.php, accessed 22 June 2011.

Siddle, R. (1996) *Race, Resistance and the Ainu of Japan*. London, Routledge.

Solomon, S., Qin, D., Manning, M., Chen, Z., Marquis, M., Averyt, K. B. Tignor, M., Miller, H. L/ (eds) (2007) *Contribution of Working Group I to the Fourth Assessment Report of the Intergovernmental Panel on Climate Change, 2007*. Cambridge, Cambridge University Press.

Svenson, K. A., Lafontaine, C. (1999) The search for wellness. In *First Nations and Inuit Regional Health Survey*. St. Regis, Quebec, First Nations and Inuit Regional Health Survey National Steering Committee, pp. 181–216.

Thompson, E. P. (1976) *William Morris: Romantic to Revolutionary*, revised edition. London, Merlin Press.

Townsend, E., Wilcock, A. A. (2004) Occupational justice and client-centered practice: a dialogue in progress. *Canadian Journal of Occupational Therapy* 71(2), 75–87.

Union of Concerned Scientists (1992) World Scientists' Warning to Humanity, www.ucsusa. org/about/1992-world-scientists.html, accessed 22 June 2011.

Walker, B. L. (2001) *The Conquest of Ainu Lands: Ecology and Culture in Japanese Expansion, 1590–1800. Berkeley*, University of California Press.

Wilcock, A. A. (1998) *An Occupational Perspective of Health*. Thorofare, NJ, Slack.

Wilcock, A. A. (2006) *An Occupational Perspective of Health*, 2nd edn. Thorofare, NJ, Slack.

Wilcock, A. A. (2010) Population health: an occupational rationale. In M. E. Scaffa, S. M. Reitz, M. A. Pizzi (eds) *Occupational Therapy in the Promotion of Health and Wellness*. Philadelphia, PA, F. A. Davis, pp. 110–121.

World Health Organization (1986) *The Ottawa Charter for Health Promotion*, www.who. int/healthpromotion/conferences/previous/ottawa/en/index.html, accessed 17 June 2011.

Yoshida, K. (2007) Meiji-zen Ainu jinkōshi (1) Higashi Ezochi [Population changes of the Ainu in the east Ainu territory of Hokkaido before the Meiji Restoration]. *Studies in Humanities and Social Sciences, Nihon University* 73, 101–128.

Yoshida, K. (2008) Meiji-zen Ainu jinkōshi (2) Nishi Ezochi [Population changes of the Ainu in the west Ainu territory of Hokkaido before the Meiji Restoration]. *Studies in Humanities and Social Sciences, Nihon University* 75, 209–235.

10 People with Disabilities and Participation: Experiences and Challenges of an Occupational Therapy Practice in the City of São Paulo, Brazil

Sandra Maria Galheigo, Fátima Corrêa Oliver, Taisa Gomes Ferreira and Marta Aoki

Participation tends to appear in the realm of utopia, as a desirable but unattainable component of reality. Even though this may seem contradictory, indeed it is only an identity made of contradiction. Utopia, by definition, does not exist, but it is a component of reality because it expresses the endless need for historic transformation. Because we are utopians, we do not bend to the miseries of the present and we always dream of something better. On behalf of all utopias, we challenge everything, even though we know that we cannot achieve it all.

Without utopia, we satisfy ourselves with the mediocrity of daily dominations and bend to current inequalities. It is not in fact an escape from reality, but a source of transformation, an actual historic dynamism which moves human progress forward and produces enthusiasm renewed by reborn hopes.

P. Demo (1988) *Participação e conquista.*

Politics of Occupation-Centred Practice: Reflections on Occupational Engagement across Cultures, First Edition. Edited by Nick Pollard and Dikaios Sakellariou.
© 2012 John Wiley & Sons, Ltd. Published 2012 by John Wiley & Sons, Ltd.

Participation, Disability in Daily Life and Access to Human Rights in an Urban and Unequal Scenario

Participation, daily life and community intervention: concepts, perspectives and challenges

Participation is a concept that has been increasingly associated with health and linked to service provision and engagement in health policy making. Participation has also been incorporated as a key concept in documents related to access to human rights by people with disabilities – documents such as the UN Standard Rules on Equalization of Opportunities for Persons with Disabilities (United Nations, 1994) and the World Federation of Occupational Therapists' (WFOT's) Position Statement on Human Rights (World Federation of Occupational Therapists, 2006).

Participation is also an important dimension in the International Classification of Functioning, Disability and Health (ICF) (World Health Organization, 2001), which has underpinned some assessment tools used by health practitioners since 2001. By creating a unified and standard language for health and health-related conditions, ICF incorporated the concepts of activity and participation in the language of health professionals, focusing on the individual capacity and performance. Thus 'activity' is defined by ICF as 'the execution of a task or action by an individual' and participation is viewed as 'involvement in a life situation' (World Health Organization, 2001: 12). Accordingly, activity limitations are defined as 'difficulties an individual may have in executing activities' and participation restrictions are considered 'problems an individual may experience in involvement in life situations' (World Health Organization, 2001: 12). The ICF considers participation as a personal component of functioning and disability but only within a limited and instrumental perspective.

As a concept, participation was initially used in the context of political activity – a meaning that came about with the rise of modern Western society (Vianna, Cavalcanti and Cabral, 2009). It referred to the idea that free and equal individuals should take part in the collective decisions that affected the building of democratic societies. However, contradictory meanings for participation have arisen through the use of the concept by various streams of social and political thought. It has been transformed across time in response to social, political, economic and historical contexts (Conge, 1988; Cortes, 2002; Gascón et al., 2005; Vianna et al., 2009).

For some, the novelty in the usage of the concept of participation after the twentieth century has been the change from political participation into social participation (Vianna et al., 2009). However, political participation has been usually associated with a universal right that can be exercised by anyone who live in democratic societies while social participation has been generally connected with the conditions of specific groups of people, namely the poor, the excluded and the minorities (Vianna et al., 2009). In the latter, participation can be seen as the opposite of marginalization, that is, a form of collective action by means of which marginalized people may be integrated in social life (Bordenave, 1983).

Social participation entails an involvement with decision making in all the aspects of daily life – not only in the public sphere but in respect to the people's private lives. Social participation in contemporary life may be harder to attain than political participation. For instance, voting for public offices became more accessible for some people than making decisions on how and where to live, and the type of services or assistance they wish for their lives (Gascón *et al.*, 2005; Vianna *et al.*, 2009).

Participation has usually been seen as positive, a value in itself. According to Demo (1988), participation, as a component of democracy, is both a means to an end and an end in itself. Basing his arguments on the challenges of Brazilian democracy, Demo conceptualizes participation 'as a process of achievement and organized construction of social emancipation' (Demo, 1989: 133). Participation is then seen as a dynamic historical process, rooted in time and place, which comprises the ideas of process, achievement/construction, organization and, social emancipation. For him, participation is only achieved as a result of the actions of the people concerned and depends on some competence in exercising a collective citizenship, which comes about by confronting historically structured social inequalities. (For a critical discussion of the concept of 'citizenship' see Galheigo, 2011.)

The discussion on social participation follows different paths, making authors argue in favour of one view or another. Ammann (1977), however, stresses that to make social participation happen three basic components – production, management and usufruct – need to coexist and interact in a continuous and interdependent way.

The debate on social participation is often associated, at a personal level, with autonomy and personal participation in social life and, at societal level, with community participation. The latter has its roots in the 1960s, when the United Nations changed their emphasis from the use of remedial initiatives to the development of the so-called 'more positive forms of action' (Hardiman and Midgley, 1982: 19). Community action that aimed at making ordinary people involved in local affairs became recognized as being more capable of solving their problems and needs than the hegemonic specialized and institutionalized approach (Midgley, 1986).

A landmark on community participation was the UNICEF/WHO Declaration on Primary Health Care (World Health Organization, 1978) at the Alma Ata Conference in 1978, which advocated the offering of basic health services in local communities and the mobilization of people to take responsibility for their own needs. As a result, community-based development strategies came to be recognized as an effective measure to tackle health and social problems in the peripheral countries.

Discussing the field of health and disability, Rifkin and Kangere (2002) argue that there are three distinct approaches to community participation adopted by planners and professionals who work in the area, namely medical, health planning and community development. The medical approach implies compliance of users of services with a top-down decision, which results in a marginal participation. The health-planning approach is based on a contributive and collaborative model guaranteeing substantial participation. The community development approach is based on a community control model, which entails structural participation. However, the authors assert that these distinct approaches 'should not be seen as mutually exclusive' (Rifkin and Kangere, 2002: 42). Emphasizing the importance of the participation process, they propose to consider community participation as a continuum that starts with information sharing, being followed by consultation and collaboration until the achievement of empowerment.

Other critical issues regarding participation, health planning and disability have also been raised. Rifkin and Kangere (2002) point out the lack of a universally accepted conceptual framework to develop participation programs for people with disabilities; the frequent unrealistic assumptions on the contribution of participation to the development of community-based programmes, and power and control issues that often cause disputes between professionals and community members. Rifkin and Kangere (2002) also criticize the assumption that communities are always truly involved with the problems of their members who are disabled and/or marginalized. They also refer to extreme poverty as a barrier to participation by isolating people at home and limiting the accessibility of people with disabilities to meetings.

Pollard and Sakellariou (2008), in a critical discussion on community-based rehabilitation (CBR) programmes, call attention to the limited participation of people with disabilities both in developing and developed countries. Active participation of disabled people was only reported in seven out of 66 CBR programs according to a WFOT survey. They argue that CBR strategies can generate dilemmas or problems given that the complexities and difficulties of implementing programmes often raise ethical concerns and class and culture issues. They also suggest that some CBR programmes may still take a remedial approach rather than develop community participation projects.

These difficulties should not be seen as impeding the pursuit of participation as the development of community strategies is an important means of improving the life of people with disabilities. Rifkin and Kangere (2002) emphasize that critical examination of what works and the exercise of flexibility in the implementation of CBR programmes are important and 'support intended beneficiaries, in their search to gain control over their own lives' (Rifkin and Kangere, 2002: 47). Pollard and Sakellariou (2008) claim that, in order to enhance community participation, some aspects should be considered, namely the political contexts where CBR programmes take place, the need for cultural awareness, the inclusion of CBR subjects in professional education and the importance of long-term planning in CBR programmes.

People with disabilities, poverty and lack of access to human rights

People with disabilities face intense processes of social exclusion. According to the World Health Organization (2005) there are 600 million disabled people in the world, of which 200 million are children. About 80% of this population lives in developing countries and only 2% has access to rehabilitation services. Latin America has 85 million disabled people, almost three million of them in Central America. Most of them are adults and need to provide personal and economic support to their families and communities. Moreover, the experience of disability may directly or indirectly affect almost a quarter of the Latin American population if considering the family, the close social network and the neighbourhood involved with the demands of care and support (Vásquez, 2006). Violence has been also responsible for an important increase of people with disabilities in Latin America, becoming a major concern for governments and the Pan American Health Organization (2008).

In different societies, people with disabilities have lower levels of income, education, employment, and access to health care, housing and transportation (Inclusion International, 2004; Vásquez, 2006; Souza and Carneiro, 2007; Organización Mundial de la Salud, 2008). In coming decades this general picture may worsen through changes in morbidity and mortality patterns caused by population aging, the rise of chronic diseases, the impact of violence, and the high levels of poverty and unemployment. The demands for a higher professional qualification due to contemporary technological changes may also hinder the integration of people with disabilities in the labour market. In this regard, the obvious limits to opportunities and the devaluing of personal and social experiences faced daily by people with disabilities are evident.

The lack of participation of people with disabilities points out to problems regarding the production, management and use of social goods, as pointed out previously. They are often left behind in regard to the production and usufruct of social goods. Their ideas and needs are heard less and they are less socially valued. People with disabilities are often treated as the objects of policies and services and are often required to meet unattainable pre-established criteria, which limit their access to social benefits, social services and the assistance they need (Almeida, 2000; Rocha, 2006).

In many countries, the serious disparities in the life conditions of people with disabilities have increasingly required society's attention and demanded initiatives from governmental and nongovernmental organizations to develop socio-economic alternatives that aim to equalize health care, rehabilitation, education and employment opportunities. Efforts should also be made in order to improve wealth distribution and access to housing and transportation and to develop solutions to environmental barriers.

Ever more disability issues have led to government regulation and specific legal provision, although they mostly remain the responsibility of charitable institutions. As a consequence, the establishment of policies and alternative care has become a matter of importance. It is believed that people should have equal access to human rights. At the same time, by recognizing their own experience of disability, people with disabilities are taking steps towards making a dialogue around their position. This removes them from a situation of social invisibility and enables them to become agents of their own life process. This new position is essential for the exercise of their human rights (Díaz, 2002; Eroles, 2002). In this sense, it is important to emphasize the importance of the 1990s debate, which culminated in the Convention on the Rights of Persons with Disabilities (United Nations, 2008) adopted by the United Nations General Assembly in 2006 and in effect since May 2008. Addressing participation as a matter of human rights may change unquestionably the focus of attention and the practices developed by practitioners although social and political realities vary across the world.

For this reason, we believe that the needs and demands of people with disabilities should be taken into account by health and rehabilitation services, educational and vocational programs and, social care initiatives in the view of the construction, assertion and exercise of their rights.

These services, anchored in affirmative policies and initiatives for the construction of participation and citizenship, can include in their agendas themes such as the right to come and go as you please and the access to transportation in order to enlarge the capacity of displacement for people with reduced mobility; the right to education and vocational training in a way that scholarship and autonomy can be truly achieved, having access to human and technological resources to support learning; the right to assistive technology to facilitate activities of daily life, including the support to claims, technical and therapeutic evaluation and follow-up. In other words, we reaffirm that when the access to rights becomes the goal of health, rehabilitation and social care services, the strategies of care and rehabilitation can be orientated to understand and support solutions to the complexity of problems experienced by people with disabilities in their life contexts. Besides, this may contribute to people's engagement in sorting out their significant daily life problems.

Therefore we agree with Saraceno (1999) to whom participation is essential in rehabilitation, a process that cannot be detached from the idea of citizenship. He argues in favour of increasing people's participation in social life by enhancing people's *contractual power*, as he names it. For that, he advocates the need of establishing network processes for social negotiation within the family, the close community, and local social and health services. Saraceno (1999) proposes three ways of promoting social participation. The first is linked to the right to have a place to call home, not just a place for people to stay in; a place for people to participate in daily activities, develop affective ties, and exercise their decision-making power in their life affairs. The second is the importance of having social relations within a close or enlarged social network (family, friends, and neighbourhood) as it is a means of enjoying life, taking care of others and being cared for. The third refers to the need to make a living, and to work in meaningful and satisfying ways, and by doing so, promoting social values.

Oliver *et al.* (2001), dialoguing with Saraceno's (1999) ideas, have been engaged on reflecting about frameworks and developing practices in impoverished urban areas in the city of São Paulo, Brazil, by keeping in mind the importance of a permanent connection between needs and rights, in order to increase life possibilities and enhance social participation. This chapter presents some of these ideas and practices, developed by the Laboratório de Reabilitação com Ênfase no Território from the Occupational Therapy Program of the Faculty of Medicine of the University of São Paulo.

The activities were developed in the area of the Jardim Boa Vista Basic Health Unit, which works with Family Health Teams and covers 19 000 inhabitants, divided into six neighbourhoods with approximately 3000 inhabitants each. Basic health units are local health services that deliver primary health care and work as the entrance door to the Brazilian health system, free of charge to all permanent residents in the country. The basic health unit where this practice takes place is located in the periphery of São Paulo, a city of over 10 million inhabitants without a specific policy for community rehabilitation. This is the richest city in the country and one of the biggest in the world. However, São Paulo has 12.9% of the population living in situations of extreme vulnerability. These conditions occur when there are families with very low income and schooling, comprising either large numbers of old people and few children or large numbers of children and young family heads (up to 38 years old). The map of social vulnerability of the city shows that families with this composition are dispersed throughout the city and are not concentrated in a single region. The area of the basic health unit to be presented in this chapter has levels of social vulnerability higher than the average for the city (São Paulo, Secretaria Municipal de Assistência Social, 2010).

Identifying the Rupture of Social Support Networks and the Social Isolation of People with Disabilities in Poor Areas of São Paulo: An Experience of Active Search

Through having to cope with an unprecedented experience of disability, people may face several difficulties that affect the individual, family and social spheres. This feeling may be the result of a condition never experienced before – being disabled – which does not allow connection between past experience and the new life condition. Thus, becoming disabled in adulthood, when people already have hold over their own life course, brings about a profound disruption of life dynamics. From this moment onwards, one has to live with a new condition, even if previous values, beliefs and self-awareness are maintained. The way people perceive themselves as having a disability will significantly influence the way they will cope with their new physical condition and the choices they make for themselves (Pereira, 2007).

People with disabilities can often face social isolation due to the lack of information, for themselves and for their families, about their needs and the possibilities for developing new physical and social skills. After becoming disabled, people struggle daily with their body's functioning and social environment barriers that become obstacles to their autonomy and integration. Contact with the outside world occurs, but it is limited. Their desires are alive but restrained. However, ruptures become more noticeable when social circulation is limited and the lack of places and opportunities to engage with other people is evident. As a consequence, it is essential to consider disability not as an individual problem but a population condition that has become more significant due to demographic and epidemiologic developments in several countries. Asserting their rights as a social group is a step to recognizing their condition as a major contemporary social problem. Using a territorial approach (Box 10.1) may help to deal with disability as a collective problem and bring people with disabilities out of invisibility and isolation.

Box 10.1   The Territorial Approach

The territorial approach is understood as an articulation of complex geographic, historic, political, cultural and ecological dimensions of a certain place. A territory is a place of belonging, where possibilities of moving around, dwelling and exchanges in economic, interpersonal and social terms are established. It is a region where problems and solutions can be better identified. The Brazilian Unified Health System also uses a territorial approach to map health issues and provide healthcare within a pre-defined area (Fonseca and Corbo, 2007).

Knowing the disability as a collective problem: territorial approach

The specialized rehabilitation services that have traditionally been in charge of assisting people with disabilities usually employ the biomedical model to understand and approach their condition. According to this perspective, people with disabilities and their families should be individually supported in order to enhance functionality, which might later contribute to their participation in social life. As a consequence many problems are overlooked by rehabilitation services because a biomedical perspective tends to simplify rather than recognize the complexity of the lives of people with disabilities.

We therefore argue that social participation needs to be promoted during the rehabilitation process. Opportunities should be established for social participation and these become the focus and not the final objective of the rehabilitation process. Fostering participatory processes requires close contact between services and people with disabilities. This approach aims to change the culture of assistance from a focus on the individual to a focus on the life context.

The territorial approach may be an operational means of objectively evaluating the conditions of production, social circulation, dwelling, and communication in their relation to people's life conditions. At the same time this is a process that requires a subjective understanding of local social representations (Monken and Barcellos, 2007). Within a territory both the meanings attributed to disability and the people's needs become essential elements for the development of proposed assistance measures. Inspired by these perspectives, we have used the active search as one of the strategies of identifying and localizing people with disabilities within a territory, considering that they have not frequently make use of local health services. Active search enables health professionals to recognize the territory and the problems of people with physical, sensorial and intellectual disabilities, as follows:

1. The identification of formal interlocutors in the services and local institutions (community agents, educators, amongst others) and informal interlocutors (local religious and political leaderships, family members and long-term dwellers) to bring together elements for assembling the local history, the social dynamics of the territory and the understanding of problems experienced by the local people with and without disabilities.

2. The mapping of existing people with disabilities within the territory – the features of local geographic areas, the distribution of vulnerable conditions and identification of high risks that may impact on the condition of disability.
3. The localization, identification and case study of the local people with disabilities, their families and other people living with social vulnerability.
4. The study of accessibility to social facilities, the home surroundings and the health services.
5. The study of local mobility of people with disabilities within the territory and outside it, including public transport (adapted and non-adapted), identification of geographic and architectonic barriers, and, access to aid equipment.

After the data collection on these topics, the results about the life conditions of the people with disabilities in the region showed the intensity of their social exclusion, characterized by isolation and confinement at home, by limited access to work opportunities, social and cultural activities, healthcare, education and rehabilitation. This extreme exclusion hampered the possibilities of social circulation, the development of autonomy and the exercise of human rights.

However essential, this is only a partial approximation of the life reality of the local people with disabilities. Identifying and locating them in their territories enabled them, their families and professionals to understand the problems they experienced better. To learn more deeply the dimensions of their everyday life, life stories were collected and contributed to develop a professional look at disability in context. These elements guided the future planning of care alternatives that could combine the unique aspects of living a life with disabilities and the similar needs and demands of the other local residents.

Knowing personal trajectories: life stories

Life story methodology is commonly used for data collection in qualitative research. It provides rich material for analysis because it allows people to tell their daily life experiences and provide interpretations for them (Cruz Neto, 1994). Through the process of actively listening, researchers can reconstruct actions and context because life stories help capture aspects of place, time, motivation and the person's symbolic system (Jovchelovitch and Bauer, 2002).

The use of life story methodology can also be a valuable professional tool because it allows an understanding of the perceptions of the people with disabilities about the life ruptures caused by the disability and the impact in their social relationships. Getting to know their life stories may help occupational therapists develop strategies for improving social exchange and participation in family and collective life.

By using this methodology in the rehabilitation process, practitioners become aware of the rich experience lived by people with disabilities, which is expressed by their feelings, needs, dreams, abilities and difficulties. This direct approach with the daily experience of disability may help the practitioners to have a contextualized view of what means to be disabled and thus act more in tune with reality, focusing their interventions on overcoming the main barriers faced by people with disability.

The information obtained may help occupational therapists build a partnership with the disabled people that anticipates the restructuring of their everyday life, contributing to more satisfactory experiences and engagement in interesting and meaningful activities. The process of telling their own stories enables them to become active participants in the transformation of their own reality.

For this reason, seeking to hear and understand how people with disability perceive their life situation before and after the onset of disability can help domiciliary assistance and the planning in accordance with their reality. The experience of telling one's own story may contribute to encouraging independence, autonomy and personal health care, the expansion of social relations and networks (at work, school, leisure, among others).

This resource has been used in the assistance provided by the teachers and the students in Practice and Service Learning. It has also contributed to research for obtaining a Master's Degree, such as the case of the collection of the life history of Mr. Shin (Ferreira, 2009) (Box 10.2).

Box 10.2   The Story of Mr. Shin (Ferreira, 2009)

Mr. Shin is a 67-year-old Brazilian man, son of Japanese immigrants, married with four children. Before the stroke, he could be considered a very resourceful person: he was a dry cleaner, a hairdresser and owner of a candy store. He also worked for four years in Japan as a manual labourer. His leisure interests – travelling, fishing, cycling – were quite diverse and constant in his everyday life and his social circle was mostly composed of his work colleagues, neighbours and family. He was 61 years old when he had the stroke that resulted in hemiplegia. He is independent in locomotion for short distances at home but needs assistance from his wife and grandson to look after the family grocery store. He can serve customers but has difficulty in receiving the goods and cleaning the store. He also appears to be dependent for some self-care activities (dressing, for example) and resents the noticeable decrease in his leisure activities and in the visits to friends and brothers. He cannot drive any more and finds it difficult to use public transport.

Besides reporting physical disabilities, the central theme in his narrative was related to the maintenance of his social activities. In his life story, the past was experienced as being free to go to different places, to act autonomously, to fall in love, to meet people and talk to strangers, co-workers, and neighbours. There was a noticeable decline in his close social network as a result of the difficulties in having access to workplaces and leisure. He noticed the detachment of friends, family and neighbours, which resulted not only in loneliness, but also highlighted the lack of strategies to restore his social support. This resulted in his withdrawal from social life. The impossibility of working caused a decline in social circulation that significantly reduced the opportunities to meet others and enjoy daily-established social relationships. Not having a job sometimes increased his frustration and increased the sense of loneliness and social isolation; moreover, with the increase in his free time, disabilities became more noticeable.

Becoming disabled has also caused a decrease in his leisure activities and spaces of circulation, now restricted to his house, and to monthly visits to his brother who lives in another city. Due to this fact and knowing his story, it is no surprise that his biggest complaint is the dependence on others for leisure activities. The experience of disability has limited his ways of sharing ideas, performing different roles, making social exchanges, building new social network and keeping the previous social and affective relations. Thus the experience of belonging to a group and to society as a whole was affected.

To enlarge the scope of assistance provided by services and health professionals beyond the treatment of the physical sequelae is an important alternative to be explored in order to increase the quality of life of people with disabilities.

The Construction of Participation in the Daily Life of People with Disabilities: Community Alternatives for Intervention

By helping to understand the living conditions of people with disabilities in comparison to other local residents, the territorial approach makes it possible to better recognize the problems experienced by them and their families. It is possible to develop strategies of intervention in the local social and health services that contribute to promote social participation in a multidimensional perspective – that is, in the family and the community spheres, encouraging autonomy by means of the daily decision-making regarding the use of time, routines, and, even the management of personal financial resources.

The intervention has had the support and participation of different social actors such as the members of family and the health team, other people with disabilities or living in vulnerable conditions, community leaders, volunteering dwellers and so forth. The students and occupational therapists from the basic health unit and the university have maintained the assistance to people in the project. The support of local churches and community centres has been important; financial resources have come from the university and other government funding. In this project, several strategies are used, namely individual care, group activities, human rights forums and social-cultural activities.

Individual care

This is a form of clinical assistance and mobilization of the people with disabilities and their families in order to promote social participation. The individual approach may be implemented both at home and in the health units. The aim is to get to know both the material and subjective conditions of living with a disability, to establish a dialogue with the perspectives of the people with disabilities and their families and to contribute to the accomplishment of activities of daily life, especially those related to self-care and self-maintenance. Practitioners also provide information regarding the access to resources, such as social benefits and assistive technology (wheelchairs, walkers or splints). The story of Adriano (Aoki, 2009) in Box 10.3 provides an example of this kind of intervention.

Box 10.3   The Story of Adriano (Aoki, 2009)

Adriano is a 29-year-old man with muscular dystrophy. When he was 16, he started having fatigue and muscle weakness, mainly in the lower limbs, making walking difficult. He wore crutches for some years and moved to a wheelchair four years ago. Adriano needs help to make transfers and perform activities such as personal hygiene and dressing. He enjoys doing painting and mosaic and is talented and demanding with the aesthetic presentation of his work, taking up to four months to complete a piece of work.

Adriano has not completed his education and doesñt know in which school year he stopped. At elementary school, while everyone else learned to read and write, he spent his time in the classroom drawing castles, cars and trucks. When he was 16, discouraged by his lack of education, he asked his mother to let him leave school because he wished to work. Then he began working in a factory, as assembler of refrigerators. In this job, he noticed the worsening of his motor performance, which led him to leave work and take disability retirement at 27 years old. His father, Mr John, was his main caretaker until 2007, when he died. Then his mother, Mrs Alzira, resumed this role with difficulty due to her health problems. Adriano lives with his two brothers, the oldest with psychiatric and drug addiction problems and the youngest with muscular dystrophy, already presenting with walking difficulty. Although Adriano receives disability retirement benefit and his mother has a pension, the family's low income prevents them from investing in other needs, such as the repairing of the wheelchair, the purchasing of equipment for respiratory physiotherapy and the payment for transport to hydrotherapy sessions.

The intervention with Adriano and his family began in 2002, when in a meeting of people with disabilities and government representatives in the local church, his mother sought out the occupational therapists to talk about her son. Adriano was getting weak and unable to walk without support, becoming isolated at home. His only occupation was watching television. The intervention started with home visits and the appraisal of his needs: a wheel chair and a proper diagnosis.

Initially, he was donated a second-hand wheelchair. Later brand-new and better suited equipment was obtained from the public health system. After months of waiting and intermediation of the occupational therapists, the diagnosis was confirmed as limb-girdle muscular dystrophy. However, this did not result in proper treatment because, due to lack of transport, or perspectives of good rehabilitation prognosis, adult patients with this diagnosis are seldom treated in specialist services.

Adriano and other people with physical disabilities living in the neighbourhood were encouraged to enrol in a program of specialized transportation to have access to the health unit. This allowed his presence in the Mosaic Group, a weekly support group for people with and without disabilities, in which he carries out mosaic handicrafts with the support of community health workers and occupational therapists. This was the first opportunity for him and his mother to break with the family isolation. His participation in the group is constant and active and his communication and social network has improved.

Encouraged by the other group members, Adriano and his mother began to participate in the activities of the Municipal Council of People with Disabilities in São Paulo. There they discuss the rights of the people with disabilities, share experiences amongst peers and enjoy events, meetings and tours sponsored by the Council. Adriano has become motivated and eager to use the city's leisure and culture resources since he joined these social groups. The needs expressed by Adriano go beyond the sphere of usual intervention, focused on disability and rehabilitation. He also wants to talk, wander and date.

Occupational therapists who work at community and territorial level can produce alternative care in rehabilitation, emphasizing community participation and access to rights, such as the reported in this story. It is important to have a dialogue between the demands presented by people with disabilities and the assistance provided by the health team, considering the community reality and its resources.

Group activities

The group activities are opportunities designed to promote the circulation outside home and the construction of collective projects. The meetings are held in health services and elsewhere in the community (schools, churches, associations). They provide opportunities for people to break home isolation and offer a place to share problems, needs and solutions among other people with disabilities, their families, community leaderships and professionals. The group activities also enable participation in social projects and in the production of meaningful objects and to experience physical activities. Participating in collective ventures is an opportunity to demystify the condition of disability and produce social value. There are different types of group activities: youth and adult support groups, bodily activities group, community therapy (Barreto, 2005), production groups (carpentry, mosaic, beading, and handicrafts), playgroups, mothers' groups, children's rights defence groups and groups for fostering the culture of peace, among others. Box 10.4 provides an example.

Box 10.4   The New Life Support Group (Aoki, 2009)

In a poor neighbourhood with 3000 inhabitants – one of those covered by the Jardim BoaVista Basic Health Unit – occupational therapists and community health workers mapped the local residents with disabilities in the neighbourhood, as well as the local resources and community leaderships. In 2005 data collection, 53 persons with disabilities were identified with a prevalence of adults (27 people) between 18 and 60 years old, with physical and intellectual disabilities. The first contacts with this population have confirmed the hypothesis of home isolation and reduced social participation. To diminish these conditions, a support group was organized with the initial support of the local community centre, used by many residents of the neighbourhood but not by people with disabilities. The centre was easily accessible without significant architectural barriers and the presence of people with disabilities there was considered a strategy to give greater visibility and awareness to disability issues.

In March 2006, the first meeting to discuss intervention alternatives took place involving people with disabilities, family members, health workers and community leaders. The outcome was the creation of a support group called New Life. The project depended on a collective effort, shared among all the people involved, and was delineated taking into account the collective needs and the existing local resources. The group coordination was carried out by two occupational therapists. Among the people with disabilities there were 10 adults – six men and four women; five of them with intellectual disability, three with physical disability and two with multiple disabilities. The participation of people with severe disabilities urged occupational therapists to seek operational support and to develop family awareness about the importance of participating in the group activities.

One of the challenges of the project was to assemble people with different profiles, considering different age groups, genders, disabilities, interests and motivations. After some experiments with handcraft activities, the group chose bijouterie due to the availability of material, easy handling, good aesthetic results and personal satisfaction with the final product. Compared with other groups, this one was unique considering its features – being heterogeneous, open, and conducted within a community centre. Within the group there were people with significant cognitive and motor difficulties; some of them with little autonomy and independence in daily activities and, poor communication skills. However, they were very receptive to taking part in the proposal.

The group was called by its members as the 'Bijou Group', emphasizing the actual experience of doing things: necklace, ring, bracelets. For the participants, the activity was motivating and promoted creativity. The group was also a place to chat and to make social and personal exchanges. Although income generation was not the main goal of the group, many referred to it as an opportunity to learn something that could be used in the future. Participants were taken to shops to buy material, which also gave them a chance to enjoy the city's facilities.

The occupational therapists who coordinated the group activities opted for a focus on the learning process of the participants by understanding that some of them had no experience in previous formal education and were considered unable to learn. Therefore, it was important to promote learning through experience (Samea, 2002) to engage the participants in the process of the production of jewellery and to facilitate their involvement in decision making (Galetti, 2004).

The experience encouraged communication and the establishment of social ties, resulting in improvements in sociability, communication and self-care. The development of social support network was also observed inasmuch as the people with disabilities and their families came to rely on the professionals, other participants and the representatives of the community centre. Improvement in communication also occurred between the group and the environment – the neighbourhood, the community centre, the health service and the city.

Being part of a group and develop social activities enabled the participants and their families to have information about social rights and the means for accessing them. They asked questions such as How can I get a publicly funded wheelchair? How can I access free bus tickets? How can I receive social benefits for people with disabilities? Where can I study? Discussion of these issues in meetings developed participants' awareness of the rights of people with disabilities. They took part in events and trips which also provided social opportunities and reduced the experience of isolation at home.

The New Life Support Group was an alternative rehabilitation approach that promoted the expansion of the social support network, resulting in better social protection. Improving social support resulted in better handling of difficult everyday circumstances, and the increase of self esteem, autonomy and quality of life.

Human rights forums

These are regular meetings in which people with disabilities, family members, neighbours, health professionals and students discuss multi-sector strategies for the access to rights such as education, health services, adapted transport, and social benefits. The participants may perceive themselves as having rights and as being part of a specific social group and community. Participants may also take part as elected members of health councils at local and municipal levels and in the Council of People for Disabilities' Rights of São Paulo. They may also be part of councils as members of work groups or attend meetings and assemblies.

The mapping of people with disabilities and the debate about their rights and their living conditions have allowed participants to submit formal requests for adapted bus services, inclusive classes for infants, and vacancies for children with disabilities in the local schools of the municipal government.

Socio-cultural activities

These are meetings that involve evening cultural gatherings (for music and poetry sharing) and regular trips to parks, recreation and cultural centres. They provide an opportunity for people to access collective spaces and to enlarge their acquaintance with the city's venues and its cultural heritage, which are mostly unknown and inaccessible for people with disabilities, their families, and residents of poor areas. Such meetings are also an opportunity to give visibility to the issues of living with disabilities both locally and elsewhere in the city.

Conclusion

Although participation is a key concept in disability and rehabilitation, scholars and practitioners express very different interpretations of it, which creates difficulty in understanding the term. The argument developed here, and the practice used as an example, are intended to give substance to the idea of participation as a collective-centred praxis. In our opinion, participation should not be approached as a personal matter but as a collective experience, which is brought about by cooperation.

However, this view of participation is socially and historically constructed and is related to the challenges faced by social and health professionals and the users of services in societies in the process of democratization, such as Brazil. Social and political experiences in the search for strategies against social inequalities throughout history have largely influenced the ideas and practices developed in the last two decades. By working to enable people to enact their rights or, in Saraceno's (1999) understanding rehabilitation as citizenship (Saraceno, 1999), practitioners recognize the need to enhance people's contractual power by means of a practice that promotes autonomy and social participation. This form of practice is a result of a collective action that permanently establishes a dialogue between people's needs and rights.

Occupational therapy is a field of knowledge and practice that seeks to encourage and equip people with disabilities and/or at risk of disruption of social support networks to develop their lives autonomously. This implies constructing and supporting alternatives for assistance in order to establish personal and collective participatory processes in the context of family, work, school and community.

The development of participatory processes, from basic care for life maintenance to the access to rights, is, for us, one of the main bases for contemporary occupational therapy in Brazil. This involves creating strategies to analyse problems and situations faced by individuals and groups, considering the complex relationships between people, their socio-cultural contexts and the historical and social processes for the establishment of human rights.

We believe that the focus on participatory processes in the development of occupational therapy assistance can encourage people to recognize themselves as being able to exercise their rights and ability to seek personal and collective ways of exercising them. Thus occupational therapy is a field of knowledge and practice that can contribute to guaranteeing human rights.

References

Almeida, M. C. (2000) Saúde e reabilitação de pessoas com deficiência: políticas e modelos assistenciais. Ph. D. thesis. Faculdade de Ciências Médicas. Universidade Estadual de Campinas.

Ammann, S. (1977) *Participação social*. São Paulo, Cortez.

Aoki, M. (2009) Reabilitação com ênfase no território – demandas de pessoas com deficiências e a promoção da participação comunitária. Master's dissertation. Faculdade de Medicina. Universidade de São Paulo.

Barreto, A. P. (2005) *Terapia comunitária passo a passo*. Fortaleza, Gráfica LCD.

Bordenave, J. E. D. (1983) *O que é participação*. São Paulo, Brasiliense.

Conge, P. J. (1988) The concept of political participation – toward a definition. *Comparative Politics* 20(2), 241–249.

Cortes, S. M. V. (2002) Construindo a possibilidade da participação dos usuários: conselhos e conferências no Sistema Único de Saúde. *Sociologias* 7, 18–49.

Cruz Neto, O. (1994) O trabalho de campo como descoberta e criação. In M. C. S. Minayo (ed.) *Pesquisa Social – teoria, método e criatividade*. Vozes, Rio de Janeiro, pp. 51–66.

Demo, P. (1988) *Participação e conquista*. São Paulo, Cortez-Autores Associados.

Demo. P. (1989) Participação e planejamento. In IPEA/IPLAN (ed) *Para a década de 90: prioridades e perspectivas de politicas publicas/Instituto de Planejamento Econômico e Social*. Brasilia, Instituto de Planejamento, pp. 129–160.

Díaz, L. (2002) Discapacidad y pobreza. In C. Eroles, C. Ferreres (eds) *La discapacidad: una questión de derechos humanos*. Buenos Aires, Espacio Editorial, pp. 82–90.

Eroles, C. (2002) Discapacidad y derechos humanos. In C. Eroles, C. Ferreres (eds) *La discapacidad: una questión de derechos humanos*. Buenos Aires: Espacio Editorial, pp. 15–39.

Ferreira, T. G. (2009) Pessoas com deficiência: condições de convivência e possibilidades de atenção domiciliar. Master's dissertation. Faculdade de Medicina. Universidade de São Paulo.

Fonseca, A. F. and Corbo, A. M. D. A. (eds) (2007) *O território e o processo saúde-doença*. Rio de Janeiro, EPSJV/Fiocruz.

Galheigo, S. M. (2011) Concepts and critical considerations for occupational therapy in the social field. In F. Kronemberg, N. Pollard, D. Sakellariou (eds) *Occupational Therapies without Borders, Volume II: Towards an Ecology of Occupation-Based Practices*. Edinburgh, Churchill Livingstone/Elsevier, pp. 47–56.

Galletti, M. C. (2004) *Oficina em saúde mental: instrumento terapêutico ou intercessor clínico*. Goiânia, Editora da UCG.

Gascón, S., Tamargo, M. C., Carles, M. (2005) *Marco conceptual y metodológico sobre participación ciudadana en salud en el MERCOSUR ampliado*. Fundacion ISALUD, primer informe de avance.

Hardiman, M., Midgley, J. (1982) *The Social Dimensions of Development: Social Policy and Planning in the Third World*. Chichester, John Wiley & Sons, Ltd.

Inclusion International (2004) *Reporte del Estado de Pobreza y Discapacidad en las Américas*. Ottawa, Inclusion International, Canadian International Development Agency.

Jovchelovitch, S., Bauer, M. W. (2002) Entrevista narrativa. In M. W., Bauer, G., Gaskell,(eds) *Pesquisa qualitativa com texto, imagem e som: um manual prático*. Petrópolis, Vozes, pp. 90–113.

Midgley, J. (1986) Community participation: history, concepts and controversies. In J. Midgley, A. Hall, M. Hardiman, D. Narine (eds) *Community Participation, Social Development and the State*. Methuen, London, pp. 13–44.

Monken, M., Barcellos, C. (2007) O Território na Promoção e Vigilância em Saúde. In A. F. Fonseca, A. M. D. A. Corbo (eds) *O território e o processo saúde-doença*. Rio de Janeiro, EPSJV/Fiocruz, vol. 1, pp. 177–224.

Oliver, F., Ghirardi, M. I., Almeida, M., Tissi, M. C., Aoki, M. (2001) Reabilitação no território: construindo participação na vida social. *Revista de Terapia Ocupacional da Universidade de São Paulo* 12, 15–22.

Organización Mundial de la Salud (2008) ¿Qué se está haciendo para mejorar la vida cotidiana de las personas con discapacidad? Preguntas y respuestas en línea, www.who.int/features/qa/16/es/print.html, accessed 28 July 2009.

Pan American Health Organization (2008) Preventing violence and injuries and promoting safety: a call for action in the Region. 48th Directing Council. Washington, DC, PAHO, www.paho.org/english/gov/cd/CD48-20-e.pdf, accessed 25 November 2008.

Pereira, R. (2007) Human handicap and self-determination: compassion and insensibility in the Vincent Humbert case. *História Ciencias Saude-Manguinhos* 14(1), 119–134.

Pollard, N., Sakellariou, D. (2008) Operationalising community participation in community based rehabilitation. *Disability and Rehabilitation* 30, 62–70.

Rifkin, S., Kangere, M. (2002) What is participation? In S. Hartley (ed.) *Community-Based Rehabilitation: A Participatory Strategy in Africa*. London, University College, Centre for International Child Health, pp. 37–49, www.asksource.info/cbr-hartley.htm, 6 October 2010.

Rocha, E. F. (2006) *Reabilitação de pessoas com deficiência: a intervenção em discussão*. São Paulo: Rocca.

Samea, M. (2002) Terapia ocupacional e grupos: em busca de espaços de subjetivação. Master's dissertation. São Paulo. Faculdade de Psicologia. Universidade de São Paulo.

São Paulo. Secretaria Municipal de Assistência Social (2010) Mapa da vulnerabilidade social, http://prefeitura.sp.gov.br/cidade/secretarias/assistencia_social/observatorio_social/mapas/index.php?p + 2012, accessed 20 August 2010.

Saraceno, B., (1999) *Libertando Identidades. Da reabilitação psicossocial à cidadania possível*. Te Corá Editora/Instituto Franco Basaglia, Belo Horizonte/Rio de Janeiro.

Souza, J. M., Carneiro., R. (2007) Universalismo e focalização na política de atenção à pessoa com deficiência. *Saúde Sociedade* 16(3), 69–84.

United Nations (1994) Standard Rules on the Equalization of Opportunities, www2.ohchr.org/english/law/opportunities.htm, accessed 28 April 2010.

United Nations (2008) Convention on the Rights of Persons with Disabilities, http://www2.ohchr.org/english/law/disabilities-convention.htm, accessed 28 April 2010.

Vásquez, A. (2006) La discapacidad em América Latina. In A. Amate, A. Vásquez (eds) *Discapacidad lo que todos debemos saber*. Washington, DC, Organización Panamericana de La Salud. pp. 9–24.

Vianna, M. L. T. W., Cavalcanti, M. L., Cabral, M. P. (2009) Participação em saúde: do que estamos falando? *Sociologias* 21, 218–251.

World Federation of Occupational Therapists (2006) *WFOT Position Statement on Human Rights*. Australia, WFOT.

World Health Organization (1978) *Declaration of Alma-Ata. The International Conference on Primary Health Care*. Alma Ata, URRS.

World Health Organization (2001) *International Classification of Functioning, Disability and Health (ICF)*. Geneva, WHO.

World Health Organization (2005) *Fifty-Eighth World Health Assembly A58/17 April 2005. Disability, Including Prevention, Management and Rehabilitation*, http://apps.who.int/gb/ebwha/pdf_files/WHA58/A58_17-en.pdf, accessed 28 July 2009.

11 Communities of Writing

Nick Pollard

Writing is one of the most popular arts activities in the UK, a field in which there has been substantial growth. It eclipses many performing and visual arts in popularity (Matarasso, 1997). Writing requires little equipment and can be practised discreetly in many different environments. While writing can be a vehicle for the private exploration of feelings and ideas, many people like to share and disseminate their writing with others, and through performance and publication have made the liberating discovery of their expressive 'voice' (Morley and Worpole, 1982).

There are many writing and publishing organizations, including some developed by disability and mental health survivors' groups. Although there are many small presses producing many different kinds of publications, a particular phenomenon within this field is that of community publishing. This chapter will explore the tradition of community publication understood by one organization in the UK, the Federation of Worker Writers and Community Publishers (FWWCP).

Evaluating the benefits of community based arts approaches presents difficulties. Newman *et al.* (2001) found impediments to comparison arose because projects are often related to specific communities and their needs, while their objectives may be wide ranging and complex. Since the 1960s community arts projects have been part of the apparatus of community development approaches to engage socially excluded groups. Participants can often express satisfaction with the outcomes of a project but it is difficult to evaluate artistic experiences in quantitative terms. The experience gained through an arts activity may be difficult to translate to something else.

Many voluntary organizations operate without funding (Clark *et al.,* 2010). Newman *et al.*'s review (2001) was concerned with professional interventions rather than those organized by voluntary or amateur groups and their search criteria excluded writing and publishing. The low cost of writing activities and some forms of publishing lend themselves to organizations that require little external funding and operate informally without the need to have a bank account, let alone professional involvement. Many writing groups begin in a corner of a café or pub, or perhaps move around members' homes, having little more formality than a place and a time to meet.

Politics of Occupation-Centred Practice: Reflections on Occupational Engagement across Cultures,
First Edition. Edited by Nick Pollard and Dikaios Sakellariou.
© 2012 John Wiley & Sons, Ltd. Published 2012 by John Wiley & Sons, Ltd.

The activity of writing is invariably inclusive of an evocation of time and space. People record or creatively translate their experiences for an audience, more often than not, a readership or a group of listeners, of whom they are aware. A poem or narrative does not take place in a vacuum but in a context in which it is about something, and produced for someone (even an imagined recipient), in forms that are influenced by other examples of cultural expression available to the author. Much of the writing that people produce in their daily lives is a product of their occupations and social roles in their community, the most common used to be postcards and shopping lists (Heath, 1983), but perhaps now they are phone texts or Facebook entries. Whether they are these brief fleeting exchanges, more reflective thoughts on paper, or something to be shared with an audience they usually concern expressions of 'doing, being, becoming and belonging' (Wilcock, 2006: 305), and often describe familiar settings.

The practice of writing, of making poems, fictions, the recording of experiences and histories is something that communities have always found ways to do. Perhaps the comparative invisibility of some forms of this literature is more due to the dominance of certain cultural expressions over those that are more vernacular, less well distributed and more ephemeral. These issues are discussed elsewhere (Parks and Pollard, 2009; Pollard and Parks, 2010). The focus of this chapter concerns the negotiation of representation through community publications, the way in which groups of people come to agree (or disagree) around local meanings. The title of this chapter concerns 'writing' but I take this word to correspond roughly with the production of narratives. It can, therefore, refer to oral narratives. The reason for this is that the discussion which follows is based not so much in the practices of high literature production, but in those which developed in the UK and other parts of the world during the late part of the twentieth century amongst a variety of community groups. These groups came from a diverse range of backgrounds, including migrants to the UK, survivors of mental distress, people with learning difficulties, people who had missed out on key parts of their education, as well as people who had gained from the greater accessibility of higher education in the post-Second World War period. Across such diversity the narratives that were shared might often be written, but many were not, and others had had to be transcribed. Accordingly it was accepted amongst these groups that writing could be produced by a range of means, and equally, that it could be published in diverse ways too, including performance.

The majority of people in these community-based writing and publishing groups wrote about their own experiences or those of their families and people around them. Particularly during the 1970–90 period, many writers in these groups were consciously producing autobiographical narratives as 'people's history', an alternative account to their experience of the history taught in schools, and part of a popular history movement (Morley and Worpole, 1982; Morley *et al.*, 2009). The FWWCP was a network of groups of people who regularly met around writing, literacy needs, local and oral history, or experiences of social marginalization.

In the local accounts of events these groups developed, people placed *themselves* in the foreground rather than key politicians, royalty, or exemplars of social movements identified and selected by others (Morley and Worpole, 1982). These autobiographical narratives, for example referring to a small part of a town, or a few streets, often generated intense local sales, and sometimes stimulated other local people to reply with their own accounts. These living histories were based not on the third-party examination of documents and secondary sources but on direct occupational experiences. They were about times and places that their authors had known themselves, written for family and friends, and perhaps other community members.

These narratives of 'unknown England' (FWWCP, 1985) have long been of great interest to me because of the wealth of local and intimate detail they contain. Over a thirty-year period I convened a writers workshop, attended FWWCP committee meetings, participated in the organization's 'Festival of Writing' and edited its magazine. I will be drawing from these experiences in this chapter. I have also conducted a couple of focus group studies with the FWWCP, some of the analysis from which is also reproduced here. I have collected and read many community publications, met their authors and shared writing with them. Thousands were produced in print runs ranging from a hundred copies to several editions of a couple of thousand. By 1982 Morley and Worpole estimated that perhaps half a million such publications existed, while Diggles (2006) later claimed a million. This is possible but the literature is so ephemeral that a full account could not be achieved. There are numerous stories in the movement of old books thrown out in shop basement clearouts, of people dying and their collections, no longer significant to present generations, going into house clearance. Time is unkind to photocopied typescripts, duplicated magazines on cheap paper, crumbling and faded books about former everyday occupations in a localized past, though some of them have been reissued digitally at www.mancvoices.co.uk for example.

This kind of writing was often stimulated by the impact of social changes on occupational experiences. Daisy Noakes (1980a, 1980b) and George Noakes (1977) wrote about the passing of a rural way of life, Moss (1986) described his work in a Bristol coal mine, while Hollick (1991), a Pullman coach attendant, and Ross (1984), a railway guard gave accounts of former types of railway work. Some accounts, particularly those describing periods before the Second World War, detail the considerable hardship many people ordinarily experienced in Britain. Childhood disease and death, the death of parents, terrible poverty and unhealthy conditions were common (Hamer, n.d.; Healey, 1980; Muckle, 1981; Noakes, 1980b; Paul, 1981a, 1981b; Wolveridge, 1981; Wheway, 1984). Working-class life has often been presented in safe historical contexts (Bromley, 1988) but these stories describe events in nearby places, in a landscape that may have altered through time and urban redevelopment, but with many features still present. They often seem very immediate.

Communities, Writing and Publishing

The FWWCP network grew to 80 writers' and publishing groups worldwide over a period of 30 years from a base of eight groups, which first met in 1976. Most of these were based in a few English towns and cities, particularly Liverpool and London, and others in rural areas. Over 30 years there were many member groups, some of which lasted only a few months, while others still continue to meet. A few, such as London Voices and QueenSpark, had been meeting for several years before the organization formed. A number originated in Workers Educational Association writing classes, part of an adult education movement with roots in nineteenth-century social activism (Fieldhouse, 1977). There were, broadly, workshops and publishing co-operatives. Most workshops met on a weekly or fortnightly basis in a community centre or an upstairs room in a pub. These usually consisted of a group of eight to 20 people who took it in turns to read from the work they were developing and receive comment from the rest.

The term 'community publishing' generally describes the means by which groups of people produce publications about and for the communities they live in. As community art forms, these produce value and at the same time enable those involved to participate socially according to the commitment they can make. The work is done cooperatively, with little remuneration for those involved, and on a non-profit basis to minimize retail costs (Mace, 1995; Philips *et al.*, 1999). While community publishing in some form (for example broadsheet ballads and broadsides) has long been possible, and people have always shared narratives about the things they do, writing about them first hand appears to have been exceptional until recently, though literate workers did occasionally write about their experiences in earlier times. With the spread of literacy in the nineteenth century a good number of working-class people were recording their lives (Vincent, 1981). The 1960s and 1970s were periods of countercultural activity and many communities in Britain had seen the growth of an alternative press enabled by cheaper printing technologies. New collectively organized local newspapers appeared and, at the time of the formation of the FWWCP, cooperatives were producing other local publications (Aubrey *et al.*, 1980; Berry *et al.*,1980; Morley and Worpole, 1982). Some of these cooperatives served a range of local writing groups, for example Bristol Broadsides, while others formed around specific writing projects, as often happened in QueenSpark, for example Osmond (1995).

Community publications take many forms from poetry, cookbooks and educational resources to community history and cultural products such as theatre and other performance. The groups involved are diverse. While Survivors' Poetry and its individual member groups are mental health user led community publishers (Smith and Burgieres, 1996), publications around the world have been developed by black writers, adult education students, disabled and homeless people (Lindsay, 1992; Madariaga *et al.*, 2001; Lorenzo *et al.*,2002; Calais DAL, 2004).

FWWCP writers were very conscious of their cultural difference with mainstream, received pronunciation, middle-class Englishness. The contributors to a key FWWCP text, *The Republic of Letters* (Morley and Worpole, 1982) did not wholly reject highbrow literature and culture, but they distanced themselves from it because it did not reflect their lived experience. In a subsequent reflection on the experience of producing The Republic of Letters the two leading editors felt that popular culture had since become more accommodating of the cultural values and experiences of ordinary people (Morley *et al.*, 2009). Class was always a contentious issue in the set of similarities and differences shared by people across the diverse FWWCP group memberships. Morley and Worpole (1982) acknowledge a certain dissatisfaction with the limitations implied by 'worker writers' in the full FWWCP title. When the network lost funding and had to regroup in 2008 as TheFED, the 'worker' was dropped, while 'community publishers' was retained. Community was something that was frequently extended by the FWWCP to other marginalized groups, such as *middle-class* black writers from the Caribbean (Courtman, 2000, 2007). The sense of being 'working class' was increasingly blurred as a consequence, and its blurring sometimes hotly contested (Woodin, 2005a, 2005c, 2007).

The personal stories in anthologies such as Bristol Lives (Bristol Broadsides, 1987), *More Bristol Lives* (Bristol Broadsides, 1988), or the two Centerprise anthologies of *Working Lives* (n.d.; 1979), published in Hackney, are some of the many examples of this connection of lived experience with place. Such narratives are expressions of the occupational identities afforded by the local environment or social conditions. Authors wrote about the things that happened to them, or their observations on the community around them. Some of the authors, such as Fred Moss (1986), also wrote longer autobiographies, and the range in the anthologies is not atypical of the range of prose produced by similar writers in other groups. The Bristol Broadsides anthologies (1987, 1988) contain pieces varying in length from a page to a few pages in which people describe scenes from their childhood, their present working or family life, experiences in the psychiatric system, or their part in particular events in the local history of the city. This intense relationship to context is evidenced in descriptions of details that are significant to a particular audience who share something of having origins in the same community, or living through the same times.

The narratives used language which was more spoken than written and carries inflexions of dialect, more usually indicated in reported speech or in the choice of particular words rather than the conscious attempt to capture the sound of dialect English through altered spelling. The varieties of dialect would become apparent when something was read aloud to an audience, as this kind of writing frequently was. The FWWCP stressed the significance of everyone's voice (FWWCP, 2006 1.1). This meant that an audience had to listen for and appreciate the context of the production of writing as a part of the content. While many people were assured performers, others often struggled to read their work, sometimes having to have others read it with them. I have even seen people 'perform' their material by playing a cassette recording, standing and holding the cassette machine to receive their applause. These approaches are ways that people who experience learning difficulties, low personal confidence or difficulty with reading or speaking can share live narratives with an audience.

Sometimes these changes are evident in the text. Louise Shore (1982) begins her book with a hesitant voice in the progress of acquiring literacy, increasing in confidence as she progresses. Autobiographical writing did not always take the form of prose, many people preferring to write poetry because it is a form of writing that can be developed around other daily occupations, as Pat Dallimore expressed in her poem 'Shush, Mum's writing!' (Morley and Worpole, 1982: 89). As some of the other selections of FWWCP writing in Morley and Worpole show, whereas most people indicated dialect through slight variations in spelling and vocabulary, Black poets frequently wrote in patois.

These communities of writing therefore were both about a peripherality or Other space, which was outside a mainstream cultural representation and at the same time located in a space that was very much a part of common experience. Social class is one the arbiters of this paradoxical positioning, outside a dominant middle-class culture and yet underpinning it through its labour and its location in the socioeconomic spectrum. The spatial otherness described in this writing about the everyday life of ordinary people, disconnected and yet connected through a continuous poetry of everyday life (Vaniegem, 1983) is in a marginal place of what both Soja (1996) and Wilcock (2006) have termed being and becoming, from which both groups and individuals have asserted their belonging. FWWCP authors quietly challenge the dominant excluding cultural perspectives with narratives of ordinary people doing everyday things in the geographical, historical and social community spaces of our present society (Morley *et al.*, 2009).

These occupations, such as that of Dallimore writing at the kitchen sink, are neither unfamiliar nor uninteresting, and wherever they are located they are instantly recognizable to audiences with a similar experience of class, yet much community publishing goes unread and unexplored. Szczelkun (1997: 5) suggests that much of this material is 'filtered out' by the middle-class values of publishers and editors, and we might contend by extension, other authors, facilitators and therapists. Barris *et al.* (1986) argue another issue, that occupational therapists' choice of treatment media is influenced most by their previous interests or exposure to activities during training; most occupational therapists lack an arts background and so therefore do not anticipate these interests in the approaches they develop with clients. Therapeutic writing remains part of contemporary occupational therapy practice (Philips *et al.*, 1999) but the once-ubiquitous Adana 85 printing machine (Hume, 1990) is no longer seen in psychiatric occupational therapy departments. Any publication would require a number of permissions before it could be issued, and these may be offputting. In my own experience so much time elapsed between putting together one client-produced magazine and obtaining permission for its distribution that the people involved lost interest.

The numbers of people who participated in writing arts activities varied around the UK – 4% in Wales and 16% in Yorkshire (Matarasso, 1997). Much writing may be hidden. The FWWCP experience is that it is common to find diaries or manuscripts in people's effects on their death, and some of these have indeed been subsequently published, for example Harris (1978) and Wren (1998). My collection of this writing contains thousands of individual pieces contributed by thousands of writers in magazines and anthologies as well as single-authored books. The FWWCP was only one of a number writers workshops networks, many organized regionally, such as the Merseyside Association of Writers Workshops (at least 24 workshops) and South Yorkshire Writers (40 workshops and writing classes), which existed in the late 1980s and early 1990s. These produced their own range of publications and could also represent large numbers of local people.

Community Publishing, Occupational Narratives and Occupational Science

My involvement in the FWWCP predated my training as an occupational therapist in the 1980s. The professional focus on the individual in clinical practice seemed to me to miss a significant connection between the individual with a critical understanding of the community. Consequently FWWCP practices in the creation, publication and performance of occupational narratives strongly influenced my position in discussing a social justice agenda in the occupational therapy profession, particularly the emerging role of negotiating needs and working with community groups (Pollard and Kronenberg, 2008; Pollard, Kronenberg and Sakellariou, 2008; Pollard, Sakellariou and Kronenberg, 2009; Parks and Pollard, 2009). These perspectives have not, so far, critically addressed the assumptions of the profession, and indeed of occupational science concerning occupation (Leibing, 2010). One of the concerns that Leibing (2010) raises is that the adoption of techniques such as writing therapeutically about everyday experience is that they become 'psychologized', made into a problem and given a focus that they do not really have. Indeed, as may be suggested by some the aspects of the community publishing movement, the dropping of the 'worker' definition and the importance of simple exchange of experiences, this is as much true for the development of an intrusive 'therapeutic perspective' as it seems to be for one based in class politics. Writing and publishing practices in the community are perceived within the movement represented by TheFED and FWWCP as expressive actions that celebrate the right to cultural dissemination (for example, FWWCP 2006: 1.1) and *not* merely 'therapeutic'. It is not the therapeutic element that this chapter addresses but whether the consciousness derived from the exploration of people's autobiographical narratives has something to offer to a critical occupational perspective. *The Republic of Letters* (Morley and Worpole, 1982) was a sharp response from the FWWCP to the work of its members being dismissed as 'therapeutic' by the then Arts Council of Great Britain. Even despite subsequent prolonged support from the Arts Council of England until 2007 this dismissal remained contentious. Many of the members of the FWWCP and TheFED felt, and still feel, themselves to be sustaining and developing opportunities and activities in order to facilitate others without any notion of 'recovery' (Pollard, 2010).

Confidentiality is a key issue with respect to the use of writing in therapeutic contexts, not only of the person doing the writing who may perhaps wish later to retract things they have published while disturbed but also with respect to other people who may be being written about. This is raised early on by Morley and Worpole (1982), where examples are given of relatives who were unhappy about aspects of their family life being published in an author's book. Goldblatt (2007) similarly describes situations where communities have been unhappy about their presentation in a local publication and yet one of the purposes of representing communities in this way is to redress a sense of imbalance in profile, an invisibility, which gives rise to marginalization. The FWWCP's therapy debate exemplifies the way in which elites dismiss and make 'other' the experiences of cultures which are unlike themselves.

Whether the communities of writing which developed into organizations like the FWWCP were a true expression of the experiences of the working class unmediated by intrusive sociologists or social reformers can be contested, in as much as there were many people involved, such as myself, from a middle-class background. Other people became professional writers as a result of the grounding they received in FWWCP workshops and so entered the middle classes. The 'working-class' expressionism became increasingly diluted over time. However, as Woodin (2005a, 2005b, 2005c, 2007, 2009) shows, there were also very strong elements of working class leadership. This class based sense of identity as an organization of 'worker writers' was largely identified through an engagement with writing about what people did, and was differentiated from a perhaps prejudiced impression that the majority of writers were either dead or concerned with the comfortable lives of the middle class. This might be debatable. The nineteenth and twentieth century were periods in which various forms of socialist novel or novels about working class social conditions flourished, through well known writers such as Charles Dickens, Emile Zola, D. H. Lawrence, Lewis Grassic Gibbon, Walter Greenwood, Catherine Cookson, Barry Hines, Stan Barstow, Nell Dunn and Keith Waterhouse to name but a few, many of whom wrote through direct experience. Some of the autobiographical forerunners of contemporary community publication might be Kitchen ([1940] 1982), Reynolds ([1908] 1982), Thompson ([1945] 1973), and Williams ([1915] 1984 and 1981). Other writers' work was more overtly politically committed, such as that by Len Doherty and Lewis Jones. However, with the exception of Dickens and Hines these writers rarely turn up in the school experience of literature education, and in the experience of the older FWWCP members literature was taught as a remote subject (Morley and Worpole, 1982). The difference the experience of the worker writer group brought was that writers and readers could affirm each others' experiences and learn from each other, to the extent that groups developed their own pedagogies (Morley and Worpole, 1982; Woodin, 2005a, 2005c, 2007, 2008, 2009).

Writing and Consciousness

As an organization the FWWCP claimed the purpose of generating a consciousness of a broadly working-class culture, an aim stated in its constitution, and influenced by some members reading of Freire's (1972) *Pedagogy of the Oppressed* and his explanation of conscientization – a critical social awareness, which resulted from dialogue, a way to 'read' and analyse social phenomena. In such a diverse network of people, however, the sense of this was diluted. Nonetheless, at a more fundamental level, the majority of people in the writing groups seemed to come because they enjoyed meeting each other and exchanging their experiences (Pollard, 2010). Through sharing narratives and being aware of the stories of other group members people could find common ground. Sometimes this is evident in the writing.

Carter (1992) refers to Manville's (1989) autobiography in his evocation of child-hood on a neighbouring street in Brighton. *Jackie's Story* ('Jackie', 1984) was pushed through the door of Centerprise because the anonymous author knew that the bookshop published autobiographical work by local people.

The recognition of commonalities across diversity is a powerful experience, although the extent to which it is sustained depends very much on its being matched with resources and organizational abilities. The FWWCP, like many other commu-nity-based and working-class organizations, was composed of small groups whose existence was precarious. The group I convened regularly experienced declines in membership, which could result in a turnout of two or three people over a month or so, especially during the summer. It was able to continue to use the local community centre for nothing because the presence of the group was thought to deter youths from vandalizing it on quiet Sunday evenings, otherwise it would not have been possible to afford to rent the room to continue meetings. Groups can be prone to a range of circumstances, which cause them to fold up such as loss of membership interest, disagreement, being overwhelmed with the tasks associated with publica-tion, or losing access to the room in which they meet. Despite this people sustain their interest; they might leave one group and turn up in another, sometimes in other parts of the country. The development of TheFED has meant an influx of new people to the movement that began with the FWWCP, but others remain from previous times. A major influence in the development of the FWWCP was its encounter with the survivors poetry movement, which affiliated in the early 1990s and soon came to be strongly represented in its leadership (Pollard and Clayton, in press).

Can Do: Affirmation and Participation

One shift in thinking about literacy has been to move away from earlier ideas of *illiteracy* to emphasize what people *can* do rather than on what they can't, ultimately to express themselves through publication. Mace (1996: 69–70), in talking about publication by literacy students advocates the practice of student publication against the ideas that:

- literacy is about 'other peoples' power' (p. 69);
- authors of texts in any public arena are 'other people';
- literacy students would only be concerned with the writing of reaction to others' demands (the proper way to write letters, fill in questions on printed forms, etc.);
- that literacy students have a deficit in their own intellectual and expressive abilities, and that this is their fault;
- 'literacy was only a small part of themselves . . . literacy means schooling . . . being literate is only about being schooled' (p. 70).

Many of these claims have potential application in other situations, for example mental health, where self esteem and confidence is compromised by disabling experiences. Freire's (1985) concern in developing literacy was not merely teaching the mechanistic ability to read and write, but to employ these skills in expressing democratic participation, in utopian liberation. Community publication activities frequently offer opportunities for people to gain in self-confidence and to recognize their own capacities as writers through the demystification of the writing and publishing process (Morley and Worpole, 1982; Pollard, 2010). They can also be vehicles for an oppositional voice (Szczelkun, 1997; Dunlap, 2007), more, perhaps, about the entertainments of folk humour and human values rather than ideology, that Bakhtin (1984: 474) calls 'pure unmixed expression . . . [of] a chorus of laughing people.' A large part of the experience is simply people enjoying writing these things because they want to say something about who they have been and who they are now, in their community (Vincent, 1981; Goldblatt, 2007).

Thus writing and community publishing, like other forms of art, is an expression of being-in-the-world (Camus, 1971; Kristeva, 1984). In Sumsion's (1999) discussion of client-centred practice, these ideas would appear to be coherent with the occupational and performance components of the model of human occupation (both feeling productive and expressing one's beliefs about the meaning of life). They also connect with the recent ethnographic and autoethnographic research methods of increasing relevance to health professions (Taylor, 2008; Muncey, 2010). These are means by which the social value of personal experiences are recognized by others. An early example was Life Story Work, where clients with learning difficulties were enabled to produce video, tape and booklets to ease their transition into the community from hospital by enabling them to communicate their individual narratives to new staff (Hewitt *et al.*, 1997). Since then digital storytelling, which has been developed with a far wider range of participants. Burgess (2006: 1) has called this facility for people who might hitherto have been media consumers to generate their own media 'vernacular creativity', a means through which people can participate in new forms of citizenship.

Perhaps disparities in wealth and power are unlikely to be seriously threatened by accessible digital technologies, which are themselves produced by major global corporations. However, the sense that one's experiences are socially valued can produce a conscientization. This doesn't necessarily require a technology but can also develop through the exchange of writer and listener roles in the publishing group (Long, 2007). Writing workshops in health service settings need not take the form of 'therapy' but still have the objectives of experiencing ownership of an organization and decision making, which can also be applied in independent community venues, something Silcock (1998a: 4) terms 'enabling practice'.

Freeing individual expression from the constraints of therapy can be important in encouraging other health benefits and pleasures (Silcock, 1998b), for example in exercising the ability to challenge others appropriately and negotiate the rules of the group. Different members of a writing group with learning difficulties in Grimsby varied in their individual ability to discuss and challenge aspects of the formation of a group project about which they were unclear or disagreed. As a collective group they were able take on and confront some issues, for example about their representation by others. Copies of all publications were shared with the group members, and while the language was often not accessible, time was made to explain what was being said, why their work was significant, and also for the researcher to simply participate in the group activities as a fellow member (Pollard, Smart and Voices Talk and Hands Write, 2005; Pollard, 2007; Pollard and Voices Talk and Hands Write, 2008). These measures are never entirely satisfactory, because the interpretation and presence remains an issue of professional power, responses to it reflect clients or users' perceptions of the health professionals' or researchers' expectations of them. Using writing as therapy threatens the writers capacity as cultural participants to negotiate identity and choice and be *authors of their own lives* (Clayburn, 1998; Natzler, 1998; Silcock, 1998a, 1998b; Philips *et al.*, 1999).

Occupational therapy has to operate in a culturally diverse society, with complex interrelations between individuals and their environments in terms of ethnicity, class and education (Pollard, Kronenberg and Sakellariou, 2008). Marginalized peoples' activities in determining their own needs and solutions may question some of the values and obligations, such as notions of 'citizenship', which are group or social demands (Philips *et al.*, 1999; Pitcock, 2000). Therapists may need to challenge themselves and the assumptions about the therapeutic value of the activities they engage in against the wider social picture, particularly so where disability is considered as a cultural response to impaired functioning in individuals where the terms are established through professional authority rather than those people who actually experience the conditions (Marks, 1999; Snyder and Mitchell, 2006). For example, a therapy programme including occupational opportunities such as voluntarism merely enables clients to 'hang with the normals' (Rebeiro and Allen, 1998: 283), thereby achieving social *acceptance*, but the social onus is that of a minority having to conform with a social majority. These forms of normalization offer vestigial integration without according equal rights (Snyder and Mitchell, 2006). Siebers (2008) suggests that the challenge lies in the fact that disability is normal, that the disabled person is neither more nor less real than someone who is nondisabled, and the challenge of cultural practices is to explain things as they are, rather than representations of something else. This is not dissimilar to the intentions of many of those involved in community publishing.

This returns us to the ideas with which we began. Writing and publication are areas long associated with maintaining identity and purpose against social and political marginalization (Davis, 1991). Rebeiro and Allen (1998) argue that the benefits of activities geared to preserve social identity may depend on not 'coming out' (p. 283) with one's mental illness, but preserving 'identity control' (p. 285). Kristeva (1984) suggests that categorization into either *madness* or *art* is a negation of the value of expression, since neither has to be taken seriously. Survivor poets aim to assert their reason through 'celebration, pride and unity' (Smith and Burguieres, 1996: 4), i.e. as themselves. Community publishing offers a vehicle for people to be 'doers and writers', not 'sitters and watchers' (Froom, 1985: 73). Community publishing and the practices of worker writing have enabled people to emerge through the written word and through publication stand witness for themselves (Ragon, 1986; Smith and Burguieres, 1996).

For the occupational therapist or scientist one vehicle for this may be autoethnography, although it is not without similar dangers to those we have explored in community publishing. Should the inner experiences of the author, perhaps an occupational therapist writing be privileged over those written about? Ethical committees have sometimes sided with the family against the publication of life story-based research (Rolph, 1998). In the small geographical spread of community publishing audiences family members have sometimes voiced suspicions about writing and strong objections to publications that may portray them to others (Morley and Worpole, 1982). Many authors prefer pseudonyms, anonymity (Morley and Worpole, 1982), or, as is evident from many survivor's anthologies, use the opportunity to construct new poetic identities.

Nonetheless community publishing may offer a means of linking social, civil and political dimensions of engagement (Roche, 1992; Szczelkun, 1997). While reciprocal relationships appear to feature prominently in its operation, the focus is on cultural expression, the production and promotion of an emancipatory literacy and history (e.g. Szczelkun, 1997). While there is a sense of mutually achieving social obligations to create, work or produce, in a diverse and accessible social and political community arena (Roche, 1992; Kymlicka, 1995; Myers *et al.*, 1998), there is a keen emphasis on answering the needs of the individual as a creator of verbal expression in a society of voices (Bakhtin, 1981; Morley and Worpole, 1982; Smith and Burgieres, 1996). In these respects, and as we have discussed earlier in the chapter, community publishing practice apparently shares similar terms and has strong parallels with occupational therapy in 'client-centredness'. In a wider set of occupation-based (rather than therapy-based) perspectives community writing and publishing may be a form of activity that people can develop to their own ends for a social awareness along a spectrum from enjoyment through to critical reflection and argument.

References

Aubrey, C., Landry, C., Morley, D. (1980) *Here is the Other News*. London, Comedia.

Bahktin, M. (1981) *The Dialogic Imagination*. Trans. C. Emerson, M. Holquist. Austin, University of Texas.

Bahktin, M. (1984) *Rabelais and his World*. Trans. H. Iswolsky. Bloomington, Indiana University Press.

Barris, R., Cordero, J., Christiaansen, R. (1986) Occupational therapists' use of media. *American Journal of Occupational Therapy* 40(10), 679–684.

Berry, C., Cooper, L., Landry, C. (1980) *Where is the Other News*. London: Comedia.

Blake, J. (1977) *Memories of Old Poplar*. London, Stepney Books.

Bristol Broadsides (1987) *Bristol Lives*. Bristol: Bristol Broadsides.

Bristol Broadsides (1988) *More Bristol Lives*. Bristol: Bristol Broadsides.

Bromley, R. (1988) *Lost Narratives, Popular Fictions, Politics and Recent History*. London, Routledge.

Burgess, J. (2006) *Re-mediating Vernacular Creativity : Digital Storytelling*, http//:eprints. qut.edu.au/3776/1/3376.pdf,. accessed 12 October 2010.

Calais DAL (2004) *Calais dal*. Roubaix, Editions Sansonnet.

Camus, A. (1971) *The Rebel*. Harmondsworth, Penguin.

Carter, D. (1992) *Just One of a Large Family*. Brighton, QueenSpark.

Centerprise (ed.) (n.d.) *Working Lives Volume One: 1905–45*. Hackney, Hackney WEA/ Centerprise.

Centerprise (ed.) (1979) *Working Lives Volume Two: People's Autobiography of Hackney 1945–77*. Hackney, Hackney WEA/Centerprise.

Clark, J., Kane, D., Wilding, K., Wilton, J. (2010) *UK Civil Society Almanac 2010*. London, National Council for Voluntary Organisations.

Clayburn, A. (1998) Letter. *Lapidus News* 6, 1–2.

Courtman, S. (2000) Frierian Liberation, Cultural Transaction and Writing from 'The Working Class and the Spades', *The Society for Caribbean Studies Annual Conference Papers*, www.caribbeanstudies.org.uk/papers/vol1.htm, accessed 12 October 2010.

Courtman, S. (2007) 'Culture is ordinary': the legacy of the Scottie Road and Liverpool 8 Writers. In M. Murphy, D. Rees-Jones (eds) *Writing Liverpool: Essays and Interviews*. Liverpool, Liverpool University Press, pp. 194–209.

Davis, A. (1991) Users' perspectives. In S. Ramon, M. G. Giannichedda (eds) *Psychiatry in Transition, 2nd edition*. London, Pluto, pp. 32–40.

Diggles, T. (2006) Foreword. *Federation 30th Anniversary Special*. Stoke on Trent, FWWCP, p. 1.

Dunlap, L. (2007) *Undoing the Silence: Six Tools for Social Change Writing*. Oakland, CA, New Village Press.

Fieldhouse, R. (1977) *The Workers' Educational Association: Aims and Achievements, 1903-1977*. Syracuse, NY, Syracuse University.

Freire, P. (1972) *The Pedagogy of the Oppressed*. Harmondsworth, Penguin.

Freire, P. (1985) *The Politics of Education*. Trans. D. Macedo. New York, Bergin & Garvey.

Froom, W. (1985) Old Swan Writers' Workshop. In B. Baker, N. Harvey (eds) *Publishing for the People*. London, London Labour Library, pp. 71–74.

FWWCP, (1985) *Once I was a Washing Machine*. London, FWWCP.

FWWCP (2006) Constitution. http://fedonline.org/fed/documents/Constitution%202006. pdf, accessed 11 October 2010.

Goldblatt, E. (2007) *Because We Live Here: Sponsoring Literacy beyond the College Curriculum*. Creskill, NJ, Hampton Press.

Hamer, J. (n.d.) *Running Away from Home*. Manchester, Gatehouse.

Harris, H. (1978) *Under Oars*. Hackney, Centerprise.

Healey, B. (1980) *Hard Times and Easy Terms*. Brighton, QueenSpark.

Heath, S. B. (1983) *Ways with Words: Language, Life, and Work in Communities and Classrooms*. Cambridge, Cambridge University Press.

Hewitt, C., Branton, P., Dunn, J., Willcocks, A. (1997) Life story work: issues and applications for learning disabled people undergoing transition from hospital to community based settings. *Journal of Learning Disabilities for Nursing Health and Social Care* 1(3), 105–109.

Hollick, B. (1991) *Pullman Attendant*. Brighton, QueenSpark.

Hume, C. A. (1990) Rehabilitation. In J. Creek,(ed.) *Occupational Therapy and Mental Health*. Edinburgh, Churchill Livingstone, pp. 333–348.

'Jackie' (1984) *Jackie's Story*. Hackney, Centerprise.

Kitchen, F. ([1940]1982) *Brother to the Ox*. Harmondsworth, Penguin.

Kristeva, J. (1984 [1974]) *Revolution in Poetic Language*. Trans. Margaret Waller. New York, Columbia University Press.

Kymlicka, W. (1995) *Multicultural Citizenship*. Oxford, Clarendon Press.

Leibing, A. (2010) Looking over the neighbor's fence: occupational therapy as an inspiration for (medical) anthropology. *Ethos* 38(2), 1–8.

Lindsay, A. (ed.) (1992) *Wrestling with an Octopus:* Stories from the Collingwood Housing Estates. Collingwood, Australia, Dight Street Tenants Council.

Long, E. (2007) *Community Literacy and the Rhetoric of Local Publics.* West Lafayette, IN, Parlor Press.

Lorenzo, T., Sanders, L., January, M., Mdlokolo, P. (2002) *On the Road of Hope: Stories by Disabled Women in Khayelitsa.* Cape Town, Disabled People South Africa, Zanepilo Disability Project, University of Cape Town.

Mace, J. (ed.) (1995) *Literacy, Language and Community Publishing.* Clevedon, Multilingual Matters.

Mace, J. (1996) The significance of student writing. In S. Fitzpatrick, J. Mace (eds) *Lifelong Literacies.* Manchester, Gatehouse Books, pp. 67–70.

Madariaga, C.A., Guajardo, A.C., Ramirez, M., Castro, O. (2001) *Neruda y el Norte Grande: del paisaje telurico al hombre.* Iquique, Fondadis.

Manville, S. (1989) *Everything Seems Smaller.* Brighton, QueenSpark.

Marks, D. (1999) *Disability.* London, Routledge.

Matarasso, F. (1997) *Use or Ornament: The Social Impact of Participation in the Arts.* Stroud, Comedia.

Morley, D., Worpole, K. (eds) (1982) *The Republic of Letters.* London, Comedia.

Morley, D., Worpole, K., Pollard, N. (2009) Class identity and the republics of letters. In D. Morley, K. Worpole (eds) *The Republic of Letters,* 2nd edn. Philadelphia, PA, New Cities Community Press/Syracuse University Press, p. 223–244.

Moss, F. (1986) *City Pit.* Bristol, Bristol Broadsides.

Muckle, W. (1981) *No Regrets.* Newcastle upon Tyne, People's Publications.

Muncey, T. (2010) *Creating Autoethnographies.* Los Angeles, Sage.

Myers, F., Ager, A., Kerr, P., Myles, S. (1998) Outside looking in? Studies of the community integration of people with learning disabilities. *Disability and Society* 13(3), 389–413.

Natzler, C. (1998) Letter. *Lapidus News* 6, pp. 2–3.

Newman, T., Curtis, K., Stephens. J. (2001) *Do Community-based Arts Projects Result in Social Gains? A Review of Literature,* www.barnardos.org.uk/commarts.pdf, accessed 11 October 2010.

Noakes, D. (1980a) *The Town Beehive – A Young Girl's Lot, Brighton 1910–1934.* Brighton, QueenSpark.

Noakes, D. (1980b) *Faded Rainbow, Our Married Years.* Brighton, QueenSpark.

Noakes, G. (1977) *To Be A Farmer's Boy.* Brighton, QueenSpark.

Osmond, N. (1995) Life after stroke: special interest book-writing groups. In M. Stuart, A. Thomson,(eds) *Engaging with Difference.* Leicester, NIACE, pp. 173–186.

Parks, S., Pollard, N. (2009) The extra-curricular of composition: a dialogue on community publishing. *Community Literacy Journal* 3(2), 53–77.

Paul, A. (1981a) *Poverty-Hardship but Happiness, Those Were the Days 1903–1917.* Brighton, QueenSpark.

Paul, A. (1981b) *Hard Work and No Consideration, 51 Years as a Carpenter-Joiner 1917–1968.* Brighton, QueenSpark.

Philips, D., Linington, L., Penman, D. (1999) *Writing Well: Creative Writing and Mental Health.* London, Jessica Kingsley.

Pitcock, R. L. (2000), 'Let the youths beware!' The sponsorship of early nineteenth century Native American literacy. *Written Communication* 17(3), 390–426.

Pollard, N. (2007) Voices Talk, Hands Write: sustaining community publishing with people with learning difficulties. *Groupwork* 17(2), 36–56.

Pollard, N. (2010) *The Federation (TheFED): A Network of Writers and Community Publishers. An Evaluative Report,* www.thefed.btck.co.uk/Media/29/Nick%20Pollard%20Research%20Papers/TheFEDevaluation25.5.10.pdf, accessed 12 October 2010.

Pollard, N., Kronenberg, F. (2008), Working with people on the margins. In J. Creek, L. Lougher (eds) *Occupational Therapy in Mental Health,* 4th edn, Oxford, Elsevier Science, pp. 557–577.

Pollard, N., Kronenberg, F., Sakellariou, D. (2008) A political practice of occupational therapy. In N. Pollard, D. Sakellariou, F. Kronenberg (eds) *A Political Practice of Occupational Therapy.* Edinburgh, Elsevier Science, pp 3–20.

Pollard, N., Parks, S. (2010) Community publishing: occupational narratives and 'local publics'. In F. Kronenberg, N. Pollard, D. Sakellariou (eds) *Occupational Therapies without Borders.* Edinburgh, Elsevier/Churchill Livingstone.

Pollard, N., Sakellariou, D., Kronenberg, F (2008) (eds), *A Political Practice of Occupational Therapy,* Edinburgh, Elsevier Science.

Pollard, N., Sakellariou, D., Kronenberg, F. (2009) Community development. In M. Molineux, M. Curtin, J. Supyk (eds) *Occupational Therapy in Physical Dysfunction,* 6th edn. Oxford, Elsevier Science, pp. 267–280.

Pollard, N., Smart, P., Voices Talk and Hands Write (2005) Voices Talk and Hands Write. In Kronenberg, F., Simo Algado, S., Pollard, N. (eds) *Occupational Therapy without Borders – Learning from the Spirit of Survivors.* Edinburgh, Elsevier Science, pp. 287–301.

Pollard, N., Voices Talk, Hands Write (2008) Voices Talk, Hands Write. In E. Crepeau, E. Cohn, B. Boyt Schell (eds) *Willard and Spackman's Occupational Therapy,* 11th edn. Philadelphia, Lipincott Williams & Wilkins, pp. 139–145.

Ragon, M. (1986) *Histoire de la littérature prolétarienne de langue française.* Paris, Albin Michel.

Rebeiro, K. L., Allen, J. (1998) Voluntarism as occupation. *Canadian Journal of Occupational Therapy* 65(5), 279–285.

Roche, M. (1992), *Rethinking Citizenship.* Cambridge, Polity.

Rolph, S. (1998), Ethical dilemmas in historical research with people with learning difficulties. *British Journal of Learning Disabilities* 26, 135–139.

Ross, E. (1984) *Tales of the Rails.* Bristol, Bristol Broadsides.

Shore, L. (1982) *Pure Running, A Life Story.* Hackney, Hackney Reading Centre.

Siebers, T. (2008) *Disability Theory.* Ann Arbor, University of Michigan Press.

Silcock, A. (1998a) Writing for health – avoiding therapy. *Lapidus News* 6, p. 4.

Silcock, A. (1998b) Implications of 'enabling practice' for writers working with people with mental health difficulties. *Lapidus News* 6, pp. 4–5.

Smith, A., Burguieres, M. (1996) *National Jamboree '96 Report.* London, Survivors' Press.

Snyder, S. L., Mitchell, D. T. (2006) *Cultural Locations of Disability.* Chicago, The University of Chicago Press.

Soja, E.W. (1996) *Thirdspace, journeys to Los Angeles and other real-and-imagined places.* Malden, MA, Blackwell.

Sumsion, T. (1999) Overview of client-centered practice. In T. Sumsion (ed.) *Client-Centered Practice in Occupational Therapy: A Guide to Implementation.* Edinburgh, Churchill Livingstone, pp. 1–12.

Szczelkun, S. (1997), *Working Press 1987-1997 Ten Years of an Umbrella Imprint for Working Class Artists Who Wished to Self-publish.* London, wORking Press.

Taylor, J. (2008) An autoethnographic exploration of an occupation: doing a PhD. *British Journal of Occupational Therapy* 71(5), 176–184.

Thompson, F. ([1945] 1973) *Lark Rise to Candleford*. Harmondsworth, Penguin.

Vaneigem, R. (1983) *The revolution of everyday life*. D. Nicholson-Smith (trans.). London, Left Bank Books/Rebel Press

Vincent, D. (1981) *Bread, Knowledge and Dreedom, A Study of Nineteenth-Century Working Class Autobiography*. London, Europa Publications.

Wheway, E. (1984) *Edna's Story, Memories of Life in a Children's Home and in Service in Dorset and London*. Wimborne, Words and Action.

Wilcock, A. A. (2006) *An Occupational Perspective of Health*. Thorofare, NJ, Slack.

Wolveridge, J. (1981) *Ain't it Grand (Or 'This was Stepney')* London, Journeyman.

Woodin, T. (2005a) Building culture from the bottom up: the educational origins of The Federation of Worker Writers and Community Publishers. *History of Education* 34, 345–363.

Woodin, T. (2005b) 'More writing than welding': learning in worker writer groups. *History of Education* 39(5), 551–567.

Woodin, T. (2005c) Muddying the waters: class and identity in a working-class cultural organization. *Sociology* 39(5), 1001–1018.

Woodin, T. (2007) 'Chuck out the teacher:' radical pedagogy in the community. *International Journal of Lifelong Education* 26(1), 89–104.

Woodin, T. (2008) 'A beginner reader is not a beginner thinker': student publishing in Britain since the 1970s. *Pedagogica Historica* 44(1–2) 219–232.

Woodin, T. (2009) Working-class writing, alternative publishing and audience participation. *Media Culture Society* 31(1), 79–96.

Wren, T. (1998) *Flying Sparks*. Brighton, QueenSpark.

12 Disability, Sexuality and Intimacy

Pamela Block, Russell Shuttleworth, Jacob Pratt, Hope Block and Linda Rammler

Overview

In this chapter we will discuss theoretical perspectives on sexuality and disability and how these relate to occupational therapy research, scholarship, practice and politics. We will discuss two autistic people who are in love and wish to be together and the negotiations, politics and policies that shape their experience of dating and intimacy. Disability shapes their experiences and occupations of sexuality and intimacy. Fulfilling their desire to be together is a time-consuming occupation not only for these two individuals but also for their families, support staff, and agency administration. What results is a complex tangle of supports and barriers, which must be collectively navigated to enable the intimate relationship's continued existence. Issues of access and the need for facilitation are central to their ability to living and loving as they choose. Our group of co-authors includes the autistic couple (Hope Block and Jacob Pratt) and Jacob's colleague Linda Rammler who is a consultant and researcher in the area of autism, with a background in special education and developmental psychology, and two anthropologists who work in occupational therapy programmes (the first author Pamela Block, who is Hope Block's sister, and the second author, Russell Shuttleworth).

Teaching Sexuality and Disability

It has been established that sex is an important life occupation and the activities of sexuality and intimacy rightly fall within the realm of studies of occupation and occupational therapy (Sakellariou, 2006a; Sakellariou and Sawada, 2006;

Politics of Occupation-Centred Practice: Reflections on Occupational Engagement across Cultures, First Edition. Edited by Nick Pollard and Dikaios Sakellariou.
© 2012 John Wiley & Sons, Ltd. Published 2012 by John Wiley & Sons, Ltd.

Sakellariou and Simó Algado, 2006a,b). The artificial binary of 'function' and 'dysfunction', so central to much of occupational therapy teaching, is rendered doubly problematic in the area of sexuality and intimacy, given the subjective nature of desire so fundamentally shaped by cultural contexts, beliefs, social structures, relations of power and individual preferences. For disabled people, the social realms of sexuality might be more complicated and difficult to navigate than the technical aspects of sex. Thus, as Sakellariou and Simó Algado (2006a) point out, OTs who become embroiled in details of positioning and energy conservation may be missing the point.

Editorials have mentioned that sexuality often does not play a prominent role in OT programme curriculae (Moores, 2008; Sengupta and Stubbs, 2008; Spencer and Wainwright, 2008). Penna and Sheehy (2000) suggest that only a minority of OTs provide sexual education as part of their practice. I (first author) have been teaching sexuality to third-year occupational therapy students for eight years. We do a series of readings and a film viewing on the topic, followed by discussions (Block *et al.*, 2005). We discuss the history of attitudes and policies concerning sexuality and disability in institutional settings such as nursing homes and psychiatric facilities as well as perceptions of family and community members. We discuss current policies and practices. We acknowledge that some people are uncomfortable discussing this subject but also the need to overcome personal discomfort in order to provide accurate information and support in this area. Every year students comment that this is an underrepresented area in their studies, yet also an area that many have encountered in various contexts during field work. The powerful nature of the topic was reinforced this year when one of my students chose it for her final project. Each year the students complete disability studies research posters as a final assignment and then participate at a juried poster session at the local Center for Independent Living (CIL). In addition to the judging, we have 'people's choice' awards based on popular vote (students, CIL staff and service recipients). In spring 2010, the poster on sexuality won by a landslide.

Historically, sexuality and disability were seen as a problem to be controlled by administrators within residential institutions (Block, 2000, 2002). In a basic example of occupational apartheid, disabled inmates were gender segregated and given little privacy or choice. Even now, the concept of sexuality as a human right is sometimes not respected as such within institutional settings or by clinicians working therein. A few years ago, one of my students commented that nursing homes were public spaces, and since sex in public spaces were prohibited, nursing home residents were forbidden to have sex. Other students have stated that their religious beliefs superseded institutional policies or client preferences. Fortunately, most students and practitioners have more nuanced perspectives. However, institutional settings meant (and still mean) increased vulnerability to sexual violence perpetrated by staff or other residents (Block, 2000). Disabled people living at home face the possibilities of overprotective parents, access barriers to finding partners, and attitudinal prejudice that they are either asexual perpetual children (parents) or hypersexual beings that are dangerous to have around (neighbours) (Shuttleworth and Sanders, 2010).

Students share stories about sexuality during fieldwork; they debate issues of informed consent and negotiating the feelings of family members and institutional policies. One told a story of two nursing-home residents with dementia who fell in love. She contrasted the heart-warming joy of the two people in love with the horror, anger and hurt of family members, including community-based spouses. Others discussed rules regarding (forbidden) sexuality in short-term psychiatric settings and how the residents flouted the rules. Others discussed hospital bedside conversations with people who had recent spinal cord injuries. Occupational therapists must be prepared for all these experiences and more. As informed practitioners we need to be aware of the diversity of sexuality and disability issues and the utility of employing diverse methodologies and conceptual frameworks for both research and practice. Different perspectives will be called for depending on the issue, and sometimes multiple perspectives will be necessary.

Theorizing Sexuality and Disability

Research in sexuality and disability still tends to be dominated by approaches that (1) perceive disabled people's sexuality as a problem to solve at the level of the individual; (2) are explicitly or implicitly concerned with treatment objectives; (3) focus on how individuals stack up on a scale of sexual functioning; and (4) view the issue of disabled sex in terms of physiological, psychological, social and relational norms derived from research with nondisabled people. This kind of research is obviously very useful for our practice with individual service recipients; however, its predominance has tended to marginalize many important everyday issues that disabled people bring up when talking about their sexual lives. It is imperative for us to be knowledgeable about the sociocultural and policy contexts that affect disabled people's everyday occupations, including that of their sexual lives.

A focus on individual function, of course is absolutely necessary at various moments in many disabled people's lives. For example, rehabilitation is crucial for those people who experience a spinal cord injury as they learn how to function, adapt and accommodate to their new physiological condition. Addressing sexual concerns is also paramount during this time and, as many researchers have argued, should be a crucial aspect in the rehabilitation process (Tepper, 1997). Thus, rehabilitation research on sexuality and intimacy for people with a range of impairments remains an important concern. Interestingly, a research focus on individual functioning does not always reinforce normative sexual practices. Using the example of the sexual rehabilitation of people with spinal cord injury again, some research with this population describes their loss of genital sensation and subsequent erotic investment in areas of the body that have retained sensory feeling (Whipple *et al.*, 1996), which shows them actually reconfiguring their relation to normative sexual functioning.

However, what are some of the important issues and perspectives that have been left out of the sexuality and disability research and by implication out of policy and practice – research that involves investigating the sociocultural and policy contexts, which can enlarge our understanding of the context of disabled people's sexual lives and can inform our practice? Several issues remain underresearched because they often make people uncomfortable – such as personal assistants or other care providers helping disabled people in some practical way to express themselves sexually (for example, buying condoms for a client, or positioning clients so they can masturbate or have sex with another disabled person). Another example of an underresearched area is the issue of some disabled people (mostly men) accessing or wanting to access sex worker services and the legal, cultural and other barriers they face when they try to do so. There has even been less research in non-Western societies on disabled people's sexual issues and the barriers that they sometimes face in trying to lead enjoyable and meaningful sexual lives. In a globalizing world, we are obliged to understand how people in other societies deal with these issues. In addition, when researchers plan research on sexuality and disability, disabled people are often not asked what the important issues are for them and/or are not included as co-researchers in some way. Finally, there has been a significant lack of theorization in sexuality and disability research, which has effectively resulted in a narrow view of our practice concerns. The effects that all this can have on our practice with clients is that certain sexuality and disability issues, therapeutic techniques and ways of looking at a particular problem appear to be cut and dried. Issues and perspectives of equal or greater significance can be neglected and maybe not even be perceived.

Research on Policy Context: The First Step in a More Progressive Practice

Ten years into the new millennium there is still a marked lack of innovative sociopolitical and cultural research in sexuality and disability – work that critically analyses social practices, public policies and cultural meanings and evaluates their impact on disabled people's sexual lives. Sociopolitical research that especially takes account of how local policies can affect disabled people's sexual lives is imperative (Shildrick, 2004; Abbot and Burns, 2007; Shuttleworth, 2007b). Policy contexts relating to such controversial issues as facilitated sex and sex work vary widely even among Western societies. For example, consider the vastly different policies concerning sex work and how this can affect disabled people's sexual access. Working as a personal assistant for physically disabled men for many years in the San Francisco Bay Area, I (second author) occasionally heard talk of some men's visits to sex workers, which was usually conveyed in hushed tones. This issue was not allowed to reach the level of public discourse because of the illegality of sex work in California. I occasionally facilitated access to sex workers for one of the disabled men who employed me and the risk involved in the situation was certainly palpable to us in terms of the often difficult process of making and maintaining reliable contacts among sex workers and their anxiety about being arrested (Shuttleworth, 2000).

In Sydney, Australia where I currently reside, sex work is decriminalized and the discourse around disabled people's access to sex worker services is public, with sex workers, disability organizations, social critics and disabled people all contributing their perspectives to the discussion. While there are still barriers to disabled people accessing sex worker services, these impediments are programmatic, attitudinal and architectural and not related to the legality of the service. However, those who attempt to research such issues as facilitated sex and access to sex worker services can encounter resistance from multiple sources including funding mechanisms, ethics committees, traditional disciplines and even some disabled people themselves.[1]

The issue of facilitated sex provides perhaps the best example of an issue that has been neglected in research and thus can be kept at arm's length in policy discussions and outside the purview of our practice. Facilitated sex is assistance with a sexual activity provided to a disabled client by a personal assistant (PA) or other provider. This assistance could include positioning the disabled person for masturbation or for sex with a partner, helping her or him undress, assisting with stimulation, transferring them to a bed or couch, transporting them to a partner's residence, purchasing condoms, or providing reminders about using birth control (Tepper, 2000; Mona, 2003). The assistance that I provided for my employer, which I described above, would also be included. To date, the United States still has no nationally based personal assistance services (PAS) programme and so services vary from state to state (Alice Wong, personal communication, 2 November 2010).

There are many pragmatic and ethical issues associated with facilitated sex in those situations in which the disabled person resides in a familial, an institutional, or a quasi-institutional setting such as a group home, or when s/he has no say in the decision of who provides their personal assistance services. Yet for those disabled people living independently in the community who control this decision and directly pay their PAs there are still a range of concerns. Most troubling is that there are no policy guidelines in place to govern sexual facilitation practice – meaning that negotiating this service with a PA is entirely up to the disabled person. Many disabled people, of course, might be reluctant to broach this subject with their PAs because of beliefs that one's sex life is a private affair and the value placed on doing things for oneself in this area (Shuttleworth, 2007b).

It is however risky to raise facilitated sex as a research and policy, and by implication practice, issue. Facilitated sex does indeed transgress the cultural view of sex as private and as an autonomous project of the self, and PAs who assist a client with sexual activity risk being seen as sexual participants and may be legally liable if payment occurs. Mona (2003) notes certain legal ramifications in her discussion of PAS in the United States, and Shildrick (2007) discusses similar legal issues relating to facilitated sex in the United Kingdom.[2] As I queried in a recent article,

Is it, then, better to leave this issue beneath the research, policy and practice radar so that only those disabled people who are bold and persuasive enough can negotiate

---

[1] Nevertheless, there is some research on facilitated sex for disabled people (Earle, 1999, 2001; Bonnie, 2002; Brown and Russell, 2005; Sanders, 2010) and disabled people's access to sex worker services (Sanders, 2007, 2010; Wotten and Isbister, 2010).

[2] Other issues that warrant concerns in regard to facilitated sex are the possibility of abuse of either the disabled person or the personal assistant, and especially for those providers from more professionalized services, the transgression of professional boundaries.

this kind of help privately with their assistants? Or should this issue be brought to the attention of researchers and policymakers with the possibility that conservative restrictions will be put in place that reflect mainstream culture's view of what constitutes a moral sexual encounter? (Shuttleworth, 2007b: 5)

Thus far, the ethical, practice and policy implications of facilitated sex have received minimal attention within research in the field.

Sexuality and Disability in Non-Western Societies

Another research issue that demands our attention as informed practitioners is how the sexuality of disabled people is viewed in other societies and any sexual health concerns that may arise. It is unfortunate that 90 per cent of research on sexuality and disability is still conducted in Western societies such as the US, UK and Canada (Shuttleworth, 2010). Those studies that do report information from non-Western societies mostly focus on disabled people's opportunities for marriage, which, while often relevant to sexual lives, cannot be considered equivalent to them (Fassin, 1991; Nicolaisen, 1995). Qualitative research attention should especially be drawn to the higher rates of STDs including HIV/AIDS in developed and especially developing countries (Groce, 2004, 2005) to enable us to understand the context, meaning and lived implications of these higher figures. Despite the limited cross-cultural research, there is growing evidence that just as in the West, disabled people's sexuality is devalued in many non-Western societies; the sexual lives of people with various impairments interacting with social institutions such as gender, marriage and class, may be restricted in various ways (Shuttleworth, 2004).

Recently Ingstad (2007) has problematized the concept of universal human rights and the agenda of the disability rights movement. She argues that cross-cultural researchers must take into account perspectives within the local context rather than assuming universal standards for human rights in relation to disabled people. One of her main points is that in the developing world where there is often rampant poverty, concepts such as independent living and accommodations for disabled people that are taken for granted in some Western societies, such as wheelchairs, may not be relevant or at least less immediately important than a more basic concern with the family's economic survival. She further cautions us not to impose forms of individualism onto the interpersonal relations of disabled people and nondisabled people in societies in which the response to disability may be more familial and communal. While Ingstad's point is crucial, we would caution against a too hasty assessment of integration within a society when further investigation may be warranted and suggest that an understanding of the dynamics of power relations should also be carried out. Godfrey Kangaude (2007) has examined the human and sexual rights contexts for disabled people in Malawi. He argues that sexual restrictions are implied, and in a sense, codified by policy documents and practice contexts, which minimize disabled people's need for sexual expression and leave it off the developmental agenda. It subsequently becomes a struggle to counter institutional precedence.

Sexual Access

Sexual access is a concept that has been employed in recent work and especially lends itself to an interrogation of the sociopolitical and cultural impediments to disabled people's sexual wellbeing (Hamilton, 2002; O'Toole, 2002; Shuttleworth and Mona, 2002; Wade, 2002; Grossman *et al.*, 2004; Kangaude, 2007; Shuttleworth, 2007a,b). In a broad sense, a research focus on disabled people's sexual access is concerned with both restrictive and inclusive aspects of sexual cultures. In terms of restriction, sexual access is not simply about physical access to negotiation contexts such as nightclubs but also includes aesthetic, psychological, symbolic, and social aspects embedded within these and other contexts of everyday life that work to deny disabled people sexual desire, desirability, relationships and wellbeing. Further, a focus on sexual access does not interrogate disabled people's sexual restrictions in terms of normative sexual identities, relations and practices, but can aim at illuminating a more inclusive access to 'sexual wellbeing' no matter its attributes/requirements. As Brown and Russell (2005) state, sexual wellbeing is 'conceptualised broadly as the capacity to enjoy and continue sexual behaviour in line with a personal and social ethic' (p. 376).

Opening the concept out in this way, links to heteronormative sexuality are severed. Of course, queers would experience forms of sexual oppression that heterosexuals do not and this aspect needs to be accounted for in any analysis (McRuer, 2006). In fact, it matters little how disabled people approach their sexuality: through culturally sanctioned, heteronormative avenues (e.g. dating, marriage); atypical (e.g. communal, BDSM)[3] and queer lifestyles; or ways of relating that emerge from their diverse socio-bodily situations (e.g. being provided personal care by a paid assistant during sexual encounters, incorporating spasticity into lovemaking) – these modalities can all nurture sexual wellbeing, provided the person can effectively contend with the specific constellation of barriers (both related to particular impairments, disability and any relevant intersections) that loom for them in the sexual domain. While this formulation will likely not satisfy those who require a thorough deconstruction and dissolution of identity intersections in order to 'envision a future in which there are no "dis/abled sexualities"' (Rembis, 2010: 56), it does provide a pragmatic, heuristic device for researchers to gauge the current sociosexual situations (degree of restriction or access to desired sexual contexts, interpersonal sexual situations, sexual and gender identities, sexual wellbeing and so forth) of people with a range of impairments.

Inclusion of Disabled People as Co-participants in Research, Writing, and Policy-Making

If we are serious about our role as practitioners with a social justice orientation, we need to support research, writing and policies that include disabled participants as

[3] BDSM is a lifestyle and the word 'is a combination of 3 acronyms, BD for Bondage Discipline, DS for Domination and Submission and SM for Sado Masochistic' (http://www.urbandictionary.com/define.php?term=bdsm).

collaborators, alerting researchers and practitioners to pertinent issues and contributing in important ways to the formulation of sexuality and disability research, policy and practice. Indeed, the critical, emancipatory orientation that lies at the core of disability studies' *raison d'être* (Barnes, 1992, 2003; Oliver, 1992; Kingsley and Mercer, 2004), and client-centred focus of occupational therapy requires that disabled people's perspectives must be central to research, policy-making and practice development in this area.

An impairment group whose participation in research on their sexual lives has rarely been elicited is people with communication/learning difficulties such as autism, learning disability, intellectual disability. Much of the research that focuses on this group has been concerned with either sexually inappropriate behaviour and perceived tendency to sexual abuse by men experiencing this condition (Wilson *et al.*,2010) or with the vulnerability to sexual abuse of mostly women (but also some men) with communication/learning difficulties (McCarthy, 1999). Hollomotz (2010) problematizes these perspectives, showing how the so-called vulnerability to sexual abuse of people with learning difficulties is at least partially constructed by their social environment. In short, Hollomotz argues that disempowerment and control in the lives of people with learning difficulties reinforces their sexual vulnerability. Most important is that some of this new research is being more articulate about how participants contributed to the project (see for example, Garbutt, 2010). We seek to add to the participatory literature in this area through the contributions of our autistic co-authors, Hope Block and Jacob Pratt.

Hope and Jacob

Hope Block and Jacob Pratt are autistic adults who met while presenting at regional and national disability conferences. Both communicate through a form of alternative and augmentative communication that is referred to in the literature as facilitated communication (FC) or supported typing. This technique involves the need for some level of physical contact between the person typing and another supporting individual to assist with motor planning and initiation difficulties. The technologies involved for this communication style can be as simple as a letter board (which Jacob often uses) and as complex as a text-to-speech device (which is Hope's preferred method).

When Hope types, her wrist, arm or elbow is in physical contact with the person helping her. It is not her preferred means to communicate when easier strategies will suffice, such as body language, vocalizations and personal signs. You can learn more about Hope and her communication strategy by visiting http://www.aina-ri.org/movies/HopeB.htm (Block, 2011). Despite a nerve-wracking fear of a new audience's disbelief, it is in public performance spaces, such as during conference presentations, where she is best able to communicate by typing. She states 'I don't see things like ordinary people and it feels like I'm out of sync with the rest of the world. I am thought of as not very smart but I am very intelligent. I am awesome at presenting at conferences, but have trouble with conversations. I don't know why

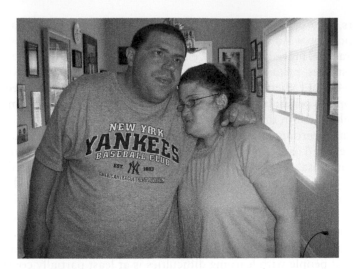

Figure 12.1 Jacob and Hope.

that is. It is odd that I have so much trouble talking to people one to one. Please realize that it is me typing not my mom. I cannot type yet without support. I am perfectly capable of my own thoughts.'

Unlike Hope, Jacob has a lot of oral language that is primarily nonfunctional. No often means yes and vice versa. When anxious, verbal diarrhoea in the form of repetitive but 'stupid' (Jacob's own term) questions abound, like 'tomorrow is Sunday?' when he knows perfectly well it is not. Jacob is also echolalic, repeating the last thing he has heard or something he was forced to repeat years ago in a speech therapy programme emphasizing oral language. None of this reflects anything at all about the myriad of thoughts swirling around his brain – thoughts both emotionally complex and vocabulary rich. To know this aspect of Jacob requires that he have access to the alphabet in either low or high tech QWERTY (standard keyboard layout) form with facilitation.

This facilitation involves skilled support for Jacob to be comfortable because for so long he was viewed as someone who was incompetent intellectually. Feedback also needs to be given to him about continuing to look at the board and to keep going if he gets stuck midword or midsentence. Although Jacob prefers to have his hand tightly grasped to provide proprioceptive input, he is capable of isolating his own index finger, crossing midline, hitting a letter target accurately, and performing many of the other skills required for supported typing with a hand tourniquetting his shirt above the elbow. He corrects misspellings with his nontyping hand, too.

Jacob states 'Without FC I would be a lost soul. I yearn to be able to type with anyone so everyone can know the depth of my thinking, my spirituality, my feelings, my understanding, and so many other sides of my complex self that one can't possibly know without typing with me. Typing does not change the fact that I am and will always be autistic, and that because of the severity of my autism, I will always flunk the standardized tests that lead me to be eligible for services provided only to those with an intellectual disability. Nonetheless, my inability to pass those tests has to do with performance barriers – the same ones that make fluent and meaningful oral language impossible.'

Eventually Hope and Jacob discovered they had feelings for each other. They began dating in late 2009 and became engaged in May 2010. Their first date consisted of sitting without support at a table in an exhibit hall at a conference and just 'being.' On their next date, in early January of 2010, Hope's staff enthusiastically began suggesting things they could do in the area, since Hope lives in one state and Jacob in a neighbouring one. Hope typed 'Why do you neurotypical people always have to do something? Why can't you just be?'

This may be a good time to note that, in the occupation of sexuality and relationships, intimacy may look very different to people who have various forms of differences in their learning or bodies that lead them to diagnoses of disabilities. As another example, Bob Williams (poet, disability rights advocate, and former Deputy Assistant Secretary for Disability, Aging and Long Term Care Policy and Commissioner of the federal Administration on Developmental Disabilities in the Office for Planning and Evaluation in the US Department of Health and Human Services under the Clinton administration), wrote a poem about two people in love in an institution. They silently prayed each day that, when staff laid them on their sides on a mat, they would be positioned so they could face each other and let their eyes speak of their loves for one another. This *is* intimacy although not, perhaps, in the way traditionally defined.

Because of communication and logistical challenges, dating for Jacob and Hope is complicated. They live several hours drive apart from each other in different states, so it is a distance relationship. Even with the support of family members and service-providing agencies, they do not get to see each other as often as they would like.

Hope

Love presides and stays alive, forever. It really speaks your heart. Without support I would never see my awesome but noisy, respectfully, handsomely, brilliant, kind and funny Jacob Pratt. Very necessary to be with my love . . . Somehow, somewhere, some way. Pretty wallflower finally has her dream. This is great . . . I am thankful for this chance. Need less reason and some awesomeness.

I love being engaged but I wish we could get married soon. It is so hard to be apart. I have another wish. Really want to just be understanding about Jacob's need to get his [undergraduate] degree first. I am so impatient. First we need a place to live and figure out the funding. We need help with [my and Pam's] father being so worried, and mom bringing me all the time to meet Jacob. It is hard for mom to drive long distances. It is weird to have your mother on dates. We can't find people to type with both of us except Linda and she is so busy. I want so much to be a wife and be with my love always. Being engaged is fun but being together as man and wife would be so much better. Really hard to be so far apart. We love each other so much and wish it weren't so hard to figure things out.

Jacob

I can't believe I finally found love. I am experiencing all new feelings that others have spoken about but I could only imagine. Shakespeare, the bible, modern day poets, all have written about this wonderful thing called love. They understated the feelings. I can't use words to describe the awesome and overwhelming feelings that overcome my mind and heart and soul but, believe me, this is the way I imagine HEAVEN WOULD BE LIKE. THE ONLY DIFFERENCE IS THAT LOVE IS GOD'S GRACE AND NOT THE SAME AS LOVING ANOTHER MORTAL IN WHOM THE HOLY SPIRIT LIVES. I am so blessed that love is in my life.

Supported dating is wonderful but it also sucks. The way it is wonderful is we have staff who are cool about our dating and our parents are too. Kind of like having approval for having a friend who your family accepts as one of its members. It allows us to see each other, because neither of us can drive or use the phone to arrange dates or even get ourselves to where we want to be. Supported dating in an ideal world wouldn't be necessary, but when you have severe movement, anxiety, communication and sensory differences [Rammler, 2007] resulting in a label of autism it is the only option for us to have the opportunity to be together.

Supported dating sucks because you are totally dependent on others to be together. Self-determination can only go so far before reality strikes. Reality includes staff thinking it is okay to cancel, or run late, or break up your plans to suit themselves. There is not a thing you can do except get frustrated, and take it out on yourself through self-inflicted pain inducing bites or head bangs, because if you don't do it to yourself you will be called aggressive and punished for being so deeply disappointed that your heart is breaking, but the outcome is worse because the punishment is another postponement.

Read Linda's respectful rules (abbreviated as an appendix). It is important for anyone providing supported dating supports to realize it's hard enough, and not make it worse by imposing their agenda on us. I wish everyone love and if you have severe autism I wish you the chance to fall and be in love. And I pray you will have the supports you need to get to where you want to be in your relationship with that special someone.

Final Thoughts

At the moment, intimacy for both Hope and Jacob involves facilitated communication to let each other know how much they love each other and why. They also discuss their futures, their current lives (e.g., college courses both took recently) and, like any other couple, may complain to each other (e.g., about the slowness of a wait unit in a restaurant). Neither has expressed any interest in physical contact except for an occasional kiss on the cheek or hug. They often choose to sit near but not next to each other. Yet, as they communicate from their hearts, it is challenging for those supporting them to 'be a fly on the wall' and to rise above feeling like a voyeur so as not to convey personal discomfort to Hope and Jacob that may limit their freedom of expression. Without support from others, such communication on their parts would be impossible. Thus their situation highlights the realities of facilitated sexuality as discussed earlier. Though the facilitation that Hope and Jacob require is, at present, on the level of logistical planning, transportation and communication, rather than sexual activities, it is already a delicate negotiation that redefines traditional notions of intimacy.

Greater levels of intimacy, particularly in the sexual arena, comprise bridges that both Hope and Jacob, their families, and other members of their support teams may have to cross eventually. It will be important for others involved in their lives to do so nonjudgmentally and in full support of what Jacob and Hope, as the involved couple, want. Resources such as Dave Hingsburger's (1990) *I Contact: Sexuality and People with Developmental Disabilities* may prove to be required reading for all concerned.

Another issue that has arisen is how soon Hope and Jacob actually may be married. If Jacob's religious orientation allowed it, he may well be amenable to living with Hope as though they were married. This would render the politics of interstate funding, reduced Social Security benefits to married couples, and other systemic logistics unnecessary. Unfortunately for Hope, Jacob believes that to do so would dishonour her. Therefore, he intends, as one of his independent study projects while he earns his Baccalaureate degree, to take on the system. In contrast, Hope's eagerness for the two of them to be together, and her personal lack of religious prohibitions, creates another level of negotiation for the couple. The take-home lesson here is that other issues beyond disability (e.g., personal values, life plans, preferences) can also intrude on sexuality and intimacy among disabled people as much as these issues affect individuals who are not disabled.

On top of negotiating practical, logistical, financial, and religious barriers, Hope and Jacob must face prejudice, discrimination, pejorative attitudes and behaviour in ignorant people in the community. Recently, as Jacob and Hope sat on a bench in a mall on a date – their facilitators dismissed and watching at a distance – they had the displeasure to hear a nearby man talking on his cell phone, passionately expounding that, 'leaving two retards alone together should be illegal.' This sort of hurtful encounter may turn out the hardest of all barriers to dismiss or overcome.

Occupational therapists are well qualified, and in most cases, well disposed to help people to negotiate this challenging terrain. It is the responsibility of educators to ensure that students receive a balanced and thorough preparation that goes beyond the physiological aspects of sex to explore emotional and cultural issues that influence the occupations of sex, sexuality and intimacy. We strongly suggest that research and scholarship engaging with these topics include the perspectives and active participation of disabled people. Hope and Jacob's experiences reveal how necessary it is to consider individual perspectives, backgrounds and desires with regard to these occupations. There are no simple answers, no cookie-cutter solutions; each situation must be approached with equal measures of respect, empathy, and creativity. On the level of policy and practice, especially in institutional settings or in helping individuals negotiate with their families, occupational therapists have the potential to play a valuable role as advocates and facilitators to help ensure occupational justice – that the rights, needs, and desires of disabled people are represented and respected. In some cases, it might be necessary to fight entrenched and repressive attitudes and policies that are decades old, if not older. Ignorance and prejudice, such as Hope and Jacob experienced at the mall, is perhaps the hardest to address and change of all the barriers discussed here. What cultural and policy changes must take place, and what roles should occupational therapists play, in order to work toward occupational justice in this realm, and a world where such experiences no longer happen? These are the questions we should be asking our students, our authority figures, and ourselves.

Appendix

An abbreviated version of the 'support staff training guidelines' used primarily to instruct Jacob's staff on how to support his dating follows. Often, dates involve family members because the logistics of coordination given other assignments, scheduled work hours, and a myriad of other factors. Another individual with a disability who is able to travel independently may accompany Hope in the near future as the 'lovebirds' take the Shoreline train to meet each other at a midway point. Fortunately, both Hope and Jacob love trains and this line is reasonably accessible to both of them.

Supported Dating
Individualized for Jacob and Hope
ALWAYS REVIEW THE ENTIRE CONTENTS UNTIL SUPPORTED DATING IS
    WELL-ESTABLISHED

Important numbers to have:
JACOB's contact information
HOPE's contact information

NOTE: Both Jacob and Hope have facebook pages. They can 'live chat' or send each
    other messages that way, too.

Planning
☐ Suggest dates/times that are mutually convenient for Jacob, Hope, and whoever is
    available to support each of them.
☐ Make sure Hope and/or Jacob don't have other commitments. (Ask them first,
    then check their calendars with them.)
☐ If either does have something else scheduled, let that person choose whether to
    maintain the commitment or see each other instead.
    ○ If they choose to see each other anyway, continue. This may require:
        ☐ Notifying whatever entity was expecting either one of them to reschedule, let
    them know s/he won't be there, etc. The responsibility for Jacob's cancellations

falls on Jacob's support staff or others and the responsibility for Hope's falls on her staff/others.

    ☐ Making sure other members of each team know of the change.

    ○ If one chooses not to see other and do whatever was originally planned instead, pick another date with each of them. *Start this process over.* (NOTE: Try to negotiate with them if the event to be missed affects health, safety, or other important life functions. Even if it does, it is still their choice.)

☐ Ask them what they want to do on the date. Use facilitated communication. They may have already communicated with each other about what they'd like to do, have new ideas, or be responsive to suggestions you offer. Support their negotiations as they jointly decide what to do. (In reality, it is often Jacob who makes the recommendation and Hope who agrees! Dates are often planned via emails.)

☐ Review the specific steps for planning dates at specific times.

It is NOT up to staff to make decisions based on what they want to do. We are all here to support Hope and Jacob lead their lives as they choose!

Additional planning for late afternoon (after 3 p.m.), evening, weekend dates

NOTE: It is really far to Hope's place but late afternoon, evening and/or weekend dates should still be planned if that is what Jacob and Hope want.

☐ Allow enough time for Hope and Jacob with their respective support to get to the meeting place before setting a meeting time.

☐ Both Hope and Jacob need rides back home so, given the distance, it is usually best to plan on both sets of support staffs to stick around. In fact, double or triple dates work well!

☐ Confirm the date, time and place right before the actual date. Do this the night before or morning. (Note that Hope's home support staff members do not work during the day all the time.)

    ○ Make sure all support staff who will be involved in supporting the date have each others' phone number in case either Hope or Jacob are sick or there is another compelling reason to reschedule.

    ○ Compelling reasons to reschedule include serious weather, serious staff illness, lack of transportation at the last minute (e.g., breakdowns, accidents).

Set dates are NEVER to be canceled/rescheduled for the convenience of staff.

Support on dates

Bring extra money just in case Jacob or Hope do not have enough. Get a receipt so you can be reimbursed. Make sure you have enough gas in your vehicle before the date. It will be okay to stop and get gas on your way back home with Jacob as long as you tell him you have to do this.

Remember what Hope said as this is paraphrased: 'You neurotypical people have a need to do whereas we autistic people are okay to be.'

Remember, it is THEIR date, not yours!!!

☐ Bring Jacob's letterboard and Lightwriter with the plug. Make sure Hope has her Dynavox. Both of them can type on a letterboard so bring a back up just in case.

☐ Bring something for each of them to use for proprioceptive input.

☐ Let Hope and Jacob change plans at the last second if they want. <u>Use facilitated communication</u>.

☐ Avoid traffic if at all possible while going on the date.

☐ Don't rush.

☐ Allow them to choose their seats. Allow them to change their minds about where they're sitting. Remember that what Jacob says may be unreliable so ALWAYS use facilitated communication to confirm.

☐ If you are there with your significant other, confirm with Hope and Jacob whether they want you to sit with them or if they'd rather sit by themselves.

☐ Be available to facilitate their communication, however.

☐ If you are at a restaurant or another place where Hope and Jacob need to communicate with other staff, ask if either of them want assistance ordering and how they would like that assistance to be provided. *Follow their instructions. You work for them!*

☐ Be ready to support any other issues that may arise (e.g., by explaining noises, movement differences, anxiety, sensory needs) to others nearby.

☐ Hope and Jacob have a right to be anywhere in public. They do not have a right to disrupt others' peaceful access to those places and, if either one continues to do so, it may be appropriate to leave (at least for a sensory break).

☐ There is a fine line between honoring Jacob's and Hope's right to be present with their autism and them truly disrupting others' rights. Here are some guidelines to help you decide:

    ○ If it is merely a case of someone else being judgmental, remember Hope's and Jacob's right to be there. It is okay to point this out gently.

    ○ If someone actually says something rude to them or you, tell them you're sorry they were 'bothered' and ignore them.

    ○ If someone has been interrupted or annoyed, apologize in addition to Jacob's verbal apology (one of his aspects of perseverative speech is to say 'I sorry' if he perceives someone to be upset with him) and explain briefly what autism is. Try to help the person understand that this is not intentional.

    ○ If someone has been hit or otherwise aggressed against, make sure they are okay. Be prepared to exchange information unless the person is certain that everything is okay.

    ○ If the environment is too noisy, at least take a sensory break. This is reason to leave if Hope and Jacob want to.

    ○ Treat other incidents (e.g., spilled glass of water, spilled popcorn, need to use the restroom, or other events) as you would for anyone else. Deal with it!

    ○ Leave if Jacob or Hope want to leave. Don't drag it out 'just because the date isn't supposed to be over.'

☐ *In a really difficult situation involving authority figures, feel free to call another member of Jacob's or Hope's team for advice.*

☐ If Jacob and Hope want to extend their date, and it is possible to do so, go ahead. Just make sure everyone else knows so they are not 'missing!'

☐ If it is not possible, negotiate with them about why not and what to do instead. Use facilitated communication.

HAVE FUN!!!!

References

Abbot, D., Burns, J. (2007) What's love got to do with it? Experiences of lesbian, gay, and bisexual people with intellectual disabilities in the United Kingdom and views of the staff who support them. *Sexuality Research and Social Policy: Journal of NSRC* 4(1), 27–39.

Barnes, C. (1992) Qualitative research: valuable or irrelevant? *Disability, Handicap and Society* 7(2), 115–124.

Barnes, C. (2003) What a difference a decade makes: reflections on doing 'emancipatory' disability research. *Disability and Society* 18(1), 3–17.

Block, P., Ricafrente-Biazon, M., Russo, A., Chu, K.Y., Sud, S., Koerner, L., Vittoria, K., Landgrover, A., Olowu, T. (2005) Introducing disability studies to occupational therapy students. *American Journal of Occupational Therapy* 59, 554–560.

Block, H. (2011) My name is Hope Block and this is about my life. Advocates in action: personal stories of celebration, www.aina-ri.org/movies/HopeB.htm, accessed 11 April 2011.

Block, P. (2000) Sexuality, fertility and danger: twentieth century images of women with cognitive disabilities. *Sexuality and Disability* 18(4), 239–254.

Block, P. (2002) Sexuality, parenthood, and cognitive disability in Brazil. *Sexuality and Disability* 20(1), 7–28.

Bonnie, S. (2002) Facilitated Sexual Expression in the Independent Living Movement in Ireland. Masters of Arts thesis, University of Leeds, Leeds.

Brown, J., Russell, S. (2005) My home, your workplace: people with physical disability negotiate their sexual health without crossing professional boundaries. *Disability and Society* 20(4), 375–388.

Earle, S. (1999) Facilitated sex and the concept of sexual need: disabled students and their personal assistants. *Disability and Society* 14(3), 309–323.

Earle, S. (2001) Disability, facilitated sex and the role of the nurse. *Journal of Advanced Nursing* 36(3), 433–440.

Fassin, D. (1991) Physical handicaps, economic practices and matrimonial strategies in Senegal. *Social Science and Medicine* 32(3), 267–272.

Garbutt, R. (2010) Exploring the barriers to sex for people with learning difficulties. In R. Shuttleworth, T. Sanders (eds) *Sex and Disability: Politics, Identity and Access*, pp. 79–98. Leeds, The Disability Press.

Groce, N. (2004) *HIV/AIDS and Disability: Capturing Hidden Voices — The World Bank/Yale Global Survey on HIV/AIDS*. Washington, DC, The World Bank.

Groce, N. (2005) HIV/AIDS and individuals with disability. *Health and Human Rights* 8(2), 215–224.

Grossman, B., Shuttleworth, R., Prinz, P. (2004) Locating sexuality in disability experience, a report from Disability Studies: Theory, Policy, and Practice, the Inaugural Conference of the Disability Studies Association. *Sexuality Research and Social Policy* 1(2), 91–96.

Hamilton, C. (2002) Doing the wild thing: supporting an ordinary sexual life for people with intellectual disabilities. *Disability Studies Quarterly* 22(4), 40–59.

Hingsburger, D. (1990) *I Contact: Sexuality and People with Developmental Disabilities*. Bear Creek, North Carolina, Psych-Media, Inc.

Hollomotz, A. (2010) Sexual 'vulnerability' of people with learning difficulties: a self-fullfilling prophecy. In R. Shuttleworth, T. Sanders (eds) *Sex and Disability: Politics, Identity and Access*. Leeds, The Disability Press, pp. 21–40.

Ingstad, B. (2007) Seeing disability and human rights in the local context: Botswana revisited. In S. Reynolds Whyte, B. Ingstad (eds) *Disability in Local and Global Worlds*. London, University of California Press.

Kangaude, G. (2007) Toward Realising Sexual Rights of Persons with Disabilities: A Challenge for Malawi. Unpublished doctoral dissertation, University of the Free State, Bloemfontein, South Africa.

Kingsley, J., Mercer, G. (2004) From critique to practice: Emancipatory disability research. In C. Barnes, G. Mercer (eds) *Implementing the Social Model of Disability: Theory and Research*. Leeds, The Disability Press, pp. 118–137.

McCarthy, M. (1999) *Sexuality and Women with Learning Disabilities*. London, Jessica Kingsley.

McRuer, R. (2006) *Crip Theory: Cultural Signs of Queerness and Disability*. New York, New York University Press.

Mona, L. (2003) Sexual options for people with disabilities. Using personal assistance services for sexual expression. *Women and Therapy* 26, 211–220.

Moores, S. (2003) The training of occupational therapists in sexuality therapy for clients with disabilities: the British perspective. *British Journal of Occupational Therapy* 66(5), 218.

Moores, S. (2008) Sexuality and health care: the training of occupational therapists. *British Journal of Occupational Therapy* 71(11), 503.

Nicolaisen, I. (1995) Persons and Nonpersons: Disability and Personhood among the Punan Bah of Central Borneo. In B. Ingstad, S. Whyte (eds) *Disability and Culture*. Berkeley, CA, University of California Press.

O'Toole, C. (2002) Sex, disability and motherhood: access to sexuality for disabled mothers. *Disability Studies Quarterly* 22(4), 87–108.

Oliver, M. (1992) Changing the social relations of research production. *Disability, Handicap, and Society* 7, 101–115.

Penna, S., Sheehy, K. (2000) Sex education and schizophrenia: should occupational therapists offer sex education to people with schizophrenia? *Scandinavian Journal Occupational Therapy* 7, 126–131.

Rammler, L. (2007) *Autism Spectrum Differences: A Supportive View*. Rocky Hill, CT: ASDI/NE, Inc.

Rembis, M. (2010) Beyond the binary: rethinking the social model of disabled sexuality. *Sexuality and Disability* 28, 51–60.

Sakellariou, D. (2006) If not the disability, then what: barriers to reclaiming male sexuality following spinal cord injury. *Sexuality and Disability* 24(2), 101–111.

Sakellariou, D., Sawada, Y. (2006) Sexuality after spinal cord injury: the Greek male's perspective. *American Journal of Occupational Therapy* 60(3), 311–319.

Sakellariou, D., Simó Algado, S. (2006a) Sexuality and occupational therapy: exploring the link. *British Journal of Occupational Therapy* 69(8): 350–356.

Sakellariou, D., Simó Algado, S. (2006b) Sexuality and disability: a case of occupational injustice. *British Journal of Occupational Therapy* 69(2), 69–76.

Sanders, T. (2007) The politics of sexual citizenship: commercial sex and disability. *Disability and Society* 22(5), 439–455.

Sanders, T. (2010) Sexual citizenship, sexual facilitation and the right to pleasure. In R. Shuttleworth, T. Sanders (eds) *Sex and Disability: Politics, Identity and Access*, pp. 139–154. Leeds, The Disability Press.

Sengupta, S., Stubbs, B. (2008) Sexuality and health care. *British Journal of Occupational Therapy* 71(12), 554.

Shildrick, M. (2004) Silencing sexuality: the regulation of the disabled body. In J. Carabine (ed.) *Sexualities – Personal Lives and Social Policy*. Bristol, Policy Press, pp. 123–158.

Shildrick, M. (2007) Contested pleasures: the sociopolitical economy of disability and sexuality. *Sexuality Research and Social Policy: Journal of NSRC* 3(3), 51–75.

Shuttleworth, R. (2000) The search for sexual intimacy for men with cerebral palsy. *Sexuality and Disability* 18(4), 263–282.

Shuttleworth, R. (2004) Disability/Difference. In C. R. Ember, M. Ember (eds) *Encyclopedia of Medical Anthropology: Health and Illness in the World's Cultures*, volume 2. New York, Springer, pp. 360–373.

Shuttleworth, R. (2007a) Disability and sexuality: toward a constructionist focus on access and the inclusion of disabled people on the sexual rights movement. In N. Teunis, G. Herdt (eds) *Sexual Inequalities and Social Justice*. Berkely, University of California Press, pp. 174–208.

Shuttleworth, R. (2007b) Introduction to special issue critical research and policy debates in disability and sexuality studies. *Sexuality Research and Social Policy* 4(1), 1–14.

Shuttleworth, R., Mona, L. (2002) Introduction to the symposium – disability and sexuality: toward a focus on sexual access. *Disability Studies Quarterly* 22(4), 2–9.

Shuttleworth, R., Sanders, T. (eds) (2010) *Sex and Disability: Politics, Identity and Access*. Leeds, The Disability Press.

Spencer, M., Wainwright, C. (2008) Sexuality and health care. *British Journal of Occupational Therapy* 71(8), 328.

Tepper, M. (1997) Providing comprehensive sexual health care in spinal cord injury rehabilitation: implementation and evaluation of a new curriculum for health care. *Sexuality and Disability* 15(3), 131–167.

Tepper, M. (2000) *Facilitated Sex: The Next Frontier in Sexuality? New Mobility*, 11(84), 20–24.

Wade, H. (2002) Discrimination, sexuality and people with significant disabilities: issues of access and the right to sexual expression in the United States. *Disabilities Studies Quarterly* 22(4), 9–27.

Whipple, B., Richards, E., Tepper, M., Komisaruk, B. (1996) Sexual response in women with complete spinal cord injury. *Sexuality and Disability* 14(3), 191–201.

Wilson, N., Parmenter, T., Stancliffe, R., Shuttleworth, R., Parker, D. (2010) A masculine perspective of gendered topics in the research literature on males and females with intellectual disability. *Journal of Intellectual and Developmental Disability* 35(1), 1–23.

Wotten, R., Isbister, S. (2010) A sex worker perspective on working with clients with a disability and the development of Touching Base Inc. In R. Shuttleworth, T. Sanders (eds) *Sex and Disability: Politics, Identity and Access*. Leeds, The Disability Press, pp. 155–178.

13 Models and Human Occupation

Nick Pollard and Neil Carver

Introduction

Model making is a relatively unexplored aspect of human occupation, not only overlooked in occupational science and therapy literature but in academic literature in general. This chapter will explore some of the value, purposes and significance of modelling from psychological, sociopolitical and materialist perspectives. It will look at the relationship of model-making occupations to adult forms of play and the representation of gendered, particularly male, identity, the formation of social networks and the understanding of objects and environments. The chapter will show that, while modelling is supported by a significant industry, modellers themselves often seem to be socially stigmatized. This marginalization emerges from a set of discourses on play and presumptions about the nature of childhood and adult occupation. While many adults initially acquire their interest in model making through childhood activities, some modellers aim to represent objects they have worked with, such as a boat or an engine. Despite this occupational link we have not been able to find a discussion in which forms of model making are explored in relation to occupations of particular social classes. The lack of researched overviews may be connected to the place of modelling activities at the periphery in popular cultural perceptions, a situation that may be partly due to their concerns with representing detailed objects in bygone worlds. The authors conclude that despite arguments that suggest the triviality of model making, it remains a valuable human occupation because it facilitates opportunities for adult play, which includes the transmission and expression of skills, values and the recognition of their complexity, appreciation of the environment, and personal reflection. Many of these skills, appreciations and reflections appear to involve vernacular elements relating to male occupations which may have been overlooked as opportunities to engage men,

Politics of Occupation-Centred Practice: Reflections on Occupational Engagement across Cultures, First Edition. Edited by Nick Pollard and Dikaios Sakellariou.
© 2012 John Wiley & Sons, Ltd. Published 2012 by John Wiley & Sons, Ltd.

especially older males, in therapeutic interventions (Ormsby *et al.*, 2010). Model making may therefore be a rich area for both occupational science and occupational therapy to pursue, both in terms of the purpose of modelling and the meaning of what is modelled.

The Social Status of Modelling

Model making usually involves the making of representations of various objects, figures and landscapes. Csíkszentmihályi and Rochberg-Halton (1981) suggest that the symbolic value of objects in general has been of more interest to, for example, psychologists, than their transactional role in enabling people to do things. King's (1996) exploration, *Remaking the World,* remains the only significant exploration of this aspect of humans in the guise of *homo faber,* the person as a maker of objects.

As an activity model making involves some exploration of form through an attempt to replicate details as realistically as possible but in a different scale, for example 76 times smaller than the original. The reason for this is so the object may be better understood or examined. For example scale models of insects are larger than real life, but those of aircraft are smaller. The materials used, such as plastics, will often differ from those employed in the original object, or 'prototype' because the prototype materials cannot be made to look effective in different scale sizes. Modelling also allows the modeller to appreciate the relationships between individual components that have to be fitted together, the relationships of one object (for example, an aircraft) with another, or even, as with a model railway, representations of distance and time.

Although it is both a profession and a meaningful hobby activity for millions, supporting a multimillion dollar modelling industry making models is sometimes disparaged as a trivial activity. Professional modellers (Association of Professional Model Makers, 2010: 2) decry a lack of recognition that prevents modellers from 'taking their rightful place at the design table'. King (1996: 207) suggests that: 'model making is an art, and sometimes art; the modelmaker, an artisan and sometimes an artist.' Nevertheless privileging artistic representation over mimetic representation has a long history. Writing about anatomical modelling Ballestriero (2010: 11) notes that: '... many wax modellers of the past centuries remain unknown because they were considered mere craftsmen; only a few are remembered as real artists'.

While King describes modelling as a 'remaking of the world' he rightfully plays down its significance alongside what he describes as 'some of the broad implications' of other 'schemes of world revision' [such as] 'revolution' or 'personal counselling' (King, 1996: 226). Compared to the goals of such 'revisions', for example justice or the reconstruction of a traumatic childhood model making may seem slight but it does, as King goes on to say, have 'its own claims to significance' (King, 1996: 226).

Model making can sometimes investigate the question 'what if?' – for example, the professionally constructed models of architectural features. The majority of modelling activity explored in this chapter, however, is concerned with replicating existing objects, often of nostalgic or historical interest and primarily as a hobby.

Although examples from the wider field of model making are occasionally referred to, most will concern the modelling of aircraft and railways in the United Kingdom and North America.

Model Making Defined

King, describes model making as (1996: 3) as 'constructing, collecting and operating tiny models of larger prototypes'; while a model is 'a re-creation of some prototype or original, generally but not always smaller and usually of materials different to those of the original.' Model making incorporates a spectrum of activities ranging from a modern folk or vernacular community occupation to a highly professional medium (Wylie, 1987; Jenkinson, 2001). King suggests: 'There appear to be virtually no objects in the "real world" that have not been re-created in reduced size and collected or operated by someone or some group' (King 1996: 3).

Professional model makers distinguish themselves from 'hobbyists' as people who '... blend a unique combination of art and science into their work of replicating, creating mock-ups, volume studies and scale reproductions of anything from a building to an automobile' (The Association of Professional Model Makers (APMM) 2010: 1). At a professional level Chaffee (2010: 1) has suggested 'great model builders' possess ten talents, paraphrased here:

1. A sense of scale.
2. The ability to visualize in three dimensions.
3. The pursuit of art.
4. The ability to sense materials when they 'talk' to us.
5. A passion for detail and the ability to do finishing work.
6. The ability to link abstract or unrelated ideas.
7. Ingenuity.
8. The ability to research.
9. The ability to interpret information.
10. The ability to balance the various factors in a project.

The Association of Professional Model Makers (2010: 1) describes the occupation of model making as 'translating and improving [model makers'] ideas into a three dimensional reality', reifying model making into a problem-solving part of the creative design process. Model makers 'wander through life thinking "I could make that"' (p. 2) – and 'are valued for their fabrication abilities and their capacity to bring about innovation' (p. 2), which they achieve through the technical mastery of specific high grade materials.

Professional modellers are generally commissioned to model objects which do not yet exist (Association of Professional Model Makers, 2010), whereas most (but not all) hobbyists try to produce 'good' or 'accurate' representations of extant objects or those lost to history. Often a 'good enough' depiction resulting from a challenge which is satisfying is more desirable to modellers than true accuracy (Jenkinson, 2001;

Lehron, 2004). Model railway gauges, for example rarely represent 'true' scale (Wylie, 1987).

Models in Early History

As an occupational activity model making can be found in many cultures and through much of history. Representational figures, sometimes combining literal features, are known from as far back as 35 000 years ago (Conard, 2009) although interpreting the meaning of these figures is speculative. Model objects, often funerary offerings representing the requirements of life, survive from ancient Egypt and China (King, 1996). Modern scale modelling appears to have its antecedents in the planning of buildings and fortifications and the study of construction techniques for ships and engineering projects. Some of the earliest surviving such models date from renaissance times (King, 1996).

The Value of Modelling to Modellers

There have been no formal empirical studies into the value of model making to model makers in academic literature. Nevertheless it seems clear that model making plays an important part in everyday life and at a simple level, is fun (King, 1996; Pearson, 2007; Booth, 2010). At the 'hobbyist' end of the spectrum, King (1996: 193) anecdotally describes modellers' responses when asked which aspect of model making they most deeply cherished. The results included 'the peace of mind that comes from accomplishment', the pleasures of accurate representation of real objects and displaying them, as well as social interaction with other modellers; either to amaze them with proficiency or to share knowledge.

This latter point is significant. The adult model maker is often portrayed disparagingly, as a socially isolated individual. This impression is possibly deepened by the remoteness of the shed, attic, or spare room in which modelling often takes place, while the pictorial evidence of Simmons (1998) and Jenkinson (2001) suggests that railway modellers may give secondary consideration to the other inhabitants of their homes. Indeed, Sutton-Smith (1997) regards model-making as one of the solitary forms of play, alongside gardening, cooking, listening to music or using computers.

Snowden, writing as an engineer for the model manufacturer Airfix (in Stanton, 2002) also concedes modelling can be a solitary activity but highlights the warmth and eagerness of the modelling community to share skills, whether through web sites or as a member of a collecting society. Beginner railway modellers are advised to join clubs in order to learn from others (Wylie, 1987; Simmons, 1998). Despite the importance of historical detail in railway layouts (Wylie, 1987; Jenkinson, 2001; Allen, 2008), a modeller may be equally concerned as to how displays may be designed for transport to exhibitions or meetings with other enthusiasts (Allen, 1979; Andress, 1988). Thus, modelling can involve many elements which Rebeiro (2001: 65) would term 'occupational spin-offs'. Many activities are connected to the activities of modelling, including the buying, collecting and selling of models, researching history, visiting locations, developing and participating in networks of modellers amongst others (Wylie, 1987; King, 1996; Jenkinson, 2001). Consequently modellers may be rightly reluctant to recognize these extensive forms of committed and involved activity as simple play activities when they seem to be related to both personal interests and forms of learning (Rieber et al.,1998). As Ward states . . . 'the hobby often derided by as the province of "anoraks" is a truly interactive hobby' (2004: 184), as much as modelling may be turning from the world, it can involve a turning to it.

Csíkszentmihályii and Rochberg-Halton (1981) suggest that the objects individuals use personally or collect express an element of their cultural differentiation. Objects have a personal connection, and often stand for, or are a 'model of' (Csíkszentmihályi and Rochberg-Halton, 1981: 43) some aspect of the environment (Wylie, 1987; Simmons, 1998). A literal example might be the souvenir with a place name on it, often a representation of something associated with a place. In a similar way, many modellers have very close autobiographical connections to the things they model (Jenkinson, 2001). Those engaged in the operation of the actual vehicles, such as railway workers (Ross, 1984; Hollick, 1991; Carter et al., 1992) or aircraft engineers (Wren, 1998) were frequently proud of their involvement and their skills. Rail and military museums display models that have been constructed by apprentices who worked on the real items they have made in miniature. King also gives examples of boatmen who model their boats, or people embellishing the modelled landscapes of their childhood 'into the picturesque' (1996: 179). Csíkszentmihályi and Rochberg-Halton (1981) describe these activities in relation to objects as interpretative – the models people make enable them to make sense of – not only to recognize but to understand their world.

Others might build models of the objects which specifically made impressions on their own personal developmental landscape – the *particular* railway, ships or aircraft. For example Gunter even produced a 'dolls house' version of the very student digs she once lived in (Booth, 2010), although she confessed she could not fully explain why she chose to model this subject. On the other hand objects such as the A3 Pacific Flying Scotsman locomotive or the Spitfire fighter aircraft are modelled because of their iconic status, part of the cultural expression of British identity. They refer to defining moments in national history, such as the Second World War Battle of Britain or the invention of the steam railway. Similar mythologies apply in other countries, for example the adulatory phenomenon that followed Charles Lindbergh's first solo flight across the Atlantic (Alcorn, 2009). Building and using such models allows some degree of vicarious participation either in the flying or driving of such vehicles or the celebration of historical events associated with them.

Some particular models, or even particular manufacturers, have even come to symbolize 'rites of passage' and occupy a special part of modelling culture. For example, between the 1960s and 1970s almost every boy in the UK constructed an Airfix kit (Ward, 2004). Such shared experiences are the subject of a growing number of nostalgic accounts of modelling plastic kits in the UK. Pearson's (2007) work on model soldiers, Ward's (1999) celebration of the kit manufacturer Airfix and his (2004) overview of 'classic kits' are good examples.

Ward implies another value of modelling by contrasting it with the so called 'passive' (and apparently solitary) pursuit of computer games, placing the 'kit' in the social context of family: '. . . for many youngsters and their parents, building a plastic kit is often a new and creative diversion from television or computer games' (2004: 184). We suggest however that modelling contains other aspects of significance in the family setting. Throughout the modelling literature there is a theme of intergenerational values and relationships (e.g. Pearson, 2007). A recent advertisement for the Hornby model railway manufacturer in the Christmas 2010 Radio Times (p. 91) depicted a father and son with a railway layout featuring modern and vintage trains, presented as a socially appropriate fatherly interest which possesses '. . . the power [. . .] to engage and the potential for years of shared enjoyment. And in today's world, that is something really special.'

This plays on the role modelling has in the development of personal identity, relationships and the transmission of values through significant others, not only in relation to internal, but also external frames of reference (King, 1996; Anning, 2002). Csíkszentmihályi and Rochberg-Halton (1981) also argue that objects often play a significant part in human socialization. Young children identify themselves with and imagine themselves in adult occupations (Erikson, 1980). An example might be gaining the ability to start and stop a toy train on an oval piece of track.

For the authors' generation, born in the 1950s, trains and planes held a particular excitement and represent culturally relevant and historically present occupations (Abrahams, 2008). Sometimes their significance is deeply embedded in family narratives, for example some of Nick's relatives worked on the railways, a background that contributed to the parental stimulation and encouragement of a railway interest. The valued experiences and reflections that the authors and many other people obtain through model making therefore relate not only to the model but also to aspects of the human occupational and cultural environment (for example railways for 180 years, aeroplanes for 100 years).

So, the building of models, for example of a railway, can be closely linked to notions of identity, where they enact some kind of relation to memory or a significant object (Jenkinson, 2001). On the other hand some modellers appear to value modelling *any* 'thing' rather than modelling a 'specific kind of thing' (such as boats) This suggests that some modellers may view the process of modelling as more valuable than the end product, although without formal research this observation is speculative.

Some modellers develop collections, for example, of prestige cars that as models are more affordable in terms of cost and space, but appear to represent a material desire for the real thing. Csíkszentmihályi and Rochberg-Halton (1981) point out that often people work for things, objects or corporate goals that are beyond their personal attainment because capitalism operates on the basis that most people do not own the means of production, and so have to hire their labour. The desire for objects is cultivated during childhood in many societies through toys, which are often linked to gender – cars for boys, dolls houses for girls, perhaps. These are part of a process of socialization through materialist values that are often linked to the growth of proper adult attributes such as responsibility, rationality and moral behaviour (Csíkszent-mihályi and Rochberg-Halton, 1981; Sutton Smith, 1997).

Adult modellers also frequently assert the educational and social value of modelling to younger people in developing the skills and attitudes necessary for the adult world of paid occupation (e.g. Simmons, 1998). This was very evident in relation to aviation when it was an emerging technology. The construction of 'solid' scale model aircraft carved from blocks of wood, a hobby prevalent until the post war emergence of plastics, was described by its advocates as an: 'educational and instructive hobby' (Elwell, 1941: 16). Solid-scale modelling involved tracing an accurate scale plan of an aircraft onto a piece of wood, then delicately carving the three-dimensional form. If too much wood was removed there was often no option but to start again. The acquisition of technique and attention to detail required offered 'fine training in patience and common sense' (Elwell, 1941: 9).

This idea was given considerably greater cogency by some through the experiences of war: 'Model plane building is more than a business or a hobby – it is education sugar- coated. And aviation education breeds 'airmindedness', from which alone can there arise the fullest appreciation of the implications of the airplane to human welfare, including military security' (Anon., 1946: 284).

A more modest educational theme concerning rail transport operations existed in the marketing of railway modelling – for example, Tri-ang Railways (1962) and Hornby (Stevens-Stretten, 1979). Ward still suggests that modelling can teach 'a modicum of history' (2004: 184) although the textless instructions in contemporary kits designed for the global market are significantly less informative than the written material that accompanied earlier kits.

Though young model makers may learn something of history, aviation or the operation of railways, it is only sometimes suggested that they will develop the skills of professional adult model makers, although Wylie (1987), Andress (1988) and Jenkinson (2001) impart professional modelling skills for those wishing to learn them. Often the anticipation is that they will be drawn to the design or operation of real aircraft or railways (for example Elwell, 1941) and develop skills valued in manufacturing industries (Parkins in Stanton, 2002).

As much as model making has been considered an enjoyable activity it has long been associated with 'rest and relaxation' (Elwell, 1941: 9) and seems capable of providing 'therapeutic' levels of distraction – even in situations of war. In the US armed forces 'Morale Welfare and Recreation Centers', according to DeMott of the Baghdad Hobby Club (2008), 'building models here in a combat zone, sure seemed to be the trick to take our minds off being here, and away from our families. It was a great stress reliever to look forward to building a model every day after missions outside the wire.'

DeMott's account of modelling resonates with what Csíkszentmihályi (1990) describes as a state of 'flow' or an optimal experience, in that the modeller can become fully involved in the activity to the extent that the sense of external stimuli is altered, including awareness of the passage of time.

Building a model kit, which has sufficient challenge but can be successfully completed allows the modeller clear and achievable goals within the technical capabilities of the individual. The outcome can be compared with the pictures in the instructions and package, the model displayed to other modellers for feedback. These themes are echoed in many other accounts of modelling throughout the literature, particularly King's (1996) account mentioned earlier. In Csíkszentmihályi and Rochberg-Halton's (1981) investigation of the relationship between people and things, one respondent refers to the lathe he keeps in the basement on which he makes components for his model aircraft. Modelling is an opportunity to demonstrate his skills in engineering, and the lathe a key object in that association with his enjoyment of his own individuality. Thus the occupational activity of modelling is connected with the continuous mastery of crafts and complex mechanisms. In building railway layouts or model airplanes the person, whether adult or child, is literally becoming through demonstrating competence in doing, 'creating self and shaping the world' (Wilcock, 1999: 77, 2006). This mastery enables the individual to acquire competencies through absorption in the model world arguably leaving real problems to work themselves through in the unconscious (King, 1996).

Critiques of Modelling

Much of this discussion so far has treated the activity of modelling as politically neutral and as having a generally positive value. Nevertheless, adult modellers often attract derision because their activities are regarded as frivolous, or as a forms of play with all its connotations of childishness. As Sutton-Smith (1997) notes, playful adult recreations originate in the exploratory activities of childhood, but are given separate ideological and rhetorical concepts that deny these connections (work is serious and adult and play is only purposeful in childhood). However, Sutton-Smith (1997) argues that play and playfulness are important elements of adult behaviour with a rich set of serious purposes and are not merely the opposite of work. While it is undeniable that many modellers like making things for fun (King, 1996; Pearson, 2007; Booth, 2010), the authors concur that what Rieber *et al.* (1998: 29) describe as 'serious play' is a valuable but often neglected aspect of human occupation. This is reflected in Van Leeuwen and Westwood's (2008) finding that the authors of psychological literature mostly explore play in children, rather than adults. The rejection of adult play and connected occupations such as modelling arises from a culture of repudiation of gendered childhood enthusiasms, which may lead modellers to be both ashamed (Marchant, 2003) and defensive of their activities.

One of the attractions of modelling is the representation both of the world as a space that can be travelled through in the vehicles that models represent and the filling of space both in the external environment and in our own homes with objects (King, 1996; Jenkinson, 2001). Simmons (1998) points out that a difference between railway modelling and other subjects is that it often concerns the representation of landscape, not just the trains in it. Consequently, another difference between railway and aircraft modelling is in the consideration of the space that a railway layout takes up. Whereas a collection of model aircraft can be placed on a shelf, model railways take up parts of the home or garden living space (Wylie, 1987; Andress, 1988; Jenkinson, 2001). Csíkszentmihályi and Rochberg-Halton (1981), Lefebvre (1991a) and Butsch (1984) remind us that this is a physical *occupation* of space with the detritus of capitalist modes of production, commodity objects that are made to be bought, sold, consumed and reproduced. It may be suggested that they have no purpose but to be displayed as representations of status (Csíkszentmihályi and Rochberg-Halton, 1981). Lefebvre may even describe them as personal fetishes – things with an abstract but not a real value. These 'badges of consumption' are some of the many representations of the way in which 'self-management of daily life' is absorbed and consumed without thinking (Lefebvre, 2005: 31). So, the experience of childhood itself becomes both commonly defined and commodified through objects such as the trainset or Airfix kit.

The making of models has become a tradition in the postwar iconography of mass consumption, but they are not the products of the traditional folk crafts that preceded them. Butsch (1984) deplores this transition from the vernacular form to the manufactured modelling experience. Even if they are invested with identity because they have been personally chosen and bought by an individual, this investment is ephemeral, and thus modelling pursuits may be dismissed by materialist critics as belonging to the fetishistic, self-indulgent and often nostalgic diversions that disguise the exploitative nature of social relations under capitalism (Lefebvre, 1991b, 2002). Many railway layouts are given names and referred to in the literature as if they are actual places or railway systems – something that may underpin Lefebvre's views. This criticism applies not only to the human occupation of modelling or the display of models in domestic spaces, but to their representation of obsolete objects and the vanished airfields or railway environments they may have been part of. Thus the consumption and commodification of modelling as an occupation is an element of the continuous social reconstruction and reproduction of space under capitalism (Soja, 1989). Railway modelling is particularly concerned with detailed representation of landscape and land uses (Wylie, 1987; Jenkinson, 2001). Accurate representation of social reality (for example signs of wear, models of people engaged in occupations) might form part of the scenery, and may contain narrative elements in the detail but is usually no more than an objective interest. The fitting of railway landscapes into spare corners of the home, garden, or even on a coffee table certainly embody the reproduction of space in Soja's terms, but actually aim to satisfy the simple visual appeal of the object moving through an outdoor scene (King, 1996).

Although it is not possible to develop the discussion further here, there are obviously some aspects of modelling that may appear to be a questionable celebration of military power and particular political doctrines. This notion is not lost on modellers (Pearson, 2007). As Baker notes in his evocative piece on the military aircraft model (1997: 32) 'its alliances are unsettled; the cozy homage it pays to lethal force is part of its attraction.' The final part of this sentence alludes to an aspect of the appeal of modelling, which Baker unfortunately does not expand on, and which remains uninvestigated. So, to return to King (1996), while it is unlikely that modelling will play a significant social or political role, it may involve a perpetuation of status quo values for good or bad, for example with regard to instilling airmindedness. To reinterpret Wilcock's (2006) occupational mantra of doing, being, becoming and belonging, model-making often represents what has been done, what was, what became of, and what belongs to the past.

The History, Scale and Nature of the Modelling Market

As a populist activity for the last hundred years modelling has long been the focus of significant business interests. For example in 1935 airplane modelling was still 'riding the Lindbergh high' following his successful translatlantic flight. With a yearly turnover of $15 000 000 the US aeromodelling industry had a potential: 'almost equal to the 1929 sales volume of the full-size aircraft industry' (King, 1996: 97). By 1946 *Aeromodeller* (p. 284) claimed 3 million youthful 'zealous followers' for this 'great scientific sport' in America, proposing that it could become an Olympic competition.

The adult hobby of serious railway modelling began to flourish in the 1930s and 1940s (Allen, 1979; King, 1996). In Britain, specialist collectors societies developed from the late 1960s as new products became increasingly adult oriented or acceptable to adults (Hammond, 1999). Today's highly detailed steam-powered model locomotives costing several hundred pounds are definitely not intended for children.

Model displays are also popular among a wider public. A contemporary example, Hamburg's Miniatur Wonderland, the world's largest model railway, claims to have attracted 4 million visitors between 2001 and 2007 (Miniatur Wunderland, 2010a).

Despite the ubiquity of modelling as human occupation throughout human history (King, 1996) it is evident that contemporary model making is a product of postwar affluence and new manufacturing technologies. This is coincident with a historic time of huge technological advances in vehicular transport and aviation. So, when plastic kits became more available after the war, they made modelling (of a variety of subjects including cars and historical figures) more accessible to nonmodellers and captured an even larger market. Ninety per cent of US males aged 12 to 15 had made one in 1959 (Butsch, 1984). Today the volume of sales is much lower but some form of commercial stability is said to exist in the sector (Ward, 2004).

Nevertheless fewer young people seem to be taking up the hobby and for some time both hobbyists and the modelling industry have expressed concerns that they need to be active in creating new cohorts of younger modellers (for example, Anon., 1957). One strategy is to produce models of varying sophistication and cost appropriate to any given age group. Another, bearing in mind the Hornby advertisement mentioned earlier, is to impress on adult consumers who in turn impress on children the idea that models are not toys and represent a lifelong hobby interest (for example, Brewer, 1970; Simmons, 1998; Jenkinson, 2001). Hornby's model railway products were made to be compatible with earlier models, the enthusiast's pocket and ability to use the available space in the home (Edey, 1979; Kedge, 1979; Lines, 1979). These compromises allowed railway hobbyists to progress from childhood games with toys to becoming modellers.

In addition, the average age of kit modellers is increasing (Parkins in Stanton, 2002) and the phenomenon of 'kids growing older younger' (Lauwert, 2008: 225) is matched by that of 'adults staying younger longer' (ASYL) (Lauwert, 2008: 233). King (1996) implies the re-explorations of childhood modelling actives may occur more widely as a motive underpinning adult modelling behaviours. He cites Jung's (1983) report of an adult episode of trying to recover something of the childhood experience of building model castles. To appeal to today's adult market many manufacturers have disassociated their products from childhood by dropping the 'toy' word from their brands (Lauwert, 2008). This enables model makers who abandoned their hobby in adolescence to reconnect legitimately with the interest as an 'adult pursuit' in later life (Ward, 1999; Stanton, 2002). These particular modellers (and those who never gave up) are a significant consumer group and represent 'down-ageing', the phenomenon of adults returning to pursuits and products from their youth (Harkin and Huber, 2004: 37). 'Down ageing' is associated with those known as 'baby boomers', born between 1945 and 1965, who are said to be the first generation to have grown up in the 'mass consumption' society (Harkin and Huber, 2004: 30).

This pattern of occupations gives rise to some controversy. Butsch (1984) describes 'traditional' aeromodelling, the building of flying models, as open to everyone because it used readily available household materials such as paper and card. The reuse of these materials offered a range of skilled modelling occupations. However, a modelling industry rapidly grew to supply modellers with items, such as preformed propellers or wheels, which made it easier to build successful models (King, 1996; Alcorn, 2009). Making modelling more accessible through the mass production of models in plastic kit form was not seen by Butsch (1984: 231) as a democratization of the hobby. On the contrary, plastic modelling involved the passive consumption of artefacts – a symptom of the capitalist (and undesirable) 'commodification' of leisure pursuits. The building of a model from already engineered parts therefore undermines traditional modelling skills.

Arguably this trend has continued through the many manufacturers catering to the relatively affluent 'downageing' market. In the 1962 Tri-ang Railways handbook, artist Terence Cuneo showed boys how to transform pristine toy trains into realistic models through painted dirt and 'weathering' details that represent the marks of use in a railway system. This is difficult to do well, requiring keen observation and a steady hand. Adult collectors can now buy their engines and rolling stock already 'weathered'.

A host of small industries now produce tiny parts (sometimes in resin or white metal) suitable for adding 'super detail' to an existing kit or to transform a mass-produced item into something apparently more personal and unique (Ward, 1999; Pearson, 2007). Although these industries are producing expensive labour-saving consumables, considerable skill is still needed to use these parts because the materials have very different qualities to the original plastic and preformed kits have to be altered (for example, Stanton, 2002). So despite Butsch's (1984) concerns, modellers still have to develop new abilities constantly to work with novel materials (for example, resin, rather than polystyrene) or devise new techniques for resolving problems (Wylie, 1987; King, 1996). These forms of 'serious play' and 'soft mastery' (Reiber *et al.*, 1998) i.e. the tinkering and 'bricolage' (King, 1996, p71) that constitute scratch building, seem to derive ultimately from experiences of 'free play' – an important developmental element of tacit learning (Parkinson, 1998; Anning, 2002) and are often arrived at through experimentation using materials that are commonly to hand. Thus, liquid plastic filler made from sprue and glue can disguise the gaps between parts of a polystyrene kit, while household rubbish like packaging and scrap wood is the basis of much model railway scenery (Allen, 1979; Tri-ang Railways, 1962).

These improvisations or bricolage challenge Butsch's (1984) assertions that important folk elements of model making, for example using materials that are to hand, have been displaced. It seems that, regardless of technological change, model-makers persist in demonstrating both improvisational and innovatory skill.

A widespread perception of these modelling industries and the occupation of modelling as a whole is that it is usually a male gendered activity. There are, however notable exceptions to this male preserve, including lifelong railway model exhibitors Vivien Thompson, author of a 1971 book on model buildings, and Shirley Rowe (1980), an expert on modelling trees. Nevertheless these exceptions seem to prove the rule. The Braun twins' initial market survey for their Miniatur Wunderland, found that men rated the model railway as the third most likely Hamburg attraction they would visit out of 45 real and proposed facilities; women rated it last (Miniatur Wunderland, 2010b).

As a social phenomenon this may derive from the extremely intense strongly gender-stereotyped interests in certain real objects, (for example, vehicles for boys and clothes for girls) that many young children show at the age of 12 months, independently of being given gendered toys or other social reinforcement (De-Loache *et al.*, 2007). Deloache *et al.* (2007) suggested that very young children show gender differences in the way they focus on stimuli in their environment, boys paying more attention to nonsocial stimuli such as cars, than girls, who pay more attention to interactions such as talking. As they develop socially, girls are less likely to have the opportunities that allow them to experiment with action-related construction toys such as Meccano or K-nex. They tend not to be given toys that give them practical experience of, for example, the use of wheels (Parkinson, 1998), although girls and women are keen collectors and modellers of dolls' houses and miniature interiors (King, 1996; Booth, 2010). DeLoache *et al.* (2007) found that these gender differences are initially acquired at 12 months old without deliberate social reinforcement, over time different activities become gendered domains.

Aircraft designer E. Lillian Todd set up a modelling society, 'the Junior Aero Club' for boys in 1908. Despite being a woman herself, girls were not included. This was possibly because she 'deferred to the wishes of the parent organization', the Aero

Club (Alcorn, 2009: 110). However, Todd herself was pressured to leave the club due to her public activities as a woman aircraft inventor, which generated some disquiet (Alcorn, 2009). The men who pursued her exclusion may have been protecting their gendered anxieties about women entering the male world of aviation. At this time women's participation in many technical and social fields was contested. A gender division appears to be maintained as evidenced in statements such as: '. . . there seems to have developed a greater dividing line between model shops staffed by model makers . . . and toy shops which often rely on girl or lady assistants who are more informed about dolls and teddy bears' (Simmons, 1998: 21).

Through such exclusions, males may have isolated themselves in their technological worlds, often concealed in attics and sheds (Simmons, 1998), perhaps only leaving them behind, as Wolmar (2007: 5) admits, when they became interested 'in girls'. Consequently children learn to reject the gendered games of the opposite sex; girls traditionally disdain boys' games because they have not until recently been given encouragement to play with technology (Reiber *et al.*, 1998). Such differences may partly explain why the literature of the predominantly female occupational therapy profession has neglected this significant set of human activities, despite a considerable interest in children and in doing (Frank, Block and Zemke, 2008). The development of 'Men in Sheds' interventions (Ormsby *et al.*, 2010) may challenge the imbalance with regard to gendered activity. These groups for older men meet in sheds to pursue activities such as woodworking and repairing or restoring items. They are a response to client perceptions that many therapeutic activities are oriented to women, with the result that men do not engage with them easily. As well as providing activities, an important objective of Men in Sheds is to provide venues for male socialization.

Conclusion: Models, Competences, Identities, and Representing Human Occupation

Though often derided in popular culture and overlooked in academic literature modelling, activities appear to offer people, particularly but not necessarily men, the means of expressing skills and competences through the skilful representation of objects. The making or controlling of models not only reflects individual mastery but complements the expression of identity. Modelling, as part of the physical expression of being-in-the-world, also expresses simple fascination with intricacy, size, and movement, elements of the wider human occupational landscape re-imagined both for private enjoyment and to share with others through social networks (King, 1996).

These models and their landscapes often arise from childhood interests as well as adult experiences and a human need to make sense of them. As a personal symbolization of the world the modelling of objects may be a meaningful element of the cultural and occupational identity of each generation (Hammell, 2004; Abrahams, 2008).

The value and purpose of model-making and its associated activities can be considered as a trivial and frivolous activity, which is materialistic and ephemeral. However these criticisms can also be applied to many other human occupations and relations with objects. People do not always need to be engaged in occupations of great and noble purpose but may enjoy the relaxation gained from smaller scale activities in the peripheral spaces of sheds, attics or spare rooms. A particular application of modelling to therapy practice may be suggested by the Men in Sheds activities, which are not very different from the kinds of social venues established for the negotiation of the many different aspects of modellers' occupations (King, 1996; Simmons, 1998).

It is evident that many people derive a lifelong interest in both making models and the objects and landscapes that they make models of, as well as the many activities such as exchanging techniques or engaging in detailed research which may support their production. Much of the literature produced so far tends to be by and for modelling enthusiasts, with the consequence that many potential themes for discussion remain as yet undeveloped, such as the uneasy relationship between occupations and their commodification. In the case of modelling, many human occupations can themselves be modelled and thus turned into commodities which can be miniature representations of 'real life' as a part of a landscape. This facility to symbolize aspects of the real environment is part of the fun, part of the serious play, and perhaps forms part of the objections others may have to the activity. Yet some valuable opportunities for purposeful and enjoyable occupation may be lost if adults cannot recognize their need for serious play, and as an occupation modelling is often absorbing, harmless, reflective and accessible.

References

Abrahams, T. (2008) Occupation, identity and choice: a dynamic interaction. *Journal of Occupational Science* 15(2): 186–189.

Alcorn, A. L. (2009) Modeling Behavior: Boyhood, Engineering, and the Model Airplane in American Culture. Unpublished PhD thesis, Case Western Reserve University.

Allen, B. (2008) Operation Desert Storm Iraqi T62-A. *Baghdad Hobby Club* 1(1), 4, http//:ipmsusa.org/, accessed 19 November 2010.

Allen, T. (1979) (ed.) *The Encyclopedia of Model Railways*. London, Octopus.

Andress, M. (1988) *PSL Complete Guide to Model Railways*. London, Guild.

Anon. (1946) quoting from unknown article in 'Planes' Editorial. *Aeromodeller*. April, pp. 283–284.

Anon. (1957), Heard at The Hanger Doors. *Aeromodeller* (July), pp. 348-349.

Anning, A. (2002) Conversations around young children's drawing: the impact of the beliefs of significant others at home and school. *International Journal of Art and Design Education* 21(3), 197–208.

Association of Professional Model Makers (2010) Definition of a model maker, www.model-makers.org/mc/page.do?sitePageId=73232&orgId=apmm, accessed 25 September.2010.

Baker, N. (1997) Model airplanes. In *The Size of Thoughts*. New York, Vintage, pp. 27–35.

Ballestriero, R. (2010) Anatomical models and wax Venuses: art or scientific craft works? *Journal of Anatomy* 216(2), 223–234.

Booth, H. (2010) Interiors: Living doll's house. *The Guardian* 21st August. http://www.guardian.co.uk/lifeandstyle/2010/august/21/dolls-house-brighton accessed 28th January 2012

Brewer, J. (1970) *Build a Model Railway*. London, Wolfe Publishing.

Butsch, R. (1984) The commodification of leisure: the case of the model airplane hobby and industry. *Qualitative Sociology* 7(3), 217–235.

Carter, D., Kent, J., Hart, G. (1992) *Pullman Craftsmen: Life in the Pullman Car Company's Preston Park Works*. Brighton, QueenSpark.

Chaffee, H. (2010) Ten Talents of a Model Builder, www.modelmakers.org/mc/page.do?sitePageId=73244&orgId=APMM, 18 November 2010.

Conard, N. J. (2009) A female figurine from the basal Aurignacian of Hohle Fels cave in southwest Germany. *Nature* 459, 248–252.

Csíkszentmihályi, M. (1990) *Flow: The Psychology of Optimal Experience*. New York: Harper & Row.

Csíkszentmihályi, M., Rochberg-Halton, E. (1981) *The Meaning of Things: Domestic Symbols and the Self*. Cambridge, Cambridge University Press.

Cuneo, T. (1962) Creating lifelike models. In Tri-ang Railways (1962) *The First Ten Years*. Margate: Cuneo, pp. 65–70.

DeLoache, J.S., Simcock, G., Macari, S. (2007) Planes, trains, automobiles – and tea sets: extremely intense interests in very young children. *Developmental Psychology* 43(6), 1579–1586.

DeMott, S. (2008) *Hello to All from Baghdad. Hobbies for Heroes*, http://www.ipmsusa.org/, accessed 19 November 2010

Edey, P. (1979) The Hornby system. In S. W. Stevens-Stratten (ed.) *The Hornby Book of Trains, 25 Year Edition. Prototypes and Models*. Kent: Rovex Limited, pp. 134–141.

Elwell, J. H. (1941) *Solid Scale Model Aircraft*. Leicester, Harborough Publishing Company.

Erikson, E. H. (1980) *Identity and the Life Cycle*. New York, Norton.

Frank, G., Block, P., Zemke, R. Introduction to special theme issue anthropology, occupational therapy and disability studies: collaborations and prospects. *Practicing Anthropology* 30(3), 2–5.

Hammell, K. W. (2004) Dimensions of meaning in the occupations of daily life. *Canadian Journal of Occupational Therapy* 71(5), 296–305.

Hammond, P. (1999) A history of collecting model trains in Britain. *Model Railway Express Mag*, www.mremag.com/articles/col-18.12.99/collectinghistory.htm, accessed 20 October 2010.

Harkin, J., Huber, J. (2004) *Eternal Youths: How the Baby Boomers are Having Their Time Again*. London, Hendey Banks.

Historic Scotland (2010) Orkney Venus Gets a Partner, www.historic-scotland.gov.uk/news_article.htm?articleid=28619, accessed 19 October 2010.

Hollick, B. (1991) *Pullman Attendant*. Brighton, QueenSpark.

Jenkinson, D. (2001) *Historical Railway Modelling*. York, Pendragon.

Jung, C. G. (1983) *Memories, Dreams, Reflections*. London, Flamingo.

Kedge, J. M. (1979) Tooling and production in the Hornby factory. In S. W. Stevens-Stratten (ed.) *The Hornby Book of Trains, 25 Year Edition. Prototypes and Models*. Kent, Rovex Limited, pp. 38–47.

King, J.R. (1996) *Remaking the World, Modeling in Human Experience*. Urbana, University of Illinois Press.

Lauwaert, M. (2008) Playing outside the box – on LEGO toys and the changing world of construction play. *History and Technology* 24(3), 221–237.

Lefebvre, H. (1991a) *The Production of Space*. Oxford, Blackwell.

Lefebvre, H. (1991b) *Critique of Everyday Life: Volume 1* Translated by John Moore. London, Verso.

Lefebvre, H. (2002) *Critique of Everyday Life: Volume 2 Foundations for a Sociology of the Everyday*. Translated by John Moore. London, Verso.

Lefebvre, H. (2005) *Critique of Everyday Life: Volume 3 From Modernity to Modernism*. Translated by Gregory Elliot. London, Verso.

Lehron, A.L. (2004) The modeling miscreant. http://www.ipmsusa.org/Features/Miscreant/Miscreant.htm accessed 28th January, 2012.

Lines, H. L. (1979) The story of the Princess and the Duchess. In S. W. Stevens-Stratten (ed.) *The Hornby Book of Trains. 25 Year Edition. Prototypes and Models*. Kent, Rovex Limited, pp. 48–53.

Marchant, I. (2003) *Parallel Lines, or Journeys on the Railways of Dreams*. London, Bloomsbury.

Miniatur Wunderland (2010a) *Wunderland Facts*, www.miniatur-wunderland.com/exhibit/wunderland/wonderland-facts/, accessed 5 December 2010.

Miniatur Wunderland (2010b) Conception of the Wunderland, www.miniatur-wunderland.com/exhibit/wunderland/wonderland-conception/, accessed 5 December 2010.

Ormsby, J., Stanley, M., Jaworski, K. (2010) Older people's participation in community-based men's sheds programmes. *Health and Social Care in the Community* 18(6), 607–613.

Parkins, D. (2002) What is Happening to Our Hobby? In Stanton, M. *Scale Aircraft Modelling*. Ramsbury, The Crowood Press.

Parkinson, E. (1998) *The Seduction of the Wheel: A Synthesis of Research Based Issues Surrounding Car-led Construction Activities of Young Children and the Relationship These May Have with Current Environmental Trends which Progressively Seek to Limit the Impact of Road Traffic*. Loughborough, Loughborough University, http://hdl.handle.net/2134/1427, accessed 25 October 2010.

Pearson, H. (2007) *Achtung schweinehund, a boy's own story of imaginary combat*. London, Little, Brown.

Rebeiro, K. (2001) Occupational spin-off. *Journal of Occupational Science* 8, 33–34.

Rieber, L.P., Smith, L., Noah, D. (1998) The value of serious play. *Educational Technology* 38(6), 29–37.

Ross, E. (1984) *Tales of the Rails*. Bristol, Bristol Broadsides.

Rowe, S. (1980) *Model Trees*. Rowe.

Simmons, N. (1998) *Railway Modelling*, 8th edn. Sparkford, Patrick Stephens.

Snowden, T. (2002) Foreword. In M. Stanton (ed.) *Scale Aircraft Modelling*. Ramsbury, The Crowood Press, pp. 4–5.

Soja, E. W. (1989) *Postmodern Geographies: The Reassertion of Space in Critical Social Theory*. London, Verso.

Stanton, M. (2002) *Scale Aircraft Modelling*. Ramsbury, The Crowood Press.

Stevens-Stratten, S.W. (1979) Scales and gauges. In S. W. Stevens-Stratten (ed.) *The Hornby Book of Trains, 25 Year Edition. Prototypes and Models*. Kent, Rovex Limited, pp. 26–31.

Sutton-Smith, B. (1997) *The Ambiguity of Play*. Cambridge, MA, Harvard University Press.

Thompson, V. (1971) *Period Railway Modelling Buildings*. Seaton, Peco.

Tri-ang Railways. (1962) *The First Ten Years* ... Margate: Tri-ang Railways.

Van Leeuwen, L., Westwood, D. (2008) Adult play, psychology and design. *Digital Creativity* 19(3), 153–161.

Ward, A. (1999) *Airfix: Celebrating 50 Years of the Greatest Plastic Kits in the World*. London, HarperCollins.

Ward, A. (2004) *Classic Kits: Collecting the Greatest Model Kits in the World, from Airfix to Tamiya*. London, HarperCollins.

Wilcock, A. A. (1999) Creating Self and Shaping the World. *Australian Occupational Therapy Journal* 46, 77–88.

Wilcock, A. A. (2006) *An Occupational Perspective of Health*, 2nd edn. Thorofare, NJ, SLACK Incorporated.

Williams, A. (1984) *Life in a Railway Factory*. Stroud, Alan Sutton.

Wolmar, C. (2007) *Fire and Steam. A New History of the Railways in Britain*. London, Atlantic.

Wren, T. (1998) *Flying Sparks*. Brighton, QueenSpark.

Wylie, J. (1987) *The Professional Approach to Model Railways*. Sparkford, Patrick Stephens.

14 Participation, Time, Effort and Speech Disability Justice

Devva Kasnitz and Pamela Block

Introduction

Who experiences speech disability? People who stutter; people with motor speech problems such as cerebral palsy (CP), amyotrophic lateral sclerosis (ALS), dystonia; people with hearing impairments, people labelled with psychological, cognitive, or developmental conditions such as autism or Down's syndrome; people with illness or injury to head, neck, chest, caused by stroke, cancer, or traumatic injury, among others; people whose chosen or imposed 'voice' is a letter board, a machine, or a human interpreter or revoicer. All these people share experiences of speech anomaly or difference that are usually considered impairments in the medical world and are usually treated as disability in the socio-cultural political world. We include in this chapter and in our work and organizing around issues of speech, people of all kinds of speech differences, whether the difference is in cause or perceived cause, in the actual functional difference in their speech or lack thereof, or in the strategies they employ to live in the world.

We speak of 'speech disability justice', an admittedly awkward phrase, to highlight a current paradigmatic shift in disability scholarship and activism from a framework that highlights not only the choice of independent living and the identification, defence, and expansion of disability rights, but human interdependence and reciprocal responsibility. In this social justice approach, full participation and citizenship for disabled people means that accommodation is not 'for' only the disabled person (see Kasnitz, 2008c). It is not as simple as a disabled person asking for or being offered something specific, an 'accommodation,' that moves them closer to parity in participation and citizenship. Disability justice stresses that we all must take on responsibilities to assure ourselves, and the most marginalized among us, maximum

Politics of Occupation-Centred Practice: Reflections on Occupational Engagement across Cultures, First Edition. Edited by Nick Pollard and Dikaios Sakellariou.
© 2012 John Wiley & Sons, Ltd. Published 2012 by John Wiley & Sons, Ltd.

agency, even within the disability rights movement. Some activists use 'disability justice' to specifically refer to disabled people who also experience racism (see Milbern, 2010). Borrowing from occupational justice, we use speech disability justice here to refer to the broadest sense of social justice applied to disability, and focused on societal and individual responsibility to and of speech impaired people, one of the most marginalized impairment groups. In oral history interviews with people with multiple impairments from cerebral palsy, including the inability to walk, transfer at all alone, or use their arms or hands, the experience of speech impairment consistently is their biggest concern and source of pain (see Shuttleworth, 2000; Zukas, 2000; Kasnitz and Shuttleworth, 2003; Kasnitz, 2005). Speech disability, that is, *the perception of anomalous impairing speech and the experience of discrimination and exclusion to which it leads in the world*, is the domain where speech-impaired people seek social justice.

This chapter is unusual in its format. It is a continuation of a decade-long conversation between two friends and colleagues in anthropology specializing in disability studies. It is written in three voices. We switch voice from Devva writing in the first person, to Pamela writing in the first person, both clearly marked with our names and indented, to us speaking together in reflection as 'we'. Devva has dystonia, a genetic movement disorder that affects all of her body and her speech, and Pamela's older sister, Hope, has autism and rarely uses her biological voice, preferring instead various *alternative and augmentative communication* (AAC) voices (Pamela's sister is a co-author of Chapter 12 in this volume). We have worked on speech impairment together, with Hope (Block *et al.*, 2008a, 2008b, 2009), with Devva's colleague and revoicer Russell Shuttleworth (Kasnitz and Shuttleworth, 2003; also see Chapter 12 in this volume), with Devva's sister (Steinberg and Kasnitz, 2011) and with many colleagues, other speech-impaired people, and allies, although much of this work is done at conferences and is unpublished (see Scheer, 2005; Kasnitz and Munger, 2010). We are organizing a Speech Impairment Research and Advocacy Interest Group within the Society for Disability Studies (SDS),[1] an organization of which Devva is the current and Pamela the past president. In our conference panels, as in this chapter, we try to take what might be called a cross-etiology ecological approach to speech disability and its phenomenological nature and political posture. As we both also study disability in global medical systems, in particular the training of medicine-related professional in general and occupational therapists in particular (Block *et al.*, 2005; Block, Frank and Zemke, 2008; Kasnitz, 2008a; Mankoff *et al.*, 2010), we look at the interface of medicine, social services and community development, with a strengths-based approach.

The goal of this piece is to introduce the readers to some of the lived experience of people with different speech and the crossroads at which we stand between exercising our rights to accommodation and access to social participation and citizenship. We understand that this will take everyone's' effort and time and it's our responsibility to use both responsibly. This approach to speech disability justice emphasizes mutual responsibility. Few issues hit deeper than communication

---

[1] For information see www.disstudies.org or contact devva@earthlink.net.

disability. Focus on speech also raises questions about language. A focus on language raises questions about cognition. A focus on cognition raises questions about competency. Without being unrealistic, we believe some of these links to be derogatory stereotypes (see Kliewer *et al.*, 2006). We either have seen loved ones or personally been through the pain of, or fear of, being labelled 'retarded' – a measure of competency we now completely reject, and not only for ourselves. In assuring that we expend and receive the effort and time it takes to truly communicate, we celebrate our interdependence. There are many factors at work in creating disability and occupational apartheid (Kronenberg and Pollard, 2005) out of difference: economic, educational, medical, technological, attitudinal, and environmental factors, and more (Frank and Kasnitz, 2011). We look today at *time* and bodily/perceptual concentration or *effort* involved in disability and occupational justice for people with speech impairment. What more precious resources do we need and offer than time and effort?

In the development of the disability rights movement, few of the voices of speech-impaired people are memorable. Prominent individuals – such as Bob Williams, the first developmentally disabled person to hold the post of Commissioner of the Administration on Developmental Disabilities (1993) under President Clinton, and physicist Stephen Hawking – are the exceptions who prove the rule. In both of these cases, their work is not about speech impairment and what you remember is not their own impaired biological voice, but the computerized voice they both eventually adopted and share, and with which they are identified and self-identify. To some the machine is their voice. Stephen Hawking refuses to switch to new voice synthesis technology. He is accustomed to his voice (as are we – so many people seem to have his same accent) even though the new software might cost him less effort and time.

To say that people with speech impairment lack 'voice' in their struggle for agency in their lives should be obvious. The institutions of speech therapy and occupational or physical therapy, are not structured to help 'patients/clients' meet each other and organize, though there are exceptions to this rule too, particularly in the practice of progressive community-based rehabilitation, occupational therapy without borders, and similar paradigms (Kronenberg *et al.*, 2005; Kronenberg and Pollard, 2005).

Perhaps the most successful speech-impaired person advocating on issues of speech impairment in the policy arena is Bob Segalman (2009). Bob is responsible for the existence of the US Federally mandated speech to speech (STS) telephone relay system which mirrors the much better known and used text to text relay for people with hearing impairments. For many reasons, while this remote telephone mediated system of revoicing is underutilized, something that the addition of video might change, face-to-face revoicing, such as Devva uses, is gaining acceptance.

What does universal design mean to people with speech differences? Many people assume technology will solve the problem yet technology designers are latecomers to studying the experience of disability (Mankoff *et al.*, 2010). Simply knowing what technology to apply, for example sound proofing, would be a good start (another tie to the hearing impairment world). But how do we slow the elevator down enough for us to actually be able to answer the basic question 'how are you mate?' (Hughes and

Paterson, 1997). Acoustics and ambient noise, any distracting visual stimuli, physical dividers, like tables that keep people too far apart or out of sightlines, the design of most microphones or phones or laptops (Kaye *et al.*, 2009; Pedlow *et al.*, 2010), are all just a few technical issues that may or may not be understood but are changeable. How do we change listeners' expectations, stereotypes, and behaviour? How does Devva say 'I'm sorry, but I have a speech impairment, you need to listen more carefully' fast enough and clearly enough to the woman on the phone from the bank who has just asked if she speaks English? (I don't. I hang up. Bob tells me to use STS.) How do we, and our allies, participate, and when is the fight worth the effort? Some people take some refuge in virtual reality (see Boellstorff, 2008), not a total solution. Answering these questions is where we learn together and from a commonality with all disabled people.

Devva:	At home I rarely speak out loud, never when I am alone. Alone I don't even vocalize at all. I conserve my energy. I even train my dogs with hand signals. But I like my biological voice, as long as I don't hear it recorded. Typing is still harder than talking and slower, unless I have the right table, chair, and keyboard on a bad speech day with no revoicer.
Pamela:	To Hope, her machine *is* her chosen voice.[2] She rarely vocalizes in public. It is a very intimate activity to her that only dear family and friends get to share. She sings. She hums, they are happy hums, angry hums, annoyed hums. They are often supported and emphasized by personal signs. Sometimes, very rarely, they are songs. When she was a child she hummed all kinds of songs but now just Happy Birthday on people's birthdays. Somewhere along the line she decided not to use her biological voice publically.

Participation and Citizenship

Participation and citizenship are common goals. What we choose, or are allowed to choose, to do to achieve them, independently or interdependently, is cultural, situational, and temporal. We learn from each other. Steeped in the most progressive part of the academic study of disability, we may have much to offer global diffusion and intensification of the independent living paradigm (DeJong, 1979) but being open to interdependent ways of achieving participation or citizenship is also important. One of our unique desires is to see what the commonalties are across all kinds of reasons for speech differences, including where and when and for how long what kind of effort is acceptable to achieve the goals of participation and

[2] Hope and all of the other individuals discussed here by Pamela, and Ephraim, Neil, and Teddy and others discussed by Devva, or both of us, have had the opportunity to review this chapter and have given their permission to be mentioned.

citizenship. The following is an example of how imposing one cultural and situational view of the limits of interdependence on another can be problematic (Kasnitz and Edwards, 2011). We offer it here to remind ourselves that despite our personal experience with speech impairment, we too may have our biases about what is acceptable accommodation that we unknowingly impose on other people with speech impairment. It's often easier to see one's internalized bias looking at something a bit more removed from the intensely personal.

Devva: This lesson was brought home to me last summer. I was teaching disability studies in a field school in Guatemala hosted by the local independent living centre. Transiciones had long tried to see the mayor of Antigua, the colonial capital of Guatemala. My American PhD student in public administration used her status as a hook and we got an appointment for our last day in town. As we shuffled and rolled to the 1700s building where he occupied a suite of upstairs rooms, at first the secretary told us our appointment was cancelled, but then they decided they would fit us in because we were two American *Professores*, but of course he could not come downstairs to meet with us but they could carry six foot Ephraim up the stairs. We two crip American women, both of whom had directed Independent Living Centers were aghast. That was not an option to us. We went to sit in the waiting room upstairs and strategize. About 10 minutes later Ephraim rolled in. He had decided that participating in the meeting was more important than our gringa sense of outrage and he let the police carry him up the stairs when we were not looking. When we got to talk to the mayor an hour later, in the waiting area, not the inner sanctum, Ephraim had his coming out as an orator and made the most eloquent comments to the mayor, every moment of which would have been such a loss had he let our sensibility rule. Although, it was something to watch four Guatemalan police, one a woman, carry him down all those crumbling 400-year-old marble steps. He had participated. His sense of self and of citizenship has never been stronger, and he is effective. I should have known better. Ephraim compromised his preferred physical accommodation (elevator or first floor) in order to have a voice. How often do I, too, compromise my preferred speech accommodation to have a voice? More importantly, this story sticks in my mind when I am speaking about speech accommodations in general. I remind myself to be careful. I try to avoid imposing my personal sense of what accommodations I will accept when, in order to participate, on my speech impaired peers.

Pamela: When a graduate student asked for captioning at a national anthropology conference, the organization was taking an extraordinarily long time to give an answer. After an initial denial, we began a game of good-cop bad-cop where the student communicated her needs and rights forcefully while Devva and I (along with some others) educated and suggested practical options, with much hemming, hawing, and helplessness (from the organization). The student finally received marginal quality captioning rationed for a few sessions, but the organization did adopt most of a disability accommodation policy and procedure we suggested. This past year, for another national anthropology organization's conference, after they included a minimal question on disability accommodation requests in their registration procedure, it still took the disabled person several extra steps and satisfaction was definitely not guaranteed. In this case, after repeated requests and compromising on American Sign Language interpreting instead of captioning, the student arrived at the conference not knowing if there would be interpreters and with lawyers' numbers in her pocket. Perhaps worse, the interpreters were instructed to stop work when conference sessions ended. The D/deaf[3] members lost their voice in-between sessions, at the book exhibit, the placement center, or in the hallway, where of course the most important conversations happen. Costs of captioning and sign language interpretation are significant. The Society for Disability Studies provides accommodations for *all* conference hours and spends tens of thousands of dollars each year on these costs, which are essential to the organization's mission, but often mean the difference between a financially profitable conference and ending the year in the red. Speech accommodations, in the form of voice interpreters, revoicers, computer-assisted speech, facilitators and so on may also fall in this category of expensive but essential to assure voice.

Chapter 10 in this volume beautifully summarizes definitions of participation and their connections to concepts of citizenship and rights (also see Frank and Kasnitz, 2011). We explore these issues for people who do not speak or speak differently and we do so looking at the elements of time and effort. Who cares where you sit on the bus if you can't get on the bus. Similarly, who cares if you can get on it if you can't ask where to catch it or where to get off before you miss your stop? As we move from talking about independence to interdependence, from function to choice in how to achieve tasks, from universal design to inclusive design, and even from participation to citizenship, we are now also moving from rights to justice.

Rights often need to be acknowledged by law and defended in policy. Justice implies mutual responsibilities toward everyone's rights. The Silicon Valley Independent Living Center strategic plan states a focus 'On a movement level, we challenge and partner with other advocates and organizations to think critically about our movement and move beyond disability rights to disability justice (focusing

---

[3] The capital *D* refers to people who identify or are identified as culturally *Deaf*. Small *d* refers to people who do not necessarily fit that category, including people who identify as hard of hearing. Neither refers to any measure of, or the nature of, the hearing loss or problem. We use the convention D/deaf as do others to be as inclusive as possible while acknowledging the importance of the distinction.

not only on what we have a right to, but also on what we are responsible for)' (Silicon Valley Independent Living Center, 2010). What responsibilities do listeners have to fundamentally change how, and for how long, they listen and the effort they expend in that activity? What responsibilities do we all have to apply our most creative efforts to ourselves and our material and social environments to minimize the effort and time, or take the effort and time it takes us all to communicate so that basic fatigue is not a crushing barrier?

The concept of occupational justice and the right to meaningful occupation is useful here (Galheigo, 2011; Stadnyk, Townsend and Wilcock, 2010). What is the experience of justice and overall participation, and of justice in the occupation of talking, for people who do not speak or vocalize, or who speak or vocalize differently? How can people assert what occupations they find meaningful if there is no appreciation of varied approaches to communication?

Experiences in Time and of Effort

Speaking is about vocalizing, that is making sound and about forming words. Some people vocalize a lot when they aren't speaking and some don't. For some the vocalization is what takes the effort; for some it's the words; for some it's both. We have noted that among our colleagues with cerebral palsy who use many kinds of AAC, from high to low tech and particularly in public, they may vocalize at the beginning just as if to say, 'Hi, I'm here, I'm the man behind the machine', then they turn to typing, or head pointing, or eye blinking, alone or with human help. The effort it takes them to do all of these tasks with rigid or involuntarily moving muscles is obvious and expected. When working with human help, reading a letter board, revoicing, speaking a prepared text, the two are a duet. The speech-impaired person articulates *with* the helper. Age and unpredictable bodies may make the effort needed, alone or in the duet, more intense. This is Devva's experience. For others, like Pamela's autistic sister, Hope, the years have been kinder.

Pamela: Years ago I remember seeing sweat and tears dripping down her face, I've seen her trembling with the effort of typing. These days it is definitely easier for her and seems to be continuing to flow more smoothly and requiring less support over time. So as you discuss how your voice continues to change, hers does too, but where your difficulty increases, hers seems to decrease overall, but with the same day-to-day fluctuations you experience.

Devva: The effort it takes me to speak has become much more obvious over the years, and I no longer try to hide it. I speak by starting sound at the end of the inhalation, forcing sound past a dysartic tongue, and running out of air at the end of a phoneme. Although I don't have CP, I have the CP 'accent' as surely as Steven Hawking has the AAC machine accent. Participation involves constant negotiation with no rest. It is exhausting.

Pamela: I have revoiced for Devva at conferences and when she recently guest lectured by skyping into one of my classes. Depending on who attends the conferences there might be many people who know Devva and are experienced at revoicing for her but sometimes it is just me. I have to agree with Devva, it is very exhausting for the revoicer too. It can also be fun negotiating things like location (so that attention remains centred on Devva rather than me and technologies (for instance, microphones, computers). Revoicing over the phone is hardest because there is no body language to help me along. If the connection is good, Skype works better. Unfortunately the connection during the guest lecture wasn't great and there was disconnection between blurry body language and facial expressions that were several beats slower than the speech. After about an hour to an hour-and-a-half I lost the ability to comprehend what Devva was saying. So we lost the thread and the students' attention.

At a recent disability studies conference in Brazil, which I attended in person and Devva attended by Skype, we had to be very creative with access technologies. One D/deaf participant could read English but could only read lips in Portuguese and Spanish. Lacking funding for captioning, all speakers, including me, presented in Portuguese. Devva and I presented jointly, we prepared our slides in English, (which the participant could read), but all spoken content was in Portuguese. When Devva had something to say via Skype, a Brazilian colleague of ours, who has met Devva, translated what she said, with me revoicing as necessary.

During monthly Society for Disability Studies phone conference call board meetings, there is constant experimentation to figure out what combination of communication strategies will work for all (or at least almost all) board members. Sometimes we used relay services for D/deaf members, sometimes chat served a captioning function. When I was president I struggled with how to both facilitate the meeting and revoice for Devva. The following year when Devva was president, the Vice President, Alberto Guzman, who is blind, chaired phone meetings for her, struggling to also listen to his computer read him the agenda and Devva's e mails and chat comments. Meanwhile, the secretary, Joan Ostrove, struggled to both take notes and revoice for Devva. We abandoned chat for regular email because the delay meant that those using it were left behind in the discourse anyhow and were also frustrated by the inability of chat systems we used, unlike email, to accept prepared text for cut and paste. Currently Devva relies heavily on email before, during, after the meeting, which is extremely time consuming for her, but deemed the best of all available options. Occasionally access needs come into conflict, as when someone using relay unknowingly introduces the sound of sirens and other street noises, making it impossible for auditory conversations to take place, or when one person best communicates through speech and has trouble reading and writing, while another has trouble speaking and best communicates by email. With almost a third of the board rotating off each year, communication strategies must be continually renegotiated.

Our friend, artist Neil Marcus, who like Devva has dystonia, in his acclaimed play *Storm Reading* (1988),[4] re-enacts his experience, with *comedia del'arte* humour, depicting his glee when the person behind the speaker in the Burger King drive up lane he has taken with his power wheelchair finally, finally, finally understands 'cheeseburger'.

Devva: On a lovely visit, we sit eating at a great round table with Neil's big opinionated family who loved to talk. In the US conversationalists take turns by overlapping sounds until one person wins the majority attention and others drop out. I realized then that we could stop any conversation. We could wave, or grunt to make it clear we wanted to speak until someone realized and helped us get everyone's attention. In that unaccustomed silence, we could take the floor and give a command speech. When we were done, the mutivoiced conversation would flow back over our heads and off onto the brain's hearing beach and merge into the next comment. Yes, we could stop any conversation, but we could enter very few.

Like the classic bit of elevator phenomenology by Hughes and Paterson (1997) who note that in that short burst of confinement with strangers, to be able to answer a courteous but formulaic question like 'how are you?' is not possible in speech-impaired time. We live in the *Star Trek* episodes (Heinemann, 1968; Taylor and Menosky, 2000) where some characters have speeded up so much, they are like buzzing gnats to the others, only in the reverse. Our speech is too slow for any polite answer. Do we participate and stop the door open with foot or wheel, or do we just smile, ignore, and contribute to our stereotypes as either dumb and dumb, or frosty?

Why do strangers assume an impairment is new and something we should talk about? In that same elevator I stand dressed to the nines with a foam cervical collar covered in purple (a knee sock, but you can't tell), to match my suede heels. The collar is embellished with an antique Mexican sterling and amethyst broach that matches my sterling earrings and belt. She asks 'Oh what happened to you?' Why would anyone think a silver and amethyst decorated purple foam collar is anything that 'happened' in any way I would/could/should answer in an elevator?

Why is it that Moses had Aaron speak for him? Did the existence of this earliest model of revoicer (or accommodation – Gracer, 2003) add extra power and memorability to his words in a world of face-to-face,

---

[4] This is a play on neurologists' reference to certain kinds of acute episodes of dystonia as 'storms'.

word of mouth communication? How important are the words that merit repetition or remote voicing, like the Greek chorus of the mute but telepathic arbiter of interplanetary peace accords in another *Star Trek* (Zambrano, 1989) with a different human voicer for different kinds of speech: emotional, intellectual, political? Am I seen as infantile, with unintelligible babble in a usual setting with no help, and occasionally feel like a skilled orator in a public space with a good revoicer where I can perform a speech? In either case, I feel the pressure from my audience to really say something if I expect them to give me the attention it takes to understand me and/or the time to wait for a revoicer to comprehend and echo my words. Why do people always start by apologizing for their hearing loss, or lack of time? Yes, I have lost some volume and they some hearing, but not to that degree. Why do they need to assure me (themselves?) that they could not understand anyone with that background noise, and that they will speak to me later, in a quieter context, and then I watch them converse at length right there with many others, and my 'later' never comes? Some I can dismiss, friends like that I don't need. But what if they are my teacher, family member, or someone I do want as a friend? I know that the issue is the degree of effort and the amount of time.

Pamela: When revoicing for Devva at conferences, sometimes I get so tired, I just want to stop but I also feel the need and desire of Devva to communicate so I keep going in session, out of session, and in private conversation, for as long as I can. At the end of one three-day conference I remember appealing to the crowd 'can someone else take a turn please?' By the end of three days many people had talked and listened to Devva enough to participate in revoicing but everyone had gotten so accustomed to me doing it. It just never occurred to anyone (even Devva and me) to suggest taking turns. And when someone did take over, I found myself listening carefully to make sure they were doing it right.

Our crosscutting approach to so many kinds of speech impairment is somewhat unusual and adds another layer of complexity. It would be easier to divide and pathologize. There are organized groups of people who stutter (perhaps mostly organized by families and allies or adults). Another somewhat organized group is those with CP, other motor speech issues, and on the autism spectrum who use technological assistance, AAC. But AAC is often used instead of speech. How different is that experience? Most of AAC users' organizing effort has been focused on sharing information and resources among themselves and technology designers. We ask what access to participation someone has if they can only speak with an overpriced machine, classed and priced as a medical device, one that frequently and unpredictably spends weeks in the shop. How would most people feel if a simple machine that should be cheap, was rationed so you had no backup? How would you even tell someone 'Sorry, my tongue is in the shop?' How many layers of backup to the ability to communicate are too many?

Pamela: My sister Hope and Jacob are engaged to be married. They are autistics in love. Hope is nonspeaking and Jacob's speech is not always under his control, so both type with human facilitation through physical contact with them (upper arm, elbow, wrist or hand, which for Hope involves only a light touch on top at times). For a more detailed explanation of facilitated communication see Chapter 12. In June 2010, Hope and Jacob presented at the SDS conference [Stubblefield, 2010]. It was Hope's second time presenting at SDS and Jacob's first. Since the conference was in Philadelphia, our parents' hometown, the room was filled not just with academic colleagues, but aunts, parents, siblings and cousins all wanting to see Hope present and meet Jacob, her new fiancé, for the first time.

I was there as well, with my 10-months-old nursing infant son. I would rush out between sessions to nurse him, or finally just bring him into sessions and nurse him there. I was also president of SDS at that time, and needed to publicly apologize and try to compensate for some major communication-accommodation-technical-difficulties that made it impossible for us to use microphones or provide live captioning. Talk about access barriers! The SDS board and the conference hosts were horrified, heart-broken, and humiliated by this basic failure to provide an acceptable level of access at a disability studies conference.

So on both personal and professional levels there was a great deal of pressure and (disappointed) expectations. On top of the global access failure, Hope was having a meltdown because her Dynavox was frozen. Mom, sister and onsite computer techies were unable to revive it, and Hope was beside herself, rocking crying, waving her arms. She was unable to give her own presentation in her own preferred manner. She was able to type (with mom facilitating) on a borrowed device and Jacob read a copy of her printed presentation while her sister (me) captioned it for the audience. I was also a discussant for the session (and still revoicing for Devva in another session we organized that day) and by the end was so emotional that I was ready to burst into tears. Jacob was composed and erudite. After the presentation he did need to leave the room once, but eventually returned to kick me out of his seat.

Hope and Jacob celebrated Valentines' Day 2011 by having a 'date' to present to a class I was co-teaching on Assistive Technology for Occupational Therapy. Mom, who usually facilitates both communication and travel, had moved to New Mexico, which meant we needed to find other people to help. Jacob's friend and colleague Linda Rammler (who facilitated for him in Philadelphia too) agreed to travel and facilitate with both of them, for this experience. Hope's friend, autistic activist Emily Titon, travelled with her from Rhode Island, meeting up with Jacob and Linda in Connecticut. While they were on the ferry from Bridgeport, Connecticut to Port Jefferson, New York I called to find out what they wanted for lunch. At this point, Hope and I got into a mediated fight (via Linda and her cell phone) about the portion sizes of her order of fries and shake accompanying a quarter-pounder with cheese. Unsurprised by my reaction, Hope was not happy with what she perceived as my controlling behaviour. She told me she'd get back at me, and did she!

In contrast to the experience in Philadelphia, in my class room she was focused and sharp. Although her Dynavox was functioning properly (for once), Hope decided to use some of the other devices that Linda had brought along. We invited the occupational therapy (OT) students to stand close so they could see Hope and Jacob use the different devices, as Linda switched back and forth from machines to letter board and back again. Hope spent the entire class making jokes at my expense, to my students' delight. She cussed like a sailor, complained that I was afraid she'd get me fired, then she told the students that I was perfectly capable of getting myself fired without her help. We next proceeded to publically rehash the MacDonald's food argument. Me: 'Eating yourself to death is *NOT* empowerment!' Hope: 'It's just a @#^&* cheeseburger!'

Meanwhile Jacob was not having such a great day. He was having breakthrough seizures and had a hard time staying calm and focused. He left repeatedly to go to the bathroom. I felt obliged to accompany him every time because I was afraid he would get lost in our confusing maze-like Health Sciences Center, but mostly because the place is teaming with health professionals who might decide he needed their help or that he belonged upstairs in the hospital psychiatric ward. My students were very pleased and impressed by the experience, which showed them a different view of autism. I was so frazzled that I somehow managed to lose my husband's $400 camera. After class we returned to my house for pizza. Hope and Jacob sat at a table by themselves for some 'alone' time, before Hope, Jacob, Linda and Emily took the ferry back to Connecticut. Just a typical Valentine's Day date! Actually it was rather typical of the coordination needed to get the two together and able to communicate with each other.

Like Devva and Neil, Hope rarely chats, though she is starting to do so with more frequency, when the expectations are there and she trusts her communication partner and facilitator. Linda Rammler notes that 'This is what can happen when nonspeaking people gain voice – everyone else forces them into a question answering mode because they are so excited to learn what the non-speaker has to say that any desire to chit-chat is quickly extinguished' (Rammler, email correspondence with author sent 12 July 2011). In general, she would much rather present.

As to effort, when I asked her in class on Valentine's Day if she would ever type independently, she said it was difficult enough to type with the current levels of human facilitation support. 'Both Hope and Jacob are working on independence – and slowly but surely gaining the necessary skills – because they are motivated by the arrogance of others who refuse to believe it is them doing the communicating' (Rammler, 2011; email correspondence with author sent 12 July 2011). And she doesn't type with most people if she can get her point across some other way. I think, in part it's what OTs call an energy-conservation technique, and also a marked enjoyment of gestural and physical communication, especially physical humour. Yet there are limitations to this preference as, according to Linda Rammler: 'experienced facilitators always validate through typing, because a problem with gestural communications is that it is not universally applied or understood. Pointing, vocalizing and bouncing while riding in the back seat can mean: "I'm about to fritz because of the traffic" or "That's the turn you were supposed to take! Do I always have to remind you, because you haven't learned the route yet?!?!?!"' [Rammler 2011, email correspondence with author sent July 12, 2011].

Anger, Advocacy, Responsibility, and Disability Justice

Devva: I rarely root for the Oscars, but *The King's Speech* hit home. Not only do I, by a quirk of fate, consider Colin Firth's only maternal Uncle and Aunt beloved friends, but I too speak better when singing, dancing, and otherwise doing strange things. Radio technology was not the king's friend, unless you consider the lack of necessity to concern himself with his visual performance. Of course, television would add those of us who twitch to the outed status of unfit rulers. We presume King George emerged at some point from his womb-like textile-draped radio studio chamber to something more intimately public than waving from a balcony. My small-town newspaper picked up the Associated Press writer Lindsey Tanner from Chicago's article titled, *'King's Speech' earns praise from kids who stutter* (4 February 2011). News columnists, researchers, therapists, and children who stutter and their parents appear in the article. The emphasis is on communicating the sense of stigma and the causes, treatments, and cures. The concept of advocacy is implicit in that the reaction of the environment directly affects the expression of the impairment. There is mention of the Stuttering Foundation of America as an advocacy organization. Tanner talks about stigma and mortification, the pain of the disorder, but not yet about anger. The article ends with a past stutterer-now-therapist's, admonition to talk about it. The wisest comment may be from a boy,

Aidan Hardy quoted as saying 'There are certain ways to help someone talk better and there are some things that most people think will help, but they don't.' In the light of *The King's Speech,* people who stutter, or used to stutter, have come out [see Hsu, 2011]. Although at times the 'overcoming' discourse is a bit oppressive, that can't be bad. It can only help my effort to build a strong advocacy community among the speech disabled. Don't tell me what I need however. Don't tell me to slow down, calm down, or breathe. Ask me what you should do. If you want to share citizenship with me, ask not for only what you think I should do to help you understand me. Ask me what you can do to better understand me and to help create an environment that supports our most effortless communication possible.

Time and Thought

Devva: Anticipation of what people think I will/am saying has long been a barrier. Without a revoicer, and even with the revoicer, people often listen long after they have lost the thread of my thought, hoping they will understand some key word that will make it all pop into focus. We lose more time running the thread backwards to the parting point. When Hope types her machine may speak word by word but then she runs the whole idea again for clarity, connecting the words. There are some advantages to this pace and repetition for both of us in a presentation. Tell them what you are going to tell them, tell them, and tell them what you told them is still a good idea. In a presentation, with a good revoicer, it gives me a world of time to think and craft my next phrase to my audience. It is less successful without a revoicer, particularly in casual conversation, and deadly in a big group, making me blubber. My speech is not consistent, few speech-impaired people's is. Stress and fatigue makes it deteriorate, and some days are just good or bad speech days with no pattern I can discern even after 45 years of practising anthropology. On the bad days and in the worst situations listeners question my intellectual capacity. Like the rabbis of the Talmud, the only way I thought I could assert my humanity is through my intellectual capacity. Hope too, who was misdiagnosed as 'retarded', asserts her independence of thought and her intelligence.

The speech/language divide is a tricky one. While there is a reasonable request for people to be able to speak in 'plain English' in order to be understood by a diverse audience, it's not that simple. In the same SDS session in NYC in 2008 [Kasnitz, 2008b] where Hope spoke, our colleague Susan Fitzmaurice and her son Teddy presented (Fitzmaurice and Fitzmaurice, 2008). Teddy, who has Down's syndrome, designs his own successful line of disability themed Tee Shirts, Teddy's Tees. They explained that, for Teddy to be interviewed by the press, Susan had to interpret to and from him, not because of vocabulary or grammar, but to contextualize questions for him. This took time the journalist did not want to take as she thought that her small-word, short sentences were enough. Similarly, she found it hard to believe that Susan's long interpretation of Teddy's short answers was not a parlour trick. None of this convinced her that with his slow lispish speech he understood the messages on his Tee Shirts. What Susan was doing, she explained, was translating from Teddy's shorthand references to other conversations and events, the metaphors and allegories that were encoded in his answers. Again, *Star Trek* does not fail us [Menosky, 1991]. In one episode Picard is marooned with a species the universal translator cannot accommodate as they speak by reference to history and myth and without knowing the history or myth the speech is untranslatable. Picard must go to the effort and take the time to learn the context of his companion's life in order to communicate.

Susan writes to us that, as Teddy matures, as his world expands further and further beyond Susan, it is often she who is lost in his conversations and needs to ask questions to get to the heart of what he is trying to communicate (Fitzmaurice, private email communication, 2011). He will reference some personal history of which she is unaware. It is not just attentive listening that is required but also curiosity and willingness to see below the surface of an unusual word in a seemingly simple sentence. It is easier to just say 'uh huh' than it is to take the time to question why that word was used and where it will lead. Too often the response to an unusual word is to think that it has been used improperly and Teddy is called 'retarded' when he is actually expressing higher level thinking than the person listening thought he could express. How much of the perception of Teddy's severe intellectual disability is simply an inability to understand his communication pattern?

Devva: It has often been suggested to me that I should speak differently. Actually, rather, that I should change my use of language and speak more 'plainly'. Many scholars resist the request to use 'plain English' to be inclusive of people with 'intellectual' differences, or people with differences in language processing. At some point it threatens their own sense of professionalism and it can confuse their unenlightened colleagues and creates significant career obstacles. For a person with multiple visible and audible differences, whose competence is so often judged by those differences, it is a bigger risk. Also, for me it would be a personal poetic loss. My speech impairment developed slowly, starting in my early twenties and changes yet today. My unexpected play of language has always been a signature family trait and a joy to me. Also, I have long been aware that my written and spoken language uses are closer to each other than are most people's. So, like my appearance, since I came out to myself as disabled – my sister says that there was no closet in which I could hide and that the only person who thought I was in a closet was me – my decision has been that if people are going to stare anyway, let's give them something to look at. Well, I do appreciate the effort and time it takes to listen to me. I share the experience of listening to people like me. I have no better innate talent in hearing/listening to different speech than anyone else. As I will reiterate, if people are going to expend the effort, I need to give them something to listen to. The medium and the message, it seems again, cannot be divided. When we all succeed in understanding me say a message such as 'There is no wall into which I can flower. I must flourish in the center of the room', my message is more likely to be remembered. Being a wall-flowering fence sitter is an option I have never had and the choice to be in the room rather than outside, often taking a visible if not a leadership role, is not courageous as I'm so often told, but comes from the sheer joy and comfort of participation when it all works out, and from the pit of frustration of exclusion when it does not. This is not to say that I don't have shy and quiet moments. Participation can be exhausting and rejection still hurts.

Conclusion

At the 2011 annual business meeting of SDS, when an old pain regarding the intersection of disability and racism emerged – part of the problem being how to be both financially accessible to poor and student disabled people of colour and cover all requested disability accommodations, and part being a request for a balanced analysis of the intersection of white and ableist privilege – Devva, who was presiding, almost lost her voice as the stress of the silence in the room exacerbated her dystonic speech, and as it deteriorated, her revoicer could barely understand her. At the same time, this most uncomfortable event also triggered 'storms', as Neil of *Storm Reading* would say, in several participants with autism or emotional processing impairments. They were effectively excluded from the debate by episodic speech impairments until we broke into small informal groups where the emotional charge dissipated and they had the time and effort they could direct to speaking so that they could participate. This unprepared-for switch in discourse tone hurt us all but has taught us much by watching who was silenced by the effort and timing of the event and how we might avoid this in the future.

Considering Hope and Jacob's two presentations, in each case unpredictable events also resulted in unexpected speaking directions due to things like technology failure and Hope's and Jacob's autistic moments or storms. These examples illustrate the stress and pressure of having only brief and rare moments to make a lasting impact, of wanting so much for a presentation to be a success that sometimes everything just collapses under the weight of the effort. Yet even these 'failures' may serve to communicate a powerful message of the struggles involved for Hope and

Jacob to communicate and how hard won are the successes. Perhaps the message was all the more clear to the OT students due to the contrast between Jacob's brilliant observations on the functioning of his brain, and his need to leave repeatedly to engage in ritualistic hand washing. This would be, as one of the editors of this volume has suggested, not just 'making do' but a creative improvisational process, a *bricolage*.

Jacob and Hope and Neil and Teddy too are no less aware, and probably better aware, of this performative value of their slow and effortful speech than are OTs, who reduce it to a static 'technique' for energy conservation, or disability studies anthropologists, such as ourselves, who apply our participant observers' eye and discourse analysis ear to the result. Their view is contextualized in the moments of *effort* in their own lives, and longitudinally in their experience of *time*, a view that all disability studies researchers and allied health professionals should emulate.

Nick and Dikaios make a similar point in chapter 1 with regard to occupational therapy's limited ahistorical and acultural approach to occupation, where human doing is only regarded in a clinical, biomedical context, an abstraction from reality. Decontextualized and stripped of a longitudinal view, meaning is lost. We have our biases too. If anthropology is not the only discipline that considers context, we are one of the best at describing it and do so longitudinally.

But, as we describe how effort through time can be exhausting, it can also be productive in providing emphasis. But, this can be ambiguous. In a letter to Helen Keller, Mark Twain refers to Keller and Sullivan as a duet: 'You are a wonderful creature, the most wonderful in the world – you and your other half together – Miss Sullivan, I mean, for it took the pair of you to make complete and perfect whole' (Twain, 2003; also see Kliewer *et al.*, 2006). Twain's admiration is genuine. The duet quality of Helen/Ann or Devva/Pam or Jacob/Linda is not unimportant, nor unintentional. All the effort and time must be justified to most otherwise inattentive and fickle and short attention-span audiences. However, although Twain may have a more complex view, do speech-impaired people really want to be seen as half of a whole, even a perfect one? Isn't the goal to be seen as a whole – interdependent yes, but whole?

Is it reductive OT thinking to make something that may be quite rich into a technical process for 'energy conservation', not to say it doesn't have that function? Maybe in the most McLuhanist way, the mode of speaking enables us to say something different or confers a different eloquence. This might be *bricolage* again. Do we want to hear a piece of music that has been played by some device (*Star Trek*'s android Data's perfect violin), or would we rather hear something live that will never be played exactly as we expect, or even may be fragmentary (Data's human comrade Riker's improvised jazz). The fragments might be more important than the piece we imagined it was going to be – does that diminish the music or is the experience of listening and playing more important? This sounds rather romantic but we are looking at issues of communication technique. It's not always about technical performance to an accepted standard; sometimes it's about flavours, quality of sound, combinations of noises, spaces, arbitrariness, invention, and circumvention.

This chapter has made a number of leaps. We ask ourselves, without minimizing the differences, can we generalize about all kinds of speech impairments, even those confounded with language issues? We ask how we apply social justice concepts to speech-impaired people's experience of disability injustices to construct a concept of speech disability justice. For whom are speech accommodations and who bears what responsibility? We have done this as a personal dialogue, our biases exposed, our stance self-reflective. To impose some order on this description of lived experience, and to do so in a way that is memorable to the audience of this book, we focus on two basic characteristics of all human occupations – time and effort. How do time and effort interact with speech impairment to create speech disability? And, how do time and effort figure into individual accommodation and group design for inclusion for speech impairment? We have no easy answers. However, when confronted with anomalous speech, we hope our readers reflect more deeply on the elements of time and effort in the task of assuring participation, the exercise of citizenship, and speech disability justice.

References

Block, P., Block, H., Kilcup, B. (2008a) Autism, Communication, and Family. Society for Disability Studies Meetings, New York City, 20 June.

Block, P., Block, H., Kilcup, B. (2008b) Autism, Communication, Family and Community. American Anthropological Association Meetings, San Francisco. 21 November.

Block, P., Block, H., Kilcup, B. (2009) Autism, Family, Meaningful Occupation and Life Transition. Society for Applied Anthropology Meetings, Santa Fe, New Mexico, 19 March.

Block, P. Frank, G., Zemke, R. Guest Editors, (2008) Anthropology, occupational therapy and disability studies. *Practicing Anthropology*, 30(3) 2–5.

Block, P., Ricafrente-Biazon, M., Russo, A., Chu, K. Y., Sud, S., Koerner, L., Vittoria, K., Langrover, A., Olowu, T. (2005) Introducing disability studies to occupational therapy students. *American Journal of Occupational Therapy* 59(4), 554–560. (Special issue on occupational therapy and disability studies.).

Boellstorff, T. (2008) *Coming of Age in Second Life: An Anthropologist Explores the Virtually Human*. Princeton, Princeton University Press.

DeJong, G. (1979) Independent living: from social movement to analytic paradigm. *Archives of Physical Med. Rehabilitation* 60, 435–446.

Fitzmaurice, S., Fitzmaurice, T. (2008) Interpreting and interpretation: Teddy's Tees. In Speech Impairment, Community Building, and Taking it on the Road, Devva Kasnitz, *Organizer and Discussant*. New York, Annual Conference of the Society for Disability Studies.

Frank, G., Kasnitz, D. (2011) The meaning of self-care occupations: perspectives for new practitioners from occupational science, anthropology and disability studies. In C. H. Christiansen, K. M. Matuska (eds) *Ways of Living: Adaptive Strategies for Special Needs* 4th edn. Bethesda, AOTA, pp. 27–45.

Galheigo, S. (2011) What needs to be done? Occupational therapy responsibilities and challenges regarding human rights. *Australian Occupational Therapy Journal* 58(2), 60–66.

Gracer, B. (2003) What the Rabbis heard: deafness in the Mishnah, *Disability Studies Quarterly* 23(2), 192–205.

Heinemann, A. (1968) *Star Trek, Wink of an Eye*. Story by Lee Cronin, directed by Jud Taylor, original air date, 29 November.

Hsu, J. (2011) *What The King's Speech Gets Right, and Wrong, about Stuttering*, http://today.msnbc.msn.com/cleanprint/CleanPrintProxy.aspx?1299028724832, accessed 1 March 2011.

Hughes, B., Paterson, K. (1997) The social model of disability and the disappearing body: towards a sociology of impairment. *Disability and Society* 12, 325–340.

Kasnitz, D. (2005) Speech impairment and disability privilege. In session. *The hidden oppression of disability privilege*, organizer, Denise Scheer, Annual Conference of the Society for Disability Studies, San Francisco, June, 2005.

Kasnitz, D. (2008a) Collaborations from anthropology, occupational therapy and disability studies. In: Block, P., Frank, G., Zemke, R. (guest eds) *Anthropology, Occupational Therapy and Disability Studies, Practicing Anthropology* 30(3), 28–31.

Kasnitz, D. (2008b) *Speech Impairment, Community Building, and Taking It on the Road.* Society for Disability Studies, New York.

Kasnitz, D. (2008c) Speaker/Sender, Listener/Receiver: Speech impairment is a two way thing. In panel: Inclusion of autism and disability, collaboration with disability studies and occupational science, and engagement of kinship and citizenship in social justice, organizer Devva Kasnitz, Annual Meetings of the American Anthropological Association, November, SF.

Kasnitz, D., Edwards, E. (2011) Authoritative discourses in disability theory, policy, and activism concepts Examples from international policy analysis an interdisciplinary conflict. Organized panel: negotiating ordinary and extraordinary discourses: Discourse within disability theory and disability activism, organizer, Michele Friedner, Annual Conference of the Society for Disability Studies, San Jose, 17 June.

Kasnitz, D., Munger, K. (2010) Panel: 'What?' Speech, voice, expression and participation: *Research goals and advocacy ideas*, Annual Conference of the Society for Disability Studies, Philadelphia, June.

Kasnitz, D., Shuttleworth R. (2003) Model of Communication Image, Communicative Power, in session: *Communicative Power: Disability, Participation, and Speech in the 21st Century*, organized by Devva Kasnitz, 16th Annual Meeting of the Society for Disability Studies, Bethesda MD, June.

Kaye, S. H., Neri M., Wong, A. (2009) *Telecommunication Needs of Californians with Disabilities: Final Report*. San Francisco, CA: UCSF Disability Statistics Center.

Kliewer, C., Biklen, D., Kasa-Hendrickson, C. (2006) Who may be literate? Disability and resistance to the cultural denial of competence. *American Educational Research Journal* 43(2), 163–192.

Kronenberg, F., Algado, S. S., Pollard, N. (eds), (2005) *Occupational Therapy without Borders: Learning from the Spirit of Survivors*. Edinburgh, Elsevier.

Kronenberg, F., Pollard, N. (2005) Overcoming occupational apartheid: a preliminary exploration of the political nature of occupational Therapy. In: F. Kronenberg, S. S. Algado, N. Pollard,(eds) *Occupational Therapy without Borders: Learning from the Spirit of Survivors*. Edinburgh, Elsevier, pp. 58–86.

Mankoff, J., Hayes, G. R., Kasnitz, D. (2010) Disability studies as a source of critical inquiry for the field of assistive technology. In *ASSETS '10* Proceedings of the 12th international ACM SIGACCESS Conference on Computers and Accessibility. New York, American Computing Machinery.

Marcus, N. (1988) *Storm Reading*, written and performed by Neil Marcus, adapted for the stage by Neil Marcus, Rod Lathim, and Roger Marcus, Presented by Access Theatre, Santa Barbara, CA.

Menosky, J. (1991) *Star Trek Next Generation, Darmok,* story by: J. Menosky, P. LaZebnik, directed by Winrich Kolbe. Original air date, 30 September 1991.

Milbern, Stacy (2010) http://blog.cripchick.com/archives/8560?utm_source=feedburner& utm_medium=feed&utm_campaign=Feed%3A + cripchick + %28poetic + propaganda %3A + cripchick%27s + webhome%29, accessed 22 July 2011. Also see http://www. democracynow.org/2010/6/23/disability_justice_activists_look_at_ways, accessed 22 July 2011.

Pedlow, R., Kasnitz, D., Shuttleworth, R. (2010) Barriers to the adoption of cell phones for older people with impairments in the USA: results from an expert review and field study. *Technology and Disability* 22, 1–12.

Scheer, D. (2005) Disability privilege: Speech impairment and its accommodations, in session the hidden oppression of disability privilege, Denise Scheer, Organizer, Annual Conference of the Society for Disability Studies, San Francisco, June.

Segalman, B. (2009) *Against the Current: My Life with Cerebral Palsy.* Verona, WI: Full Court Press.

Shuttleworth, R. (2000) The Pursuit of Sexual Intimacy for Men with Cerebral Palsy, *PhD Dissertation*, University of California, San Francisco-Berkeley.

Silicon Valley Independent Living Center (SVILC), *Values, Vision and Mission, Final Document*, San Jose, California, 19 March 2010.

Stadnyk, R., Townsend, E. A., Wilcock, A. (2010) Occupational justice. In C. Christiansen, E. A. Townsend (eds) *Introduction to Occupation: The Art and Science of Living*, 2nd edn. Thorofare NJ, Prentice Hall, pp. 329–358.

Steinberg, N., Kasnitz, D. (2011) Disability, speech, and judaism: 'Will you be my Aaron?' in a panel: Speech Communication Differences, *Society for Disability Studies*, San Jose, California, June.

Stubblefield, Anna (2010) Organizer, Communicative Trust and Care, Panelists: Sandra McClennen, Jacob Pratt, Hope Block, Derrick Johnson, Jenn Seybert, and Discussant Pamela Block, Annual Conference of the Society for Disability Studies, Philadelphia.

Taylor, M., Menosky, J. (2000) *Star Trek: Voyager, Blink of an Eye,* season 6, episode 12, directed by Gabrielle Beaumont, original air date 19 January 2000.

Twain, M. (2003) Letter to Helen Keller from Mark Twain. Helen Keller Kids Museum Online, www.afb.org/braillebug/hktwain.asp, accessed 20 July 2011.

Zambrano, J. (1989) *Star Trek Next Generation, Loud as a Whisper,* directed by Larry Shaw, original air date, 9 January 1989.

Zukas, Hale (2000) Oral history, http://bancroft.berkeley.edu/collections/drilm/collection/ items/zukas.html, accessed 22 July 2011.

15 A Society Founded on Occupation

Nick Pollard and Dikaios Sakellariou

While some professional commentators have tried to reduce occupation to a containable set of descriptors, others have explored concepts of holism and complexity that broaden definitions. A description of human occupation that is about 'doing, being, becoming and belonging' (Wilcock, 2006) is very broad, almost without capacity for definition; what aspect of human life is *not* about these dimensions?

Society is dependent on occupations that have a functional element of not only contributing to the social fabric but also facilitating distinctions. In some societies there may be little need to make a clear distinction between work and leisure, but in others this is much more evident. Andre Gorz (1982: 81), in his critique of Marxism, argued that individuals attempt to separate their work life from 'real life', but this is not a distinction that really emerged until the industrial era with the rise of leisure (Flanders, 2006). Gorz goes on to argue that 'becoming' in the sense in which Marx (1973) used it is about the autonomous use of free time, rather than work, which is for many people the means by which activities of free time can be materially afforded. Thus, for example, an aim of feminism, in the sense of women's liberation, is the achievement of individual freedom for everyone, irrespective of gender (Gorz, 1982). The achievement of this, however, depends on practicalities of enablement. To be independent of the need to work under the conditions of capitalism, people need to have the time away from passive consumption and instead develop the skills or 'tools for conviviality' that Illich (1975, 1978) claims are necessary for 'useful unemployment'. As discussed in Chapter 2, conviviality is used by Illich to describe a condition of communal felicity in which groups of people cooperate for mutual benefit in pleasurable activities. Gorz closes his book with appendices offering a utopian vision of cooperative farming and building projects, small-scale industries based in communities, enabled by, and enabling increased autonomous time.

Politics of Occupation-Centred Practice: Reflections on Occupational Engagement across Cultures, First Edition. Edited by Nick Pollard and Dikaios Sakellariou.
© 2012 John Wiley & Sons, Ltd. Published 2012 by John Wiley & Sons, Ltd.

One of the interesting ideas that Gorz uses (1982: 88), from Raymond Bahro, is the claim that 'what people in the developed countries need is not the extension of their present needs, but rather the opportunity for self-enjoyment in doing, enjoyment in personal relations, concrete life in the broadest sense.' A society that allows people more time for interpersonal activity, Gorz maintains, is one that has a better work life balance and also one that is more creative and productive. This theme of orientation to human values and needs has been reiterated by Max-Neef's discussion of economic theory (Max-Neef, 2010).

This idea is a familiar one to current occupational therapists (e.g. Frank 1995) and to people from whom the early professional pioneers of occupational therapy took inspiration, such as Ruskin and Morris. Their arts and craft movement drew on an idealization of aspects of the renaissance and the development of craft guilds. Although this was not an idealization of the social conditions of the renaissance, the importance of the period for figures such as Morris was that it marked a point where he felt that commerce began to detract from craftsmanship (Morris, 1890/2011). However, the popularity of Morris designs shows that he had a certain gift for commerce and the growing consumer market himself.

Ruskin's *Sesame and Lilies* (1865/2002), a very popular book amongst the nineteenth-century middle classes, had earlier set out similar values as underpinning the relations between men and women. In Britain the movement of masses of people from the country to the cities in search of work and a living had been a feature of life for well over a century, but little had happened to address the widespread problems of displacement, slum housing and wretched social conditions that served the combination of capitalist growth and swelling consumerism (see Chapter 2). As the accounts of working-class people who lived through that period such as that of Hewins (1982) or a group of interviewees from Hackney (Centerprise, n.d.) describe, disease and injury, disability and poverty were rife. Fear of them was ever present. The old and vulnerable went to the workhouse, and from there to a pauper's grave.

In *Sesame and Lilies* Ruskin attacked the poverty of the working people as the product of capitalist greed, but his principled proposals for change were based in moral arguments and reform. While he recognized the capacities of women, his advice to them was contradictory, urging them to be a strong moral force in the home but to be submissive. He discussed many of these ideas with his friend Octavia Hill, the housing and social reformer, to whom he loaned money for her slum improvement projects but expected a return on his investment. Hill in turn was an influence upon Elizabeth Casson, one of the founders of occupational therapy in the United Kingdom. As a young woman, prior to her later medical training, Casson worked as a housing manager at Red Cross Hall, part of Hill's project in Southwark to improve tenants' conditions, which included gardens and arts-based leisure activities. It is possibly here that she first came to value occupation, although perhaps the physical condition of the people she worked with may have led to her subsequent medical training. In the course of encountering boredom amongst psychiatric patients she became interested in the potential of occupation, although Wilcock (1999) notes that she recognized that occupation was vital to health as well as mode for treatment.

Such women were able to develop the precursors to occupational therapy because of their particular social, economic and political position. By the mid-nineteenth century middle-class women formed a large minority in Britain. As a good number of the eligible middle-class men were drawn into the service of the British empire (Trollope, 1994) where they could often live well and cheaply, and obtain sexual services (Gilmour, 1994), many women were deprived of opportunities for marriage. At the time women were conventionally expected to be supported by their husbands, and were not prepared to find partners beneath their social position or be employed as governesses for the children of those who were able to marry. Modern occupational therapy (as opposed to antecedents such as moral treatment) evolved from the philanthropic concerns and social transformation ideals that arose in the nineteenth and early twentieth century (Wilcock, 1999, 2002; Frank, 1992; Frank and Zemke, 2008). Koven (2002) claims that Ruskin's work appealed to the popular evangelical spirit amongst these mid-century women, and was the inspiration to their social actions as reformers. Hill, for example, believed that women who like herself did not marry had a duty to be philanthropists (Jones, 2011); such women found themselves a social purpose through philanthropic or missionary occupations (Trollope, 1994) became increasingly connected with demands for women's rights, but were perceived as a social problem, threatening the stability of the middle-class way of life. Hill herself recognized this argument, and advocated a quiet and discreet approach to her reform work, which did not stand in the way of dominant male interests; none the less she was one of a group of women social reformers who intervened with their middle-class values in the lives of the working classes (Jones, 2011). While there may be some criticisms about the imposition of values, none the less Hill was intrepid and overcame considerable opposition from all levels to provide spaces and opportunities for balanced occupation and better living conditions (Wilcock, 1999). Although their practical social vision contained many conservative elements consistent with the philanthropic ideals of their era (Jones, 2011) they remain the great aunts of present day concepts of occupational justice (Wilcock, 1999).

Yet neither occupational justice, nor the linked concept of occupational deprivation (Whiteford, 2000) have really developed an explicit political dimension in relation to the consequences they describe. At first glance this might seem unusual, given that occupational therapy, nursing and social work were among the professions that were developed to deal with the problems of an industrial society, but in their pioneer form they were a part of a spectrum of responses to the social problems of a gender-imbalanced middle-class whose surplus women needed something to absorb their energies. The women who developed these professions chose to work with, rather than work against the forces in their society, and therefore one aspect of their achievement is that they broadly accepted the status quo in order to make the gains they did (Frank, 1992).

Occupation and Codependency

Occupation is an inherently political aspect of human life. It is not simply expressed as an individual characteristic, dependent upon personal abilities and desires.

Rather, it generates and is generated by opportunities, the engagement in a dialectical relationship with the socio-political context in relation to which it has to be understood and 'read'. As in the example of middle-class women in the nineteenth century, access to occupation is regulated on the basis of class, gender, age or other arbitrary characteristics that serve as building blocks for power differentials and create opportunities. This regulation turns access to occupation into a form of commodity, and people abide by rules and principles in order to preserve their access. For example, in Chapter 2 we also suggested that some of the values of early occupational therapists may be linked to the rising era of mass consumption. This is not merely a matter of following rules and principles but reading and interpreting them so as to understand how to manipulate and use them.

In Chapter 4 we considered the examples of Alex from *A Clockwork Orange*, and *Billy Fisher* from Billy Liar, who as adolescents are negotiating their paths through an adult world which they are not prepared to accept. Updike's Rabbit tetralogy (1991, 2006) commences with its protagonist Harry 'Rabbit' Angstrom at the same stage in his life, and follows his narrative through to his death where he has to resolve his relationship with his wife and son, Nelson.

Rabbit exhibits many human faults. Much of the narrative concerns the issues that arise through his difficulties in meeting the expectations of others; he does not follow rules and principles much of the time and neither do many of the other people around him. Much of what Rabbit achieves may seem to be purposeless and meaningless. He is haunted by guilt at the various infidelities and failures to take responsibility through his life, continues to harp on his adolescent success as a basketball player, despite his increasing weight and lack of fitness in middle age. He recognizes that as a father he has passed these failings on to his son, Nelson, who also has considerable difficulties with attaining maturity. Many of the other characters in the novels exhibit similar flaws and anxieties, which propel them into collision with each other. The reader of the novels is able to 'read' the situations that Rabbit stumbles through 'without reading'. Updike seems to suggest that material striving might be as much as any of Rabbit's readers may themselves expect out of life. The novels can thus be interpreted as showing something that is fairly typical of Western society since the early 1960s, and in which people are shown to be no more than human, managing to carry out occupations in spite of themselves. Society does not collapse, and a form of good-enough structure prevails, even if it lacks greater ideals because consumer values have made moral values less certain.

Perhaps this continuity of occupation is possible because many of the occupational activities in human society are co-dependent on the stability of other social structures (Stockhammer and Ramskogler, 2008). The interrelationships between these supporting structures are complex. For example, the maintenance of care services through local government requires a series of budgetary arrangements to ensure that services are sustained and can be accessed by the public who continue to demand the availability of these facilities. Despite all the effort which societies put into managing some of the structures (for example the British National Health System (NHS), which is one of the largest employers in the world) it is probably a Sisyphean task to attempt to understand them as a whole. In fact successive governments have failed to do so, despite the continuous assertion that the NHS is a priority for policy initiatives. The initiatives have frequently made the task of dealing with structural problems harder (House of Commons Health Committee, 2009).

The NHS interfaces with numerous other supporting structures. These include professional bodies and unions supporting the roles of the various categories of workers, higher education facilities and training organizations, numerous suppliers of equipment, pharmaceutical products, foods, uniforms and contractors for services such as building maintenance, and utilities such as power and water. Each of these aspects is peopled by individual workers, who, like Rabbit or Billy Fisher, are plotting their own occupational furrow with a greater or lesser degree of capacity. Whatever may seem to be a priority at the macro level of organization, in delivering something like the NHS, may not be so significant at the micro level amongst the employees, who as Hammell reminds us (2007, 2010), may be more concerned with personal needs.

The Ownership of Occupation

While Hammell (2007) challenges the bold claims made by occupational therapy professionals with regard to concepts such as client centeredness and other principles, the divergences between the reality, practice and a theoretical ideal arise for a number of reasons. Much socioeconomic power is concerned with the ownership and control of the mechanisms through which access to occupation is distributed (employment in industry and services, access to legislative, religious, educational and leisure facilities and the nature and form of the occupations which take place in these facilities). This complex of mechanisms or hegemonic institutions has arisen over time through the development of capitalism as a product of human trade and technologies. Gorz (1982) supposes that society is founded on occupation, structured through occupation, and is determined through the material relations of occupation. This is not entirely so. Felipe Fernandez-Armesto (2000) describes how communities developed and were shaped according to the environments in which they settled and this in turn formed the basis for material relations. Different kinds of terrain support different approaches to the problems of human survival and eventually making settled communities. The colonization of raw territory is itself occupation. While occupation, whether of raw territory or of aspects of production involves what Hegel (1942) described as a process of appropriation, of making it your own, it none the less is a process that is determined by what is environmentally possible.

The earliest human narratives of these events are stories very concerned with proper observance of ritual, taboo and *geis* (a form of taboo based in a personal destiny akin to the story of Achilles' heel, or Baldur and the mistletoe) and matters of precedence and dominance as a daily aspect of human occupation in the relationships which took place between tribal groups. For example the context of such accounts as the *Tain bo Cualnge* (*The Cattle Raid of Cooley* – Taylor, 2005) is about a close relation to the land, food sources, and the other resources it provided for sustaining the occupations of Iron Age society. The cycle of stories involves a complex social context of ritual observances, and much of the plot is based around the pressures of destiny and fate.

The discovery of a good food source, and the decision to cultivate it, probably necessitates settlement nearby so that it can be tended. In turn this requires the organization of a range of occupations that Gorz (1982) and Illich (1975) would recognize – the building of accommodation, finding food and water supplies, obtaining warmth and getting rid of rubbish so as not to contaminate your living area. However, it eventually involves larger numbers of people who are concentrated into denser communities, creating problems of supply, transport, and distribution of resources (Fernandez-Armesto, 2000). Rules become established about who does what, how people relate to each other and how things are allocated. Occupations become defined. In the science fiction novel *Dhalgren* (1974/2001), Samuel Delaney explores what happens when the structures of society break down. Ignored by the rest of America, from which it is cut off by some undefined disaster, the city of Bellona has rapidly deteriorated into chaos, but a new set of social relationships and principles begins to emerge. Property relations are organized on a more feral and tribal basis, and groups of people compete for the dwindling resources.

This novel is one of many written against the background of civil unrest and a sense of collapse in middle-America during late 1960s and early 1970s. These events and the conflicts they expressed were reflected around the world in both reactionary and popular protests and attempts at revolution (e.g. the civil rights movement; Prague and Paris, 1968; the beginning of the troubles in Northern Ireland; demonstrations against the Vietnam War), causing many people to question the direction in which society was moving, indeed the very basis on which society was founded. It is perhaps worth revisiting in terms of the current anxieties about socioeconomic, cultural, and political disparities that continue to exist in many Western societies, such as the economic crisis of 2008, and the UK riots of 2011, or their role in conflicts in Iraq, Afghanistan, and the Arab uprisings of 2011.

Unlike the *Rabbit Redux* section of Updike's Rabbit tetraology (Updike, 2006) *Dhalgren* takes a largely underclass perspective (despite the references to Chomsky and others in the university linguistics syllabus), which graphically confronts many personal/social boundaries and the way in which diversities continue to be acknowledged. With a vernacular boldness Delany provides an anarchic perspective of society and the structure of occupation, which in some respects echoes the broadsides, ballads and Newgate confessions described by Linebaugh (1991) and the heteroglossaic significance of articulating them discussed in Chapters 6 and 11. Occupation and the way it is stratified is so often understood in these cultural forms as being concerned with the monopoly of a particular economic group over property relations, as Linton Kwesi Johnson (1980/2002: 41), one of the poets who emerged from the early worker writer movement wrote: 'mi know dem have work, work in abundant/yet still, dem mek mi redundant'.

The ownership of resources including the ownership of the power to ascribe relative value to culture determines the distribution of occupation and access to meaningfulness in what an individual is able to do (see Chapters 3, 5, 8, 9, 10, 11). This is a point that Fanon explores in *The Wretched of the Earth* (1990). In this he describes the destructive consequences of French colonization of Algeria for the indigenous population and draws from it inferences for all acts of territorial occupation as a total colonization, which is interiorized as well as experienced externally. The occupation of the land by one group of people denies the use of that territory or its resources to another group of people giving rise to occupational injustices (Townsend and Wilcock, 2004). Social roles develop and status emerges, with consequent effects in how resources are distributed and needs are determined (Illich, 1975, 1978). Whereas inequalities may be naturally determined through the might and dominance of particular individuals in a group, as society develops they become reinforced through the construction of strata of socially determined rules and principles. These are concerned with the maintenance of a society, which Illich has termed them 'manipulatory tools' (1975: 22).

As a consequence of these inequalities all societies are inherently unstable as their powerful hegemonies attempt to balance affairs so that they retain their power and others try to obtain a better share. Stockhamer and Ramskogler (2008) offer some economic theories about the characteristics of Western societies in recent decades, showing how developments such as increased prosperity for workers in the postwar period for some economies produced conditions in the 1970s where workers exerted their power and in return businesses retaliated by reducing their investments. But these issues are part of a mesh of global and more local influences. As instabilities have entered the economy as a result of influences such as property price bubbles, the hegemonic forces have intervened to preserve financial interests, whereas interventions to preserve workers from rising unemployment have not been so readily available.

The worker is free to trade work as a commodity to the owners of business or to offer to participate in activities, but workers do not own these places and usually have to accept the owner's terms to enter them legally or legitimately participate in the activities carried out there. Owners also determine wages for work or the price of leisure occupations. If this price is unacceptable, the worker does not work, because the maintenance of unemployed surplus labour ensures that the supply of labour always exceeds the demand. Alternatively, the worker cannot buy access to the leisure occupations operated by the business sector. One of the cultural conflicts of the development of modern societies has concerned the control of leisure into sanctioned or licensed forms – which are often then operated as a business (Illich, 1975; Flanders, 2006).

Despite the notion of a constitutional democracy in which the people may have the power to vote an administration in or out every few years, the negotiation of the power to determine access to occupation frequently takes place in shareholder meetings, on the stock exchange, and in the boardroom, amongst the owners of businesses. Therefore the decision-making processes preserve power amongst those in business and government; the worker has less knowledge to work with in order to position a bargain for wages or other resources. Numerous commentators have argued that this process alienates people from their occupational engagements in society, not merely with regard to work (Illich, 1975; Max-Neef, 2010; Whiteford and Townsend, 2010) and that measures are needed to make the workings of society more democratically accountable. Suggested initiatives include a refocusing on human needs and satisfiers and facilitating greater participation in decision making (Max-Neef, 2010; Whiteford and Townsend, 2010), simplifying processes to a human level and reducing demand (Illich, 1975; Frank, 1996), and encouraging dialogue by encouraging access to knowledge (Freire, 1972).

Throughout this book we have explored how the complexity of social structures and their interfaces presents a challenge to the acquisition of this knowledge. As we have argued earlier, it is impossible to expect people to develop a total understanding of social processes and structures, but an occupational literacy should facilitate people in negotiating their respective expertise. In despotic political situations discourse is controlled and limited so that real discourse is restricted to those in power. Any threat to the status quo is a threat to the economic basis and occupational pattern of the whole society. Arendt (1958/1998) argued that people with no access to political discourse can be reduced to *animal laborans* – they only have access to needs-driven and survival related occupations, a position of slavery or serfdom. Yerxa (2000: 91) wrote:

> A person may be viewed from different perspectives according to emphasis; for example, *Homo sapiens* (wise), *Homo symbolicus* (symbolic), *Homo faber* (tool maker), *Homo ludens* (player) and so on. The Latin root, *occupacio*, means to seize or take possession. I take this to mean that *Homo occupacio*, the occupational human, is seized by his or her occupations and in so doing takes possession of his or her world.

To be in the condition of '*Homo occupacio*' requires that people and the communities to which they belong are empowered – that they have occupational rights on which their well being depends (Hammell, 2008). The logic of Yerxa's statement is that people have the knowledge to combine these perspectives and that they are able to read and interpret their use in the pursuit of their occupations. The operation of these occupations in a way that is mutually beneficial requires occupational justice.

Occupational Justice

Occupational justice is a concept that refers to the right of all persons to engage in desired meaningful and dignified occupations according to their needs, desires and capabilities without being restricted by factors such as race, disability, illness, gender, poverty or other characteristic (Townsend, 1993; Townsend and Wilcock, 2003). Essentially it is the right to meaningful occupation, which is chosen, and answers the needs of individuals or their communities.

In Chapters 3 and 5 we briefly reviewed Max-Neef (2010) matrix of human development needs and satisfiers, which had been postulated in response to the argument that progress was determined by economic growth. An occupational justice perspective would incorporate an assessment of needs and satisfiers and understandings of the way that people organize their societies to meet these occupational concerns (Whiteford and Townsend, 2010). This is necessary because opportunities to be through doing are essential to human life (in Chapter 7 we queried the use of 'meaningful' and 'purposeful' occupation since this may confer external values to individuals and communities). Consequently people have a fundamental right to occupations through which they can express themselves. The realization of occupational rights is, however, at odds with much of the current direction of globalized development, if not the history of capital.

Determining Needs

In *Common Sense*, a pamphlet written at the beginning of the capitalist era, Thomas Paine (1776/1986) railed against the power of the British monarchy and the dubious hereditary rights of kings whose vested interests in retaining power determined the rights of every other individual. He called for an American republic, but in the growth of the new order he proposed was based on a concern for preserving property, a radicalism that was set out with a set of accounts for building a navy to defend it. Paine supposed that the natural state of human beings was to form a society founded on a law of common interests rather than principles defined by ruffians posing as kings. He supposed that industry will prove to be a means of liberation and self determination, but could foresee how in the following century the American 'robber barons' were to build their corporate and industrial power and the British and European commerce Paine decried was to develop a similar pattern as the world economy developed. Paine's works themselves were popularly taken up to fuel the protest against this new capitalist order (McCann, 1982).

Modern capitalism appears to have developed from serf and slave societies, towns and cities in which stimulated by markets and opportunities for trade, people began to develop specialized skills and produce goods and commodities for exchange (Bloch, 1965a, 1965b). The development of crafts largely occurred in relation to local environmentally determined needs, for example in the forms of agriculture or architecture (Fernandez-Armesto, 2000). People might need to have particular tools and it is often more efficient for individuals to buy something made for the purpose rather than try to make their own tool or cloth, especially where the making of such items requires additional equipment.

Older artisan activities involved a sense of craft, an expertise developed both through experience and a socially transmitted exchange of technique, which was, in part, peer assessed through observation of the skill an individual had acquired Gorz (1982) (see Chapters 8 and 13). No matter how elementary, almost everything individuals do toward their doing, being, becoming and belonging is connected with their physical occupation of the environment, a territorial sense or a personal space, which has to be negotiated with others (see Chapter 8). Consequently because people from the areas all around the towns and cities came to negotiate these issues, the language of the town became the lingua franca, and the common languages of trade became the languages of commerce. However, in the materialist development of power and the bureaucratic technocracies that support it by surveying, quantifying, collecting and distributing goods resources and aspects of these processes themselves eventually override the interests of the people. Linebaugh (1991) explored how property relations were asserted through the redefinition of work and forms of payment, and this relationship was reflected in the dialectics of the law and crime, each with its own specialized literacy. The wealthy wrote in the forerunner of received English; the poor, where they could write, did so in cant vernaculars that often required translation.

The holders of office may claim that their procedures have been developed to serve the people, but the control passes to a smaller specialized group. Thus, Gorz (1982) asserts, materialist progress is assumed to be better: efficiency, speed, performance are values that are not questioned because they appear to serve power. Gorz agrees with Illich (1975) that the price of serving progress is that people lose control over their occupations, and no longer exert power but become its servants. If the rhetoric of healthcare policy has become one of choice (Department of Health 2005, 2010, 2011) then such statements belie the realities surrounding individual decision making. The space, temporal and physical, in which we live *our* lives, and experience *our* care, *our* health, or assume the right to have *our* say (as in the 2005 Department of Health policy) is determined, not by anything we have voiced, but by power itself. This denial of power except to a few pervades every aspect of occupation, and so contributes to occupational injustice, because it compromises opportunities for participation. The point that Max-Neef (2010) makes with regard to human needs is that the material expression of power has become such a force that it threatens the sustainability of the planet and the people living on it. The scale of such a force and the market logic driving it is immense, and the individual does not have an effective alternative perspective to present. Making real decisions becomes impossible because the future seems unalterable.

The pervasive logic extends into healthcare systems, which many governments are concerned with limiting because of the tendency for rising costs (Department of Health, 2006; Greer, 2010). This is due to factors such as advances in the technology of care combined with the rise in numbers needing care through an ageing population. As a consequence healthcare reform is as prominent on political agendas as it may have been through recent history but there is now a sense of urgency and conflict between governments trying to implement changes, professional, client and carer groups trying to defend their interests.

The different forces on the field of battle have different strengths. Occupational therapists as suggested by their description as allied health professionals, or formerly as in the UK 'professions supplementary to medicine' (National Archives, 2011) are not amongst the foremost combatants because their role is not depicted as an essential element of service provision. Many countries have been unable to invest in occupational therapy and the numbers employed per client vary considerably between different systems. As people employed in the delivery of interventions that have been part of the client's expectations, they can be caught between their own sense of powerlessness and the bewilderment the client also experiences. This may contain elements of injustice, because economic determinants may be locally applied so that a patient in one geographical area can receive treatment that is denied to a similar patient in another, but other factors may also determine how interventions are allocated. Often the occupational therapist occupies a position in which decisions must be deferred to other specialists or to financial managers, but this is not necessarily about power alone. Clinical decision-making processes are complex and require reference to other professional groups. The potential for conflict and collaboration between different professional groups and individuals in the various processes of managing care are multiple, because each individual operates to some extent on predetermined values arising from a combination of personal and professional beliefs and education (Atwal and Caldwell, 2003; Coombes and Ersser, 2004; MacDonald *et al.*, 2010).

It could be inappropriate and potentially dangerous to take autonomous action on behalf of a client, even in the pursuit of justice, without having agreed a process with others such as the client's family, or the other members of a professional team. This does not always mean that consultation produces justice, or that the outcomes reflect an agreed process. Changes in healthcare procedures with regard to discharges have not always included the clients' opinions, while the professional advice of some team members has been overridden and procedures have been delegated to junior team members with less experience (Atwal and Caldwell, 2003; Bowman, 2006; Connolly *et al.*, 2009). As experienced from the client perspective, the question 'when can I go home after treatment?' might be rephrased as 'do I have the right to return to my own home after treatment?' The right to go home is to be determined by a group of professionals who need to ensure that clinical procedures are being correctly followed, but are also concerned to reduce costs, retain their jobs through efficiencies and prevent litigation arising from poor decisions, perhaps to secure further con-tracts for their department by demonstrating good and efficient outcomes.

These situations represent a series of decisions that may have little to do with the client experience. A response such as 'well, first we need to do some assessments to make sure you'll be alright' might be interpreted as 'No.' In an ageing society, although occupational therapists may feel that their role has been reduced to merely discharge planning (Bowman, 2006), that role might prove to be a key one in the exercise of grey political rights and justice. In ageing societies where older people are increasing and may through their financial assets as well as their voting power be enabled to exercise more power there may be more demands for effective inclusion in decision making, and the justice to support the appropriate satisfaction of their occupational needs.

Perhaps there is a long way to go before the profession can realize the ambition of the American Occupational Therapy Foundation (AOTF) which in 2001 set up the Institute for the Study of Occupation and Health (AOTF, 2001). The AOTF envisaged a society where occupational therapists will

> have as an internalised mandate of occupational therapy the promotion of equal opportunity for access to resources needed for full societal participation and the promotion of inclusion of all individuals in participation. The therapist perceives the reduction of poverty; the stabilization of the population; the achievement of a sustain-able, natural environment; and the empowerment of women as problems that fall within

the practice domain of occupational therapy insofar as these problems relate to the domain of societal health.

(Gillette, 2002: 700)

This is a vision of a profession working for an occupational just society, but progress towards realizing this goal calls for the development of tools for successful navigation in the political environment within which occupational therapy operates (e.g. Frank, 1995).

Choice and Contradiction

Perhaps it is due to its philanthropic beginnings that occupational therapy is still sometimes presented as a vocation, as an approach not just to activities of daily living but to life itself (Watson, 2004). As professionals we model this through our professional behaviour and enact it as therapeutic tools in the ongoing process of assessment, planning and implementing our client centred interaction with clients (Hagedorn, 2000). The problem-solving strategies that form the basis of the treatment plan are directed, therefore, to individual needs. Although through codes of practice that recognize the need for antioppressive practice or which call for the acknowledgement of cultural needs there is an accommodation of features at a broader social or community level, the problems posed by the experience of disability remain with the individual. This produces a professional dichotomy, a contradiction, which as some critics (such as Abberley, 1995) have pointed out, can prove so difficult to reconcile that disabled people themselves are blamed for their own disabling experiences. If people are reluctant to comply with treatment they find irrelevant this can be unquestioningly labelled as a lack of motivation, whereas professionals are reluctant to explore possible deficiencies in their own practice.

But right should not always be assumed to be totally on the side of the client. It is possible that if clients were paying directly for the services they received they might be more likely to discuss the rationale for treatment and their reasons for discontinuing aspects they found unhelpful. If people are referred to a freely available service it is inevitable that some of them will consider that they do not actually need it and so, for example, will not show up for appointments. Choice is a principle that has been embraced by governments of all the dominant hues in British politics with the personalization of care and the drive towards the development of social enterprises in recent health policy (Department of Health, 2005, 2006, 2010, 2011). This might seem perfectly sensible but for the problems that are clearly revealed in Hewins' stark narrative (1982) of early twentieth-century poverty, and which continue wherever there is impoverishment. In the early part of the last century people often had to choose between paying the doctor, paying the rent, or starving; a particularly graphic account of this dilemma is given by Healey (1980). Recent UK research suggests that despite increases in life expectancy, the disparities between the experiences of rich and poor that were so evident in the 1930s still exist (Thomas et al., 2010). The choice is not available for some people unless provision is in place to guarantee a minimum standard of income and education in order to know enough to access services or not.

Occupational therapy is directed to rehabilitation so that people can regain former roles or acquire new occupations, so it is clear the profession has a value in preserving earning and other convivial capacities that enable people to support themselves and others around them. This situation describes part of the political dilemma of occupational therapy. Its effectiveness depends on *being seen to be effective* (both being 'seen' and 'being seen to be effective') in order for an understanding of its benefits to be achieved at the levels of popular awareness (over and above client/taxpayer), amongst colleagues in other health disciplines and by financial managers of services (e.g. Bowman, 2006). Occupational therapy is based around a concept so fundamental and replete with potential power yet it is taken for granted. Occupational therapy – it's common sense, everyone knows that. Don't they?

However, occupational therapists themselves have to begin to think occupationally. If the origin of the profession is in social transformation, then it has a tendency for reform in which social relations might be renegotiated at a superficial level rather than calling for substantial changes by challenging the status quo that produces occupational injustices. Frank and Zemke (2008, Frank, 1992) point out that despite professional origins in reform, the influential early occupational therapist Eleanor Clarke Slagle was able to draw on Republican Party connections to align the emergent profession with the military and medical interests of the First World War. Yakobina and Harrison-Weaver (2008) trace the relationship of the development of the profession, particularly with regard to techniques in hand therapy, to the history of conflict in the twentieth century. Consequently the profession adopted a position closely allied to medicine and clinical rehabilitation approaches. The development of technical solutions, while fundamental to the way in which the profession is valued can at the same time obscure some of the other questions about the nature of occupation surrounding the technological advances. This development away from the roots in Hulme House and Christian socialism may be a further reason for the lack of a critical apparatus that it can use to address political questions of occupation.

In this discussion we have considered how political issues occur in the broad domain of macro events resulting from economic and policy changes, and at the same time many individual occupational outcomes are effected or not at the individual level, often focused on immediate concerns such as family or personal needs. We have also considered how a sense of occupational literacy arises from recognizing a relationship between these factors of needs and the wider influences around them, and that often people work for their own needs or those of their family or friendships rather than larger principles. In Chapter 3, we also considered that any tools for occupational literacy have to be simple rather than adding to the social distances created by professional specialization. The 3P archaeology exercise (Pollard *et al.*, 2008) is about identifying congruence and incongruence between our personal and professional values and political actions. It will bring to the surface conflict and cooperation situations that one may need to come to terms with in order to understand one's readiness to engage in activities that foster what Townsend and

Wilcock (2003) have termed 'occupational justice' and address issues of what Kronenberg and Pollard (2005) call occupational apartheid.

The 3P archaeology exercise asks therapists (but the questions can be applied to anyone) to begin with the personal dimension of their values, which explores what individuals bring with themselves into the profession and their potential as therapeutic tools. Unless, as professionals, we know what we can bring into the therapeutic environment, into the transitory space between the therapeutic environment and the community, and thus into the community itself, we will not be able to facilitate occupation effectively. This is not necessarily about competence in discrete skills relating to specific occupations – although these can often prove to be important in proving the value of the individual as a professional, but about being able to draw on the skills of the community. Everyone has something significant to contribute to this process in their own ways but our actions may also be motivated by personal needs and interests. Rather than ignore these motivations, by recognizing and engaging with them individuals can be enabled to contribute and to perform as social actors in the political environment. By exchanging accounts of this contribution and engagement, thus creating a dialogue, individuals can develop the narrative history of their community, i.e. a community of people from whom they can draw support, and through which they can obtain reflective detachment about their involvement in the evolution and implementation of occupational approaches and strategies. This can be the basis of a process of occupational literacy and a fuller participation toward occupational justice.

One way of viewing this process of occupational literacy is to see it as part of the development of an occupational therapy 'cell' working for goals within the wider environment. An occupational literacy tool already widely employed amongst occupational therapists to further their own knowledge is the journal club. This workshop for sharing and interpreting reading can be the basis for other knowledge exchanges. Making strategic and political goals clear enables people to discuss them more objectively and identify them as collective tasks, but also to recognize that the personal investment they put into them is often more about learning the political process rather than the goals themselves and building resilience. Similarly, when goals are achieved it is important to dissect and evaluate successful strategies. The political, social and economic environment in which people are engaged and participate in is actually an experimental arena and no-one can never be absolutely certain what will work and what won't, or even why, until after the event (Stockhammer and Ramskogler, 2008).

The Professionalization of Doing

We have already touched on some of the aspects of the historical development of occupational therapy that may affect how the profession conceptualizes and promotes human occupation. A considerable aspect of this history concerns its strongly gendered nature, which continues to have implications for the future development of the profession and its capacity to address occupational needs and therefore occupational justice. Occupational therapy has historically developed in such a way that it has both nurtured and due to the need to be perceived as conforming to larger medical and scientific principles, also rejected domestic skills and occupations (Pollard and Walsh, 2000). It has delegated other aspects of occupation to technical instructors in ways that have reinforced social class divides within the profession, especially as technical instructors and occupational therapy assistants faced barriers in attaining professional qualifications. Woodwork departments, for example, were often maintained as a largely male preserve in the OT departments in which the first author worked, where female occupational therapists entered in passing and few female clients would have entered to make something themselves. Male occupational therapists on the other hand would sometimes be conjoined to work with male clients on occupations connected with sports, woodwork or gardening, within a narrow interpretation of what male occupations are, reinforced by a professional matriarchy. The development of Men in Sheds projects in Australia and by the UK charity Age UK has been partly in response to a perception that therapeutic services are largely oriented to women and to a lack of research into men's occupational activities in retirement (Ormsby *et al.*, 2010; Age Concern Cheshire, 2010).

This perception is not without foundation. Dow-Royer (2010), commenting on the development of the profession in the US, but very redolent of other parts of the Western world, has traced how many aspects of gender and socialization contribute to the predominance of women in occupational therapy. This has affected the profession in many ways. The difficulty of developing a sufficient number of therapists educated at doctoral level, the preference for teaching and syllabus development over research, the relatively short time spent in practice before moving into education, a culture of deference and sexism in a variety of administrative educational and clinical situations in which men dominate, have all contributed to an educational and training process in which a strongly gendered professional culture is reinforced both without and within. These same factors have made it very difficult for occupational therapy to assert its position against competing professions and their academic structures.

However, in recent years the development of degree rather than diploma entry to the profession in the UK has necessitated, or encouraged, the growth of theoretical and rhetorical education over pragmatic training. Dow-Royer (2010) points to disinterest amongst practitioners for academic training, which arises through an earlier pedagogical tradition of locating occupational therapy training in liberal arts colleges (in the UK occupational therapy education took place in NHS-run schools, which did not enter the university system until the 1990s).

The practical has lost out in the prevailing academic demand, perhaps because the dominant research paradigm has favoured objective measures which do not adequately address the lived experience of people (Cook and Chambers, 2009). This presents a problem in that many people, for example those experiencing psychoses, lack access to valued social roles and opportunities in a stigmatizing society. The thrust of occupational engagement is not only about acquiring skills but about the literacies that underpin social engagement and relationships, and the acquisition of such literacies is not simply a task for the client or service user but wider society.

Occupational therapy education has moved away from crafts and their importance has been diminished since the early 1990s (Tubbs and Drake, 2007). The apparatus of woodwork rooms and potteries has gone. Occupational therapy education does not encourage occupational literacy – it no longer involves forms of apprenticeship in learning about weaving and types of wood, the correct preparation of paper in order to make it suitable for watercolours, or the maintenance of equipment. It has lost all this complexity in doing (Tubbs and Drake, 2007) to acquire a further stage in the professionalization of doing. The pursuit of professional status entails being a further stage removed from the actualities of occupational engagement.

Always a middle-class profession, one of the goals of occupational therapists has been to obtain better recognition from those further up in the hegemony (Wilcock, 2002; Dow-Royer, 2010), a move that takes them further from the people with whom they mostly work, and further embeds them in the culture of the hegemony operated by employers. Occupational therapists feel they have needed to do this in order to do their job better and secure better access to the resources controlled by their employers through the acquisition of power. But the acquisition of power is often for its own ends rather than for some altruistic purpose. Occupational therapists have also often been in competition with other elements of the hegemony – other professions also seeking their own position of power in order to practise as they desire.

Occupational Literacy and Occupational Justice

Without an occupational literacy that is capable of interpreting the consequences of this power struggle in terms of class and cultural impact there can be no occupational justice. A female gendered profession or a strongly middle-class profession has to recognize how these tendencies create certain emphases in concepts and theories (see Chapter 2). To practise, a profession must be empowered, and the process of obtaining power entails distancing itself from others and from a native knowledge of the competencies that operate in these contexts. This has the effect of diminishing the capacity of the profession for occupational literacy and for class and cultural competence.

On the other hand, the client needs the professional power of the occupational therapist to secure the resources and facilities to which the therapist is a gatekeeper. This binary position is not necessarily antithetical because it can provide the means of conflict and cooperation that have to operate in balance, or alliance, for clients' needs to be met. Clients are unlikely to be experts in their condition, or at least while many clients are able to acquire expert knowledge this often relates to the specific aspects of their condition, but not the broader perspective that informs professional knowledge of the resources and interventions available.

Consequently, the profession has to balance on a wire between the demands of professionalism and the necessity of maintaining power and expertise and the ability to facilitate the client from this position, with the need to be able to relate effectively to the client's realities and interpret them in a way that leads to competence.

Occupational therapy also needs to be independent of the other hierarchies in the hegemonic structures in which it operates and on which it depends to be able to use occupational literacy to arrive at occupationally competent judgements that enact occupational justice. Its practitioners need to realize and put into effect the full power of the concept of occupation as a specific component of social justice. This entails having the ability to address and exercise them in ways that are accessible to others, through alliances with our clients. These alliances combine a professional and a lay occupational literacy as a two-pronged discourse that is dynamic and interactive.

Occupational literacy, therefore, is not a literacy that is read one line at a time, but a process of interpreting and synthesizing. Because of its heteroglossic nature it is more of an orchestration for multiple voices and instruments in which the elements can relate to others through indications of repetition or syncopation, and in which clear movements can be discerned.

References

Abberley, P. (1995) Disabling ideology in health and welfare-the case of occupational therapy *Disability and Society* 10(2), 221–232.

Age Concern Cheshire (2010) *Every Man Needs a Shed*, www.ageconcerncheshire.org.uk/shed.htm, accessed 9 March 2011.

American Occupational Therapy Foundation (2001) Introducing the Institute for the Story of Occupation and Health. *American Journal of Occupational Therapy*, 55(6), 693–694.

Arendt, H. (1958/1998) *The human condition. Chicago*, University of Chicago Press.

Atwal, A., Caldwell, K. (2003) Ethics, occupational therapy and discharge planning: four broken principles. *Australian Occupational Therapy Journal* 50(4), 244–251.

Bloch, M. (1965a) *Feudal society. 1 The growth of ties of dependence*. (L.A. Manyou, trans.). London, Routledge.

Bloch, M. (1965b) *Feudal society. 2 Social classes and political organization*. (L.A. Manyou, trans.). London, Routledge.

Bowman, J. (2006) Challenges to measuring outcomes in occupational therapy: a focus group study. *British Journal of Occupational Therapy* 69(10), 464–472.

Brown, D. (1978) *Hear that Lonesome Whistle Blow*. London, Chatto & Windus.

Centerprise (ed.); (n.d.) *Working Lives Volume One: 1905–45*. Hackney, Hackney WEA/Centerprise.

Connolly, M., Grimshaw, J., Dodd, M., Cawthorne, J., Hulme, T., Everitt, S., Tierney, S., Deaton, C. (2009) Systems and people under pressure: the discharge process in an acute hospital. *Journal of Clinical Nursing* 18, 549–558.

Coombes, M., Ersser, S. J. (2004) Medical hegemony in decision-making – a barrier to interdisciplinary working in intensive care? *Journal of Advanced Nursing* 46(3), 245–252.

Cook, S., Chambers, E. (2009) What helps and hinders people with psychotic conditions doing what they want in their daily lives. *British Journal of Occupational Therapy* 72(6), 238–248.

Delaney, S. R. (1974) /2001) *Dhalgren*. New York, Vintage.

Department of Health (2005) *Our Health, Our Care, Our Say*. London, Department of Health.

Department of Health (2006) *No Excuses. Embrace Partnership Now. Step Towards Change! Report of the Third Sector Commissioning Task Force*. London, Department of Health.

Department of Health (2010) *Equity and Excellence: Liberating the NHS*. London, Department of Health.

Department of Health (2011) *Health and Social Care Bill 2011*. London, Department of Health.

Dow-Royer, C.A. (2010) Scholarship in occupational therapy faculty: the interaction of cultural forces in academic departments. *Open Access Dissertations*. Paper 230, http://scholarworks.umass.edu/open_access_dissertations/230, accessed 10 March 2011.

Fanon, F. (1990) *The Wretched of the Earth*. London, Penguin.

Fernandez-Armesto, F. (2000) *Civilizations*. London, Macmillan.

Flanders, J. (2006) *Consuming Passions. Leisure and Pleasure in Victorian Britain*. London, HarperCollins.

Frank, G. (1992) Opening feminist histories of occupational therapy. *American Journal of Occupational Therapy*. 46(11), 989–999.

Frank, G. (1995) Crafts production and resistance to domination in the late 20th century. *Journal of Occupational Science* 3(2) 56–64.

Frank, G., Zemke, R. (2008) Occupational therapy foundations for political engagement and social transformation. In N. Pollard, D. Sakellariou, F. Kronenberg (2008) (eds) *A Political Practice of Occupational Therapy*. Edinburgh, Elsevier Science, pp. 111–136.

Freire, P. (1972) *Pedagogy of the Oppressed*. Harmondsworth, Penguin.

Gillette, N. (2002) A vision of society in the twenty-first century. *American Journal of Occupational Therapy* 56(6), 699–700.

Gilmour, D. (1994) *Curzon*. London, John Murray.

Gorz, A. (1982) *Farewell to the Working Class*. London, Pluto.

Greer, S. L. (2010) *State authority and health care delivery in the United States and United Kingdom*. University of Michigan, www.britishpoliticsgroup.org/greer%20bpg%20paper%201-4%20(Chicago%2015%20AD)pdf, accessed 16 March 2011.

Hagedorn, R. (2000) *Tools for Practice in Occupational Therapy*, Edinburgh, Churchill Livingstone.

Hammell, K.W. (2007) Client-centred practice: ethical obligation or professional obfuscation? *British Journal of Occupational Therapy* 70(6), 264–246.

Hammell, K.W. (2008) Reflections on . . . well-being and occupational rights. *Canadian Journal of Occupational Therapy* 75, 61–64.

Hammell, K.W. (2010) Contesting assumptions in occupational therapy. In M. Curtin, M. Molineaux, J. Supyk-Mellson (eds) *Occupational Therapy and Physical Dysfunction*. Edinburgh, Churchill Livingstone/Elsevier, pp. 39–54.

Healey, B. (1980) *Hard Times and Easy Terms*. Brighton, QueenSpark.

Hegel, G. W. F. (1942) *The Philosophy of Right*, Oxford, Oxford University Press.

Hewins, A. (1982) *The Dillen: Memories of a Man of Stratford-upon-Avon*. Oxford, University of Oxford Press.

House of Commons Health Committee (2009) *Health Inequalities*. London, The Stationery Office.

Illich, I. (1975) *Tools for Conviviality*. London, Fontana.

Illich, I. (1978) *The Right to Useful Unemployment*. London, Marion Boyars.

Koven, S. (2002) How the Victorians read Sesame and Lilies. In Ruskin, J. *Sesame and Lilies*. D. E. Nord (ed.). New Haven, Yale, pp. 165–204.

Kronenberg, F., Pollard, N. (2005) Overcoming occupational apartheid: a preliminary exploration of the political nature of occupational therapy. In F. Kronenberg, S. Simo, N. Pollard (eds) Occupational therapy without borders. Oxford, Elsevier/Churchill Livingstone, pp. 58–86.

Jones, C. (2011) Octavia Hill (1838-1912) *HerStoria* magazine, www.herstoria.com/discover/octavia.html, accessed 9 September 2011.

Johnson, L. K. (1980 /2002) Inglan is a bitch. In *Mi Revalueshanary Fren: Selected Poems*. London, Penguin, pp. 39–41.

Linebaugh, P. (1991) *The London Hanged Crime and Civil Society in the Eighteenth Century*. London, Penguin.

Lukes, S. (1993) Three distinctive views of power compared. In M. Hill (ed.) *The Policy Process: A Reader*. London, Prentice Hall.

MacDonald, M. B., Bally, J. M., Ferguson, L.M., Murray, B.L., Fowler-Kerry, S.M., Anonson, J.N.S. (2010) Knowledge of the professional role of others: a key interprofessional competency. *Nurse Education in Practice* 10, 238–242.

Marx, K. (1973) *Grundrisse*. Harmondsworth, Penguin.

Max-Neef, M. (2010) The world on a collision course. *AMBIO* 39, 200–210.

McCann, P. (1982) Review: radicalism and education in Britain. *History of Education Quarterly* 22(2), 233–238.

Molineux, M., Whiteford, G. (2006) Occupational science: genesis, evolution and future contribution, In E. Duncan (ed.) *Foundations for Practice in Occupational Therapy*, London, Elsevier, pp. 297–313.

Morris, W. (1890 /2011) *News from Nowhere*, www.maxists.org/archive/morris/works/1890/nowhere/nowhere.htm, accessed 6 June 2011.

National Archives (2011) *Professions Supplementary to Medicine Act 1960* www.legislation.gov.uk/ukpga/Eliz2/8-9/66/crossheading/Establishment-of-a-council-and-boards-for-certain-professions-supplementary-to-medicine/enacted, accessed 6 June 2011.

Ormsby, J., Stanley, M., Jaworski, K. (2010) Older men's participation in community-based men's sheds programmes. *Health and Social Care in the Community* 18(6), 607–613.

Paine, T. (1986 /1776) *Common Sense*. London, Penguin.

Pollard, N., Kronenberg, F., Sakellariou, D. (2008) A political practice of occupational therapy. In N. Pollard, D. Sakellariou, F. Kronenberg (2008) (eds) *A Political Practice of Occupational Therapy*. Edinburgh, Elsevier Science, pp. 3–20.

Pollard, N., Walsh, S. (2000) Occupational therapy, gender and mental health, an inclusive perspective? *British Journal of Occupational Therapy* 63(9), 425–431.

Ruskin, J. (2002) *Sesame and Lilies*. D. E. Nord (ed.) New Haven, Yale University Press.

Stockhammer, E., Ramskogler, P. (2008) *Post Keynesian Economics – How to Move Forward*. Department of Economics Working Paper Series, 124. Inst. für Volkswirtschaftstheorie und -politik, WU Vienna University of Economics and Business, Vienna.

Taylor, S. (2005) *The Complete Cattle Raid of Cooley/Tain bo Cualnge*, http://vassun.vassar.edu/(sttaylor/Cooley/HoundSlaying.html, accessed 6 June 2011.

Thomas, B., Dorling, D., Davey Smith, G. (2010) An observational study of health inequalities in Brita in: geographical divides returning to 1930s maxima by 2007. *British Medical Journal* 341 c3639 doi:10.1136/bmj. c3639.

Townsend, E. (1993) 1993 Muriel Driver Lecture. Occupational therapy's social vision. *Canadian Journal of Occupational Therapy* 60(4), 174–184.

Townsend, E., Wilcock, A. A. (2003) Occupational Justice. In C. T. Christiansen (ed.) *An Introduction to Occupation: The Art and Science of Living*. Upper Saddle River NJ, Prentice Hall, pp. 243–273.

Trollope, J. (1994) *Britannia's Daughters. Women of the British Empire*. London, Pimlico.

Tubbs, C., Drake, M. (2007) *Crafts and Creative Media in Therapy*. Thorofare NJ, Slack.

Turner, A. (2002) History and philosophy of occupational therapy. In A. Turner, M. Foster, S. Johnson (eds) *Occupational Therapy and Physical Dysfunction, Principles Skills and Practice*. Edinburgh, Churchill Livingstone, pp. 3–24.

Updike, J. (1991) *Rabbit at Rest*. London, Penguin.

Updike, J. (2006) *Rabbit Redux*. London, Penguin.

Watson, R. (2004) New horizons in occupational therapy. In Watson, R., Swartz, L. *Transformation through Occupation*. London, Whurr, pp. 3–18.

Whiteford, G. (2000) Occupational deprivation: global challenge in the new millennium. *British Journal of Occupational Therapy* 63, 200–204.

Whiteford, G., Townsend, E., Hocking, C. (2000) Reflections on a renaissance of occupation. *Canadian Journal of Occupational Therapy* 67(1), 61–69.

Whiteford, G., Townsend, E. (2010) Participatory occupational justice framework (PJOF 2010): enabling occupational participation and inclusion. In F. Kronenberg, N. Pollard, D. Sakellariou (eds) *Occupational Therapies without Borders: Towards an Ecology of Occupation-Based Practices*. Edinburgh, Elsevier/Churchill Livingstone, pp. 65–84.

Wilcock, A. A. (1998) Doing, being and becoming. *Canadian Journal of Occupational Therapy* 65, 248–257.

Wilcock, A. A. (1999) Creating self and shaping the world. *Australian Occupational Therapy Journal* 46, 77–88.

Wilcock, A. A., Townsend, E. (2000) Occupational terminology interactive dialogue, *Journal of Occupational Science* 7(2), 84–86.

Wilcock, A. A. (2002) *Occupation for Health, Volume 2: A Journey from Prescription to Self Health*. London, College of Occupational Therapists.

Wilcock, A. A. (2006) *An Occupational Perspective of Health*. Thorofare, NJ: Slack Inc.

Yakobina, S. C., Harrison-Weaver, S. (2008) War, what is it good for? Historical contribution of the military and war to occupational therapy and hand therapy. *Journal of Hand Therapy* 21, 106–114.

Yerxa, E. J. (2000) Occupational science: a renaissance of service to humankind through knowledge. *Occupational Therapy International* 7(2), 87–98.

Index

Politics of Occupation-Centred Practice: Reflections on Occupational Engagement across Cultures, First Edition. Edited by Nick Pollard and Dikaios Sakellariou.
© 2012 John Wiley & Sons, Ltd. Published 2012 by John Wiley & Sons, Ltd.

Printed and bound by CPI Group (UK) Ltd, Croydon, CR0 4YY

09/10/2024

14571434-0001